The Complete Guide to Reflexology

Ruth Hull

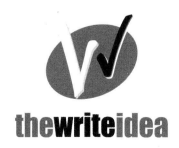

thewriteidea

Published by The Write Idea Ltd
84 Hertford Street
Cambridge
CB4 3AQ
01223 847765

First published August 2011
Reprinted October 2013
Reprinted April 2015
Reprinted September 2017

ISBN 978-0-9559011-3-3

Set in 10/12.5 Sabon.

Printed by Replika Press, India.

Contents

The editorial team

Author

Ruth Hull is a freelance writer who specialises in natural health. Born and educated in Zimbabwe, she completed a degree in Philosophy and Literature before studying and practising complementary therapies in London. She now lives in South Africa and is married with two children.

General editor

Greta Couldridge has worked within the industry for many years, starting her career in a salon environment, before moving to teaching posts in further education colleges where she progressed to a management role. Throughout this time she worked as an external verifier and examiner before accepting a position with an awarding body developing qualifications and teaching and learning materials.

Greta is continually developing her skills, technical knowledge and keeping abreast of changes within the industry by attending workshops, courses and conferences.

Publisher

Andy Wilson has worked in the publishing industry for 23 years, setting up The Write Idea in 1991. Most recently he has worked with one of the leading international awarding bodies, helping to set up their publishing division and co-producing a number of successful text books.

Acknowledgements

The publishers would like to acknowledge the professionalism and dedication of the editorial team without whose hard work and enthusiasm this book would not have been possible. We would also like to thank the following for their valuable contributions to the development of this book:

Cathy Joubert for the photographs of the hands and feet

Lisa Kirkham for the page and cover design

Vicky Slegg for the illustrations

Tammy Vermaak for the photographs of the case studies

The Wellcome Trust Photo Library for the pathology images

Glenys Underwood and Susie Jennings for their invaluable help with pre-publication reviews of the draft pages.

From the author
This book is dedicated to my brother Ryan and to his indescribable strength: '...somewhere, nobody knows where, a sheep which we have never seen may or may not have eaten a flower ... Look at the sky. Ask yourselves: Has the sheep eaten the flower, yes or no? And you will see how everything changes...' *The Little Prince*, Antoine de Saint-Exupery.

Introduction

This book is for anyone studying reflexology with any of the major awarding bodies. It presents all the information necessary to gain a thorough understanding of the subject in a clear, accurate and easily absorbed format. We have tried to strike a balance between a friendly, informal tone and serious academic content.

We hope you will enjoy using this book and would welcome any feedback, good or bad, which will help us to improve it in subsequent editions.

All of the illustrations in this book are available to order in large format for use as teaching and revision aids. For further information on these and forthcoming publications please contact us on 01223 847765 or email enquiries@writeidea.co.uk.

1 What is reflexology?

Reflexology is a gentle, non-invasive therapy that encourages the body to balance and heal itself. It involves applying finger or thumb pressure to specific points on the hands and feet. These points are called 'reflexes' and they reflect, or mirror, the organs and structures of the body as well as a person's emotional health. In this way, the hands and feet are 'mini maps' or 'microcosms' of the body that can be used to encourage holistic healing.

In this chapter you will learn more about what reflexology is, where it comes from and how it works.

Student objectives

By the end of this chapter you will be able to:

- Describe the history of reflexology
- Explain the theory of reflexology
- Describe the different theories as to how reflexology works
- Explain how stress affects our bodies and how reflexology can help counteract the effects of stress
- Describe the benefits of reflexology
- Explain when it is not advisable to give reflexology treatments.

The History Of Reflexology

Ancient times: Egypt, China, India

Healing the body through working the hands and feet is an ancient art that dates back to a variety of cultures. The earliest evidence of hand and foot massage was discovered in Egypt in the tomb of Ankhmahor at Saqqara. The tomb dates back to approximately 2330BC and is sometimes referred to as the 'physician's tomb' because of all the medical reliefs it contains. Some of these reliefs depict people receiving hand and foot massages, asking that the massages 'give strength' and also 'do not cause pain'.

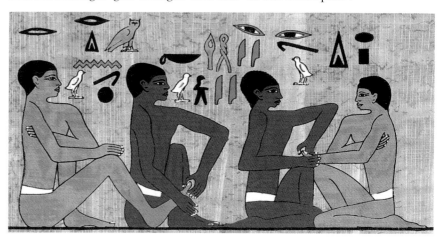

The ancient Chinese worked the hands and feet to help maintain good health and prevent disease. They developed traditional Chinese medicine (TCM) which incorporates acupuncture, acupressure, herbalism and exercise and is based on the medical text *Huang-di Nei-jing*, or the Inner Classic of the Yellow Emperor. This text, commonly referred to as the *Nei-jing*, is thought to have been compiled between 300 and 100 BC.[1] Fundamental to TCM is the theory that one's 'vital energy' or 'life force' runs through 14 major meridians, or channels, in the body. Twelve of these meridians either begin or end in the tips of the fingers and toes and massage to these areas stimulates the flow of energy and clears congestion in the meridians, thus encouraging harmony in the body. Turn to page 225 to explore the meridians and reflexology in more depth.

Evidence of working the hands and feet to improve health is also found in traditional Ayurvedic medicine. Ayurveda developed in India and is considered to be the oldest recorded system of healing, dating back approximately 5000 years. The word *ayurveda* is a Sanskrit word meaning the 'science of life'[2] and it encompasses not only physical health, but also spiritual and emotional wellbeing. Foot massage (*padabhyanga*) plays a significant role in Ayurvedic medicine.[3]

In addition to the ancient cultures of Egypt, China and India, the importance of massaging the hands and feet to ensure good health was passed down through the oral traditions of the Native American and African tribes.

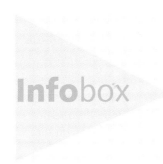

In perspective
A well-known example of how a zone on the body can reflect the health of an organ is when the pain produced by a heart attack is often felt as if it is coming from the left arm. The explanation for how this occurs is quite simple – sensory nerves from the skin, muscles and organs enter the spinal cord together as bundles, or plexuses, and often share nerve pathways in the spinal cord.

Zone Therapy: Dr William Fitzgerald

Reflexology is based on the theory that the body can be divided into zones and that imbalances in one part of the zone can be addressed through working another part of the zone. This is a very old concept that was first written about in the 16th century when two European doctors, Dr Adamus and Dr Atatis, published a book on the subject.

In the 1890s an English neurologist, Sir Henry Head (1861–1940), discovered that certain areas or 'zones' of the skin reflected the state of specific internal organs and that if there was an illness in an organ there would be sensitivity or pain in its corresponding zone on the skin. These zones became known as 'Head zones'. He also discovered that massage, heat applications or injections to the skin zone could help the internal organ.

Another Englishman, Sir Charles Scott Sherrington (1857–1952), undertook pioneering work in neurophysiology which paved the way for our understanding of the nervous system and reflexes. Sherrington was an English physiologist who won the Nobel Prize in Physiology/Medicine in 1932 for his work on neurophysiology, especially spinal reflexes and the physiology of perception, reaction and behaviour. He also published *The Integrative Action of the Nervous System*.

Although Head discovered the skin zones of the body, it was an American surgeon, Dr William Fitzgerald (1872–1942), who founded zone therapy as we know it today. Dr William Fitzgerald was the senior ear, nose and throat surgeon at St Francis Hospital in Hartford, as well as a physician at the Boston City Hospital and had experience working in hospitals in both London and Vienna. In his work Fitzgerald discovered that the body could be divided into ten zones and he could alleviate pain in one area of a zone by applying deep pressure to another area of the zone, usually on the hand. He went as far as being able to perform minor operations without the use of anaesthetics by applying pressure to specific points on his patients. Whilst doing this, Fitzgerald discovered that pressure to specific points not only anaesthetised corresponding areas, it also removed the cause of the pain and so 'healed' the patient.

Fitzgerald worked closely with a colleague, Dr Edwin Bowers, and together they became the forefathers of modern reflexology. They wrote a number of publications on zone therapy including *To Stop that Toothache Squeeze your Toe* (Bowers) and *Zone Therapy or Relieving Pain at Home* (Bowers

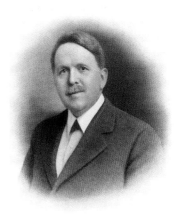

Dr William Fitzgerald

Did you know?
Dr William Fitzgerald used some remarkable aids to apply pressure to his patients' hands – he used metal combs, elastic bands, clamps and even clothes pegs.

and Fitzgerald). In 1917 their book *Zone Therapy* was published. Together, Fitzgerald and Bowers 'developed a unique method of convincing their colleagues about the validity of the zone theory. They would apply pressure to the sceptic's hand then stick a pin in the area of the face anaesthetised by the pressure. Such dramatic proof made believers of those who witnessed it.' (Dougans)[4]

An American physician, Dr Joseph Shelby-Riley, and his wife Elizabeth further developed zone therapy and published a number of books on the subject. Working with Riley was a therapist called Eunice Ingham and it was she who finally developed what we know as modern reflexology.

From zone therapy to reflexology: Eunice Ingham

Eunice Ingham (1889–1974) is often referred to as the 'mother of modern reflexology'. She took Fitzgerald's theory of zone therapy and used it to develop reflexology. Through her experiences she discovered that once you place the ten zones of the body onto the feet you can then place all the organs and structures of a specific body zone into the corresponding zone on the foot. In her own words, Ingham used zone therapy as 'a principle of dividing the body into ten zones, aiding us in our ability to locate the reflexes in the feet relative to every part of the body'.[6] In this way she developed the 'footmaps' of the body that form the basis of reflexology.

In addition to mapping the body onto the feet, Ingham also discovered the theory of crystal deposits and established that an alternating pressure on the feet has a stimulating effect on the body while a continual, uninterrupted pressure has a more numbing or anaesthetising effect.

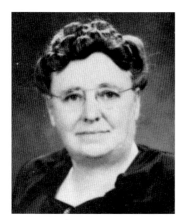

Eunice Ingham

Reflexology as we know it is based on Ingham's discoveries: mapping the body onto the feet, the theory of crystal deposits and the importance of alternating pressure. All of these discoveries were developed through hours of hands-on experience. In the early 1930s she began to develop her theories, 'she began probing the feet … finding a tender spot and equating it with the anatomy of the body … mapping ever so carefully the zones of the feet in relation to the organs of the body' (Byers).[7] Ingham dedicated the rest of her life to researching reflexology and bringing it to the general public. She wrote two books, *Stories the Feet Can Tell Through Reflexology* and *Stories the Feet Have Told Through Reflexology*, and her nephew, Dwight Byers, now continues to write about and teach the Ingham method.

Modern reflexology

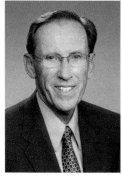

Dwight Byers

Until the 1960s, reflexology was practised primarily in the United States. However, in 1966 an English woman, Doreen Bayley, trained with Eunice Ingham and then introduced reflexology to the United Kingdom. In the 1970s a German woman, Hanne Marquardt, also studied with Ingham and then took reflexology to Germany. Both women went on to publish significant books on reflexology. Modern reflexology is also becoming increasingly linked to traditional Chinese medicine and meridian therapy is now being taught in many reflexology schools.

In the classroom
Modern reflexology is still evolving and different methods are taught in different schools. To better understand the method of reflexology you are studying, create a 'family tree' in which you trace the main influences of your reflexology. Include in it the classical historical figures as mentioned in this book and then develop it further by adding the modern 'pioneers' who have influenced the method of reflexology you are studying. At the end of the tree list any bodies, associations or organisations that govern the practice of reflexology in your area and ensure you understand any voluntary or statutory regulations you need to be aware of.

The Theory Of Reflexology

*'Put your feet together and you will see they are
the same shape as your body.'*

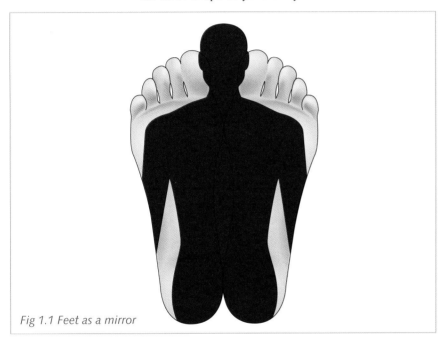

Fig 1.1 Feet as a mirror

The fundamental concept of reflexology is that the feet and hands are mirrors of the body and that through applying direct pressure to specific points on them the body can be restored to homeostasis. To understand this concept it helps firstly to divide the body into what reflexologists call 'zones'.

Study tip
According to the Oxford Dictionary, homeostasis is 'the physiological process by which the internal systems of the body are maintained at equilibrium, despite variations in the external conditions'.[8] The term was first coined by a man called Walter Cannon and it comes from the Greek *homoios* meaning 'same' and *stasis* meaning 'standing' and it defines the body's ability to maintain a steady equilibrium, or balance, within specific ranges of temperature, pH and body fluid concentration. Because the body is continually adjusting to maintain homeostasis, some people now use the term 'homeodynamics' instead of homeostasis.

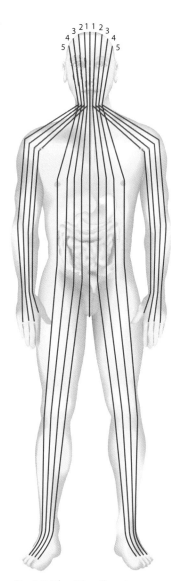

Fig 1.2 The 10 reflexology zones

Study tip

Remember that zone 1 starts in the middle of the body. The big toe or thumb is zone 1 (which can be further subdivided into five zones), the second toe or finger is zone 2, the third zone 3, the fourth zone 4 and the little toe or finger is zone 5.

The ten longitudinal zones

> *The human body can be divided into 10 longitudinal zones and 'constant, direct pressure upon any part of a particular zone can have an anaesthetising effect on another part of that same zone'.* Kunz & Kunz.

Look at your feet and imagine lines running up from each of your toes, all the way up through your body to your head and then down into each of your fingertips. You will notice that there are ten lines running from your feet to your head and ten from your head to your hands. These are the ten longitudinal zones and they form the basis of zone therapy.

Founded by the American physician Dr William Fitzgerald, zone therapy is based on the principle that the body can be divided into ten energy zones or pathways. These run the length of the body from the toes to the top of the head and then down into the fingers or vice versa. Fitzgerald described these zones as 'ten invisible currents of energy'[9] with five zones running either side of the median line. This means that five zones run from the right foot through the right side of the body and five zones run from the left foot through the left side of the body and the centre of each toe forms the centre of each zone.

It is important to note here that the big toe and thumbs are subdivided into five zones each. You will learn shortly that these structures represent the head reflex and because all ten zones run into the head (see figure 1.2), the reflexes of the head must also represent these zones. Thus, there are five zones in the left big toe and thumb because these structures represent the left side of the head and there are five zones in the right big toe and thumb because these represent the right side of the head.

So what does this all mean in relation to reflexology? Quite simply, the energy in each zone needs to flow freely and be uncongested. If the energy cannot flow then there will be congestion in a zone and this will cause an imbalance in the body. Imbalances lead to disease.

Congestion in a specific zone in the body is reflected in the corresponding zone on the foot or hand and a constant, direct pressure on the foot zone will have an anaesthetising effect on the body zone. For example, the shoulders are found on the outer edge of the body which is zone five. If your client has a sore right shoulder you should be able to feel this congestion in the outer edge of your client's right foot (zone five). You can then apply pressure to the corresponding area and work it until the congestion goes. This will help to alleviate the pain in your client's right shoulder.

Reflexions

It is important to be aware that the organs of the body are usually spread across many zones. Therefore, it is necessary to decongest all the zones of the feet during a treatment. This is done through the technique of 'zone walking' (see page 86).

The transverse zones/body relation lines

The ten longitudinal zones will help you to locate reflexes on the hands and feet. In addition to these, there are transverse or horizontal zones that will further help you to locate the organs and structures of the body. These zones were developed by Dwight Byers and Hanne Marquardt and are also referred to as 'body relation lines', 'latitudinal zones' or 'horizontal cross-zones'.

To be able to recognise the transverse zones start by looking at your own body. Your head is attached to the rest of your body by a slim neck. You then have wide shoulders which taper down to a central waistline before expanding into your hips and legs. Essentially, you can trace the following horizontal lines across your body (see fig 1.3 on the next page):

Shoulder line – above your shoulder line is your head.

Diaphragm line – this line is not so easy to see, but it can be felt as it is your diaphragm muscle which curves below your rib cage and separates your thorax from your abdomen. Between your shoulder line and diaphragm line is your thorax.

Waist line – between the diaphragm line and waistline is the upper abdomen.

Pelvic line – between your waist line and pelvic line is your lower abdomen and below your pelvic line is your pelvis.

Each of these lines divides the body into *body cavities*. These are spaces within the body that contain organs and structures that relate to specific functions and are generally innervated by the same nerve plexus or bundle. The table below shows the body cavities and their contents in relation to the transverse lines of the body.

BODY CAVITY	CONTENTS
Cranial cavity	Brain
Shoulder line **Thoracic cavity**	Thymus, trachea, 2 bronchi, 2 lungs, heart, oesophagus
Diaphragm line **Upper abdomen**	Stomach, spleen, liver, gallbladder, pancreas, adrenals, portion of the kidneys
Waist line **Lower abdomen**	Portion of the kidneys, small intestine, most of the large intestine
Pelvic line **Pelvic cavity**	Portion of the large intestine, urinary bladder, reproductive organs

These transverse zones not only help you to locate the different organs and structures of the body, they also provide a basis for your reflexology treatment. For example, if your client is suffering with eye strain, the entire head zone will need to be worked because the eye strain can affect the rest of that zone causing headaches, etc.

Note: some professional associations and awarding bodies do not acknowledge the diaphragm line but it is very useful as a guide when carrying out a treatment.

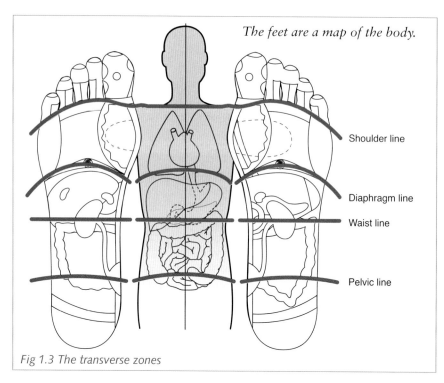

The feet are a map of the body.

Shoulder line

Diaphragm line

Waist line

Pelvic line

Fig 1.3 The transverse zones

The reflexes of the body

Now you have an understanding of the zones of the body try dividing the hands and feet into similar zones. Once you have done this, take the structures and organs from each body zone and place them in the corresponding zones on the hands and feet. In doing this, you will discover that they are mirrors of the body – every organ and structure can be located on the hands and feet in the exact same zone where they are found in the body. This is the basis of reflexology.

In reflexology, the term reflex refers to a reflection in miniature that, when stimulated, stimulates the organ or structure which it reflects. For example, when someone has a headache a therapist can apply pressure to the reflex point for the head (the big toe or thumb). When this pressure is applied, the client usually feels some degree of sensitivity or pain, indicating that there is congestion here – this congestion is the headache. If the reflex point is stimulated correctly, the headache should either lessen or disappear.

Reflexions

Have you ever developed a headache after stubbing your big toe? The reflex for your head is your big toe. After wearing high heels for a long time do the arches of your feet ache? Does your back ache at the same time? The reflex for your back is the arch of your foot.

All the organs and structures of the body are reflected anatomically in the hands and feet and those to the right of the median line will be found on the right hand and foot while those to the left will be found on the left hand and foot.

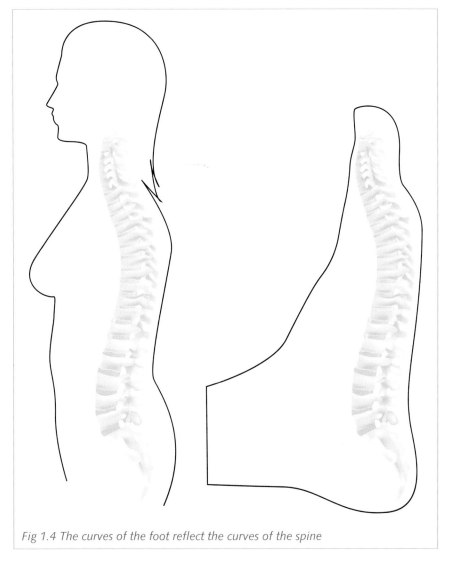

Fig 1.4 The curves of the foot reflect the curves of the spine

Note: The reflexes of the hands and feet are covered in depth in chapters 2 and 3.

The theory of crystal deposits

Once you start working with the reflexes on the hands and feet you will begin to feel different sensations under your finger tips, the most obvious being when you come across what feel like grains of sand. These are actually called crystal or crystalline deposits and indicate congestion in a reflex. Eunice Ingham first discovered these crystal deposits and taught the importance of working them out. In her book, *Stories the Feet Can Tell Through Reflexology*, she talks of 'rubbing or grinding these small sharp needle-like crystals into the muscle tissue'[10] and also said that 'as we work this out we are giving nature a chance to carry away the waste matter and restore the normal circulation to the affected part or parts'.[11]

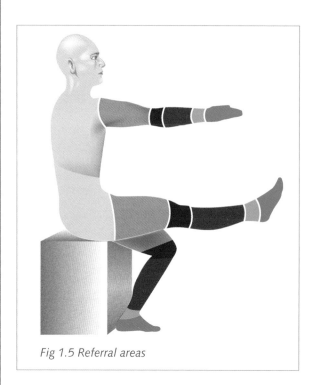

Fig 1.5 Referral areas

Referral areas

Different to the reflexes of the hands and feet, but still of great importance, are the referral areas of the body. Anatomically, our upper and lower bodies are similar:

- Our upper body includes the shoulder girdle, the long humerus, the elbow, two smaller forearm bones (ulna and radius), the wrist and then the hand.
- Our lower body includes the pelvic girdle, the long femur, the knee, two smaller shin bones (tibia and fibula), the ankle and then the foot.

Because these structures are so similar, we can actually use the upper and lower bodies as referral areas for one another in times of pain or trauma. For example, if the right ankle is damaged and cannot be touched, you can help relieve the pain and encourage healing by massaging and working the right wrist.

The body's referral areas are as follows:
- Shoulders = hips
- Arms = legs
- Elbows = knees
- Wrists = ankles
- Hands = feet

How Does Reflexology Work?

'The why and wherefore I am not prepared to explain, I only ask that you try it out.' Eunice Ingham

Now that you know the theory behind reflexology, you may be asking yourself how does it actually work? This is a difficult question to answer as there is no scientific proof that massaging your big toe can relieve your headache. However, there are many documented case studies that demonstrate the effectiveness of reflexology. The China Reflexology Association has thousands of case studies while two American reflexologists, Barbara and Kevin Kunz, have established the Reflexology Research Project which guides and documents current research into the therapy.

There are a number of different theories regarding how reflexology might work and we will touch on them briefly here. Although none of these theories have been established as fact, and are still subject to debate, they all have a few things in common – namely that reflexology helps to relax a person, helps the body cope with stress and improves the circulation of both blood and lymph. These effects will be discussed in more detail as having a thorough knowledge of them will help you to understand how reflexology actually works.

Current theories and philosophies

The pain gate control theory

When you bump your knee, what is your first reaction – to rub it? Rubbing an area that is sore is one of our most instinctive reactions to pain and it always seems to help. In the 1960s Ronald Melzack, a Canadian psychologist, and Patrick Wall, a British doctor, wrote an article for Science magazine entitled *'Pain Mechanisms: A New Theory'*. In this article they proposed the Gate Control Theory of Pain which changed the way many scientists viewed pain. Later they wrote the book *'The Textbook of Pain'* and although some details of their theory have since been proven to be incorrect, it is still considered one of the most influential theories ever written on pain. A pain researcher, Dr. Bruce Dick says, 'Melzack did for pain what Einstein did for physics.'[12]

One of their concepts that may give an indication of how reflexology has such an analgesic effect was their proposal that rubbing an area stimulates large diameter sensory fibres while pain stimulates small diameter sensory fibres. The signals from both types of fibres enter the spinal cord together and if the signals from the large diameter (pressure) fibres are of a greater magnitude than from the small diameter (pain) fibres then a 'gate' will be closed that inhibits the further transmission of the pain signal. An example of how this concept is put to use in a medical environment is transcutaneous electrical nerve stimulation (TENS) which is commonly used for pain relief.[13]

Another concept that Melzack and Wall proposed which is applicable to all holistic therapies is that pain is not merely a biological phenomenon. Rather, it is influenced by a person's psychological state and their environment. Dr Melzack said, 'There are examples of soldiers at the battlefront who have suffered severe injuries, but they feel no pain initially. What they know is that they're still alive, they've escaped death, and the brain might process pain almost as a good thing. Then you might see someone with mild gas pain who is experiencing it as intolerable pain because his close friend is dying from stomach cancer and that's what he's thinking about.'[14] This concept emphasises the importance of treating a person holistically by focusing not just on their physical ailments, but also their spiritual and emotional states.

The placebo effect theory

In many clinical trials for new drugs, the drugs are tested against placebos. A placebo is a completely ineffective pill, for example a sugar pill, that has no pharmacological action on the body. However, it has been found that these pills do, surprisingly, affect the people who take them. For example, in 2002 a trial was carried out that 'compared the herbal remedy St. John's wort against Zoloft (a drug). St. John's wort fully cured 24% of the depressed people who received it, and Zoloft cured 25% – but the placebo fully cured 32%.' (Vedantam)[15]

The effects of placebos are thought to be primarily subjective and due to the recipient's expectation – if you have a headache and take a pill for it, you expect the headache to go. What has been found is that a person's

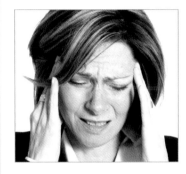

expectation of what the pill or placebo will do is enhanced by the positive language of the giver and the effect the pill has on other people who are given it.

So how does this explain how reflexology might work? Let us consider a client, Jane. Jane is suffering with migraines and hears from a friend that reflexology helped relieve his migraine symptoms. Jane also knows a woman at work who felt she was successfully treated for depression through reflexology. So Jane goes to a reflexologist knowing two people who the therapy has helped. Jane's reflexologist is a very positive, caring person and by the end of the session Jane has complete faith that her migraines will improve. The chances are that her migraines will improve. Whether it was Jane's positive expectations or the actual therapy that helped her migraines is debatable.

Many sceptics claim that reflexology only works through the placebo effect. However, current research into the placebo effect is beginning to recognise it as a valid therapy. Dr Hilary MacQueen, a senior lecturer in Health Studies at the Open University, wrote an article questioning the validity of reflexology. Her conclusion was as follows, 'Initially dismissed as an example of poor research practice and patients' gullibility, the placebo effect is now being seriously studied, with some surprising results. When a patient believes that they will get better, specific changes in brain activity can be seen by scanning and other techniques, and the level of the changes seems to be linked to the amount of improvement reported by the patients. We are learning more and more about the body's ability to heal itself, and it may turn out that the placebo effect is an incredibly powerful one, and underlies not just reflexology but many other therapies too.'[16]

The energy theory/electromagnetic theory
The theory that good health is based on the unimpeded flow of energy through the body, and that reflexology stimulates this flow, is one of the most popular theories used to explain reflexology. The founder of zone therapy, Dr William Fitzgerald, believed that 'the human body is an electro-mechanism'[17] and he called the ten longitudinal zones 'ten invisible currents of energy'[18]. Eunice Ingham, who is commonly referred to as the mother of reflexology, wrote 'There is only one disease, physical or mental, and its name is congestion'[19].

All living and non-living things consist of matter and the smallest unit of matter is the atom. Atoms are made up of a nucleus containing positively charged protons and neutrally charged neutrons and a cloud of negatively charged electrons circling the nucleus. Atoms can lose, gain or share electrons with other atoms and when this occurs, a chemical reaction takes place. Thus, 'electron interactions are the basis of all chemical reactions.'[20] Another term for 'electron interactions' is 'electrical processes', or, in reflexology terms, 'energy'. All body processes are fundamentally electrical processes.

Reflexologists believe that the human body is 'a dynamic energy system in a constant state of change' (Dougans)[21] and that energy flows through the body in specific channels or pathways. If there is a blockage or congestion in this flow of energy then the body will be in a state of 'dis-ease'. Through

In the classroom
To understand the concept of energy, rub your hands together as fast as you can for about thirty seconds to one minute. Then slowly move your hands a few centimetres away from each other and then back towards each other without letting them touch (imagine they are connected by an invisible spring, each end attached to each of your palms, that you are opening and closing). After a few inward and outward movements you will begin to feel what you may describe as a 'fuzz', 'magnetism' or 'electric pull'. This is energy!

applying pressure to specific points on the hands and feet, reflexologists can decongest the blockage and encourage the smooth flow of energy. This helps the body to heal itself and return to a state of health.

This concept of energy is not only confined to reflexology. It is, in fact, the fundamental concept of many modalities of healing. In acupuncture and acupressure energy is called *Qi* or *Chi*, in shiatsu it is *ki* and in yoga it is *prana*. What all these therapies have in common is that energy, our 'life-force', needs to flow through the body. When it does not flow, we become ill.

Some reflexologists have developed the energy theory further by focusing on the way in which the earth's electromagnetic field is intertwined with our own energy fields and how it regulates our body clocks. A very well-respected reflexologist, Inge Dougans, wrote: 'We as living organisms inhabiting this sphere are in turn electromagnetically intertwined with the energies of the earth'[22]. Reflexology is thought to strengthen our energy fields so we can cope better with environmental stresses. Dougans also quotes Ann Gillanders, another well-known reflexologist, 'The body is based on an electrical circuit and like normal circuits has negative and positive poles. Reflexology is a method of contacting the electrical centres in the body and has been used for centuries to create a smooth flow of vibratory energy through the body by contacting various points in the feet which relate to various organs, glands and cells.'[23]

The therapeutic relationship

The concept of energy, as discussed above, also forms the basis of the theory of the therapeutic relationship. However, this theory takes it a step further by proposing that healing in reflexology is based on an energetic interaction between three energies – the energies of the client, the therapist and the universal life-force.

When clients come for treatments, their bodies are often imbalanced and their energy is not flowing freely. The therapist becomes a catalyst for change in the clients' bodies and, using reflexology as a tool, encourages them to be aware of their bodies, take responsibility for their health and use their own energies to heal themselves. What is fundamental to this theory is that it is the clients who heal themselves – the therapist only facilitates the healing.

In order to be good reflexologists, therapists need to remain detached from their clients. This is only achievable if they are self-aware, balanced and centred. Therapists who bring their own problems into the relationship, or who become too personally involved, can, even unintentionally, impose their own beliefs or attitudes on the client and interrupt the natural flow of energy. Rituals such as washing the hands under running water, deep breathing and self-cleansing exercises also help therapists achieve detachment from their client.

The third energy needed, that of the universal life-force, is the natural healing energy that is present throughout the universe. It should flow freely everywhere and in everyone. However, its flow can become impeded and this causes ill health or imbalances. The therapeutic relationship encourages the free flow of this energy, but it can only flow freely when the therapist remains detached and the client takes responsibility for their own health.

The endorphin/encephalin release theory

For us to feel the sensation of pain a number of processes need to occur in our bodies. When, for example, we touch a hot stove pain is transmitted as a nerve impulse from sensory pain receptors in our hands (the peripheral nervous system) to our spinal column and brain (the central nervous system). Certain chemicals, called neurotransmitters, are essential for this nerve impulse to be transmitted. One such chemical is called substance P and it is found in sensory neurons, spinal cord pathways and parts of the brain associated with pain. Substance P stimulates the perception of pain.

Two other neurotransmitters act on substance P, either suppressing it or blocking it, and consequently inhibit the sensation of pain. These neurotransmitters are enkephalins and endorphins and they are often referred to as the body's natural painkillers. Enkephalins have very strong pain-relieving effects, 200 times stronger than morphine,[24] and suppress the release of substance P. They are found in the thalamus, hypothalamus, parts of the limbic system and spinal cord pathways that relay pain impulses. Endorphins are found in the pituitary gland and inhibit pain by blocking the release of substance P. In addition to their pain-relieving effect, enkephalins and endorphins have been 'linked to improved memory and learning; feelings of pleasure or euphoria; control of body temperature; regulation of hormones that affect the onset of puberty, sexual drive, and reproduction; and mental illnesses such as depression and schizophrenia' (Tortora & Grabowski)[25].

Reflexology is thought to increase the release of enkephalins and endorphins. Although these two neurotransmitters were only discovered in the 1970s, earlier in the century Dr William Fitzgerald emphasised the importance of stimulating the pituitary gland reflex to block or suppress pain.

The autonomic and somatic integration theory/proprioceptive theory

Two American reflexologists, Barbara and Kevin Kunz, developed a theory of how reflexology works based on an understanding of the autonomic and somatic nervous systems. The core concept of their theory is that reflexology interrupts, conditions and educates the body's response to stress by causing predictable reflex actions.

So how is this done? Because our nervous system is so complex, it helps to divide it into sub-systems, two of which are the somatic (voluntary) and autonomic (involuntary) nervous systems. The somatic nervous system consists of sensory neurons carrying information from the skin, the special senses and the limbs to the central nervous system, and motor neurons carrying messages from the central nervous system to the skeletal muscles. Buried within muscles and tendons are specialised sensory nerve receptors called proprioceptors. They monitor any internal changes in the body brought about by muscular activity and movement. The somatic nervous system allows us to be aware of our surroundings and control our skeletal muscles voluntarily.

On the other hand, the autonomic nervous system consists of sensory neurons carrying information from the viscera to the central nervous system and motor neurons carrying messages from the central nervous system to smooth muscle, cardiac muscle and glands. The autonomic nervous system controls all the automatic or involuntary processes of our internal body. These two systems are constantly working together to ensure homeostasis within the body.

When explaining their theory, Kunz and Kunz wrote: 'Pressure to the feet causes predictable reflexive actions within the nervous system. Both the internal organs of the autonomic nervous system and the neurons of the somatic-motor nervous system respond specifically to pressure applied to the feet.'[26]

The lactic acid/U-bend theory

The feet are sometimes referred to as the 'U-bend' of the body because they are the furthest point in the circulatory system from the heart and, like a U-bend in a plumbing system, they trap all the body's debris. In reflexology, this debris is thought to be calcium crystals, lactic or uric acid or lymphatic deposits. These accumulate in the feet and, like a clogged up plumbing system, prevent the body from working properly.

Eunice Ingham first discovered these crystal deposits. She believed they gathered at the nerve endings in the feet and affected not only nerve transmission, but also circulation. She wrote, 'We are all familiar with what the effect of sand or gravel would be in a garden hose, yet we expect our body to function properly regardless of obstructions in the delicate nerve endings'[27]. During a reflexology treatment these crystals can be felt in specific reflexes (they feel like small grains of sand) and they correspond to congestion in the reflex. For example, a person with stiff shoulders will have crystals in their shoulder reflex. A reflexologist applies pressure to these crystals and works them out until they cannot be felt any more. In this way they decongest the reflex and help to relieve the stiffness in the shoulders.

The meridian theory

The meridian theory of reflexology is based on traditional Chinese medicine and is the same theory that underlies acupuncture and acupressure. A very brief overview is given here as it is discussed in more detail on page 225.

The Chinese believe that life is activated by an energy force known as Qi or Chi. Qi is our 'vital force' or 'life force' and it flows through the body in energy pathways called meridians. Any congestion in a meridian manifests as an imbalance or disorder in the body. Twelve of the fourteen major meridians of the body either begin or end in the hands and feet and so reflexologists can apply pressure to points on these meridians. This improves energy flow, enhances bodily functions and is also a form of preventative health care.

The nerve impulse theory

It is estimated that the feet contain over 7,200 nerve endings which are all stimulated through reflexology. To understand the nerve impulse theory it helps to first have an understanding of the basic functioning of the nervous system.

The nervous system is made up of millions of nerve cells that all communicate with one another to control the body and maintain homeostasis. These cells detect what is happening both inside and outside the body, interpret these events and cause a response. This whole process can be broken down into three functions – sensory, integrative and motor.

Sensory receptors gather information on what is happening both inside and outside the body and transport this information to the central nervous system (the spinal cord and brain). A stimulus, such as pressure to an area of the foot, is picked up by sensory receptors and converted into a nerve impulse that travels up sensory nerve fibres to the spinal cord. Before entering the spinal cord, these nerve fibres join up with many other fibres forming a network of nerves called a plexus. Nerves at this plexus can come from skin, muscles, glands or organs of different areas of the body. Once inside the spinal cord, most impulses are transported to the brain where they are analysed, processed and interpreted. Some impulses, however, are interpreted in the spinal cord itself. These are called reflex-arc responses. Once a decision has been made, the brain sends a motor response, which is another nerve impulse, down motor nerve fibres to an area of the body that needs to respond to the initial sensory impulse. This can be a gland or a muscle.

The neural pathways described above are physical pathways that can be impinged upon by many things, for example tight muscles. The electro-chemical transportation of the nerve impulse itself can be impeded or slowed down by other physiological factors. Reflexology is thought to 'stimulate or fine-tune this sensory apparatus and its neural pathways' (Choudhary)[28] and to help clear the nerve pathways so nerve impulses can be transported efficiently. According to Dwight Byers, 'A short circuit is often caused by tension putting pressure on a vital nerve plexus or even a single nerve structure supplying a vital organ. As tension is eased, pressure on the nerves and vessels is relaxed, thus improving the flow of blood and its oxygen-rich nutrients to all parts of the body.'[29]

Embryo containing the information of the whole organism theory (ECIWO)
The basis of the ECIWO theory is that every cell and every functional part of the body, no matter how large or small, is a microcosm (or in reflexology terms, a map) of the whole body. This theory was initially founded by Professor Yingqing Zhang, an acupuncturist who discovered that the whole body could be stimulated by working the side of the second metacarpal of the hand.

The theory has now been further developed by reflexologists, and is becoming increasingly popular with modern reflexologists due to developing research in the fields of human physiology, embryology, histology and biophysics. A Danish reflexologist, Peter Lund Frandsen, has written much on the ECIWO theory and in his work he shows how every individual cell knows what is going on in the rest of the body and is able to communicate with other cells. Frandsen wrote: 'Exciting, not the least for us as reflexologists, is the emerging understanding of the human body as a giant network of interconnected parts, all constantly aware of each other, all constantly talking to each other, communicating in order to co-operate.'[30]

Stress And Its Effects On The Body

'It does not matter whether one is working on a meridian, or a reflex, or a nerve pathway, or an energy line…Whatever is transmitted by the technique is powerful and potent to the body. Reflexology achieves homeostasis of all the systems of the body through the reduction of the effects of stress and by giving complete relaxation to the recipient.' Beryl Crane[31]

The primary effect of reflexology is that it is deeply relaxing. Go for a few treatments yourself and you will soon discover just how relaxing it is – you may even fall asleep during your treatments!

When the body is relaxed, it starts to heal itself. This can be explained scientifically through the effects of the parasympathetic nervous system which only functions when the body is relaxed. To understand this better, let us first take a look at what stress is and what it does to our bodies.

Stress and the 'fight or flight' response

'Anxiety seems to be the dominant fact … and is threatening to become the dominant cliché … of modern life. It shouts in the headlines, laughs nervously at cocktail parties, nags from advertisements, speaks suavely in the board room, whines from the stage, clatters from the Wall Street ticker, jokes with fake youthfulness on the golf course and whispers in privacy each day before the shaving mirror and the dressing table. Not merely the black statistics of murder, suicide, alcoholism and divorce betray anxiety … but almost any innocent, everyday act: the limp or over-hearty handshake, the second pack of cigarettes or the third Martini, the forgotten appointment, the stammer in mid-sentence, the wasted hour before the TV set, the spanked child, the new car unpaid for.' Time Magazine[32]

A wide, general definition of stress is that it is a 'stimulus that provides a response'.[33] However, the Oxford Dictionary defines it as 'a demand on physical or mental energy'[34] and it can be caused by a wide variety of factors, often differing from person to person. These factors can be physical stressors such as exercise, fasting, temperature changes, infection, disease, emotional disturbances or fright. They can also be due to one's lifestyle, for example living or working in a negative environment, alcohol or drug abuse, smoking, poor diet, lack of exercise and tension, anxiety or worry.

 No matter what the cause of the stress, our bodies respond to it by going into what is known as the 'fight or flight' mode. This is a state in which the body prepares itself to either fight or run away from the stress. Both of these responses have the same physical requirements – the skeletal muscles of the body, especially those in the arms and legs, need energy in the form of glucose and as much blood as possible to enable them to either run or fight. Other systems of the body, such as the digestive system, do not need to be functioning optimally so they tend to shut down. Two systems, the sympathetic nervous system and the endocrine system, play vital roles in our response to stress.

Physical indicators of stress

- Feeling hot and sweaty or flushed
- Feeling your heart beating or palpitations
- Breathlessness, lump in the throat, shallow breathing
- Dry mouth
- Constipation, diarrhoea, flatulence, indigestion, nausea
- Muscle tenseness, tight jaws, grinding of teeth
- Clenched fists, hunched shoulders
- General aches and pains
- Night cramps
- Restlessness, hyperactivity, biting nails, drumming fingers, tapping feet
- Often tired, lethargic, fatigued, totally exhausted
- Sleeping difficulties
- Frequent headaches
- Frequent illnesses such as colds and upset stomach
- Feeling faint
- Cold hands and feet
- Frequent urination
- Overeating or loss of appetite
- Increased cigarette smoking or alcohol consumption
- Loss of interest in sex
- Sense of urgency in everything one does

Mental indicators of stress

- Feeling distressed and often worried or upset, tearful, deflated, helpless, hopeless or hysterical
- Being withdrawn, unable to cope, anxious, depressed
- Being impatient, easily irritated and aggravated – often angry, hostile or aggressive
- Feeling frustrated, bored, inadequate, guilty, rejected, neglected, insecure, vulnerable
- Loss of interest in one's appearance, in health, in diet
- Low self-esteem
- Lack of interest in other people
- Sense of trying to do too many things at the same time, feeling rushed and failing to finish one task before moving onto the next
- Feeling you have so much to do that you don't know where to start
- Difficulty in thinking clearly, unable to concentrate or make decisions
- Being forgetful
- Lack of creativity, being non-productive and inefficient
- Prone to making silly mistakes and having accidents (spilling and dropping things)
- Being hypercritical, inflexible and unreasonable
- Over-reacting to situations

How the nervous system responds to stress

Think back to when you studied anatomy and physiology – the nervous system is organised into the central nervous system (CNS) consisting of the brain and spinal cord and the peripheral nervous system (PNS) consisting of the cranial and spinal nerves. The PNS is then divided into the somatic or voluntary nervous system and the autonomic or involuntary nervous system. The somatic nervous system allows us to control our skeletal muscles voluntarily while the autonomic nervous system controls all the automatic or involuntary processes of our body such as the functioning of smooth muscle, cardiac muscle and glands. The autonomic system is further subdivided into the sympathetic nervous system and the parasympathetic nervous system.

The sympathetic nervous system responds to changes in the environment by stimulating activity and using energy. For example, it dilates the pupils, increases the heartbeat and stimulates the adrenal glands to secrete adrenalin into the bloodstream. All of these changes prepare the body to react quickly and strongly to environmental changes, in other words, it prepares the body for 'fight or flight'. However, it is important to note that in enabling the body to react quickly to external changes, the sympathetic nervous system also decreases activity in areas that are not important in the fight or flight response. The most obvious area is the digestive system as the digestion of food is not important when one needs to react quickly to a threat. So, for example, peristalsis in the large intestine is reduced and the secretion of saliva is inhibited.

The table on the right highlights some of the opposing effects of the sympathetic and parasympathetic nervous systems.

SYMPATHETIC STIMULATION	STRUCTURE	PARASYMPATHETIC
Pupil dilated	Iris muscle	Pupil constricted
Vasoconstriction	Blood vessels in head	No effect
Secretion inhibited	Salivary glands	Secretion increased
Rate and force of contraction increased	Heart	Rate and force of contraction decreased
Vasodilation	Coronary arteries	Vasoconstriction
Bronchodilation	Trachea and bronchi	Bronchoconstriction
Peristalsis reduced, sphincters closed	Stomach	Secretion of gastric juice increased
Glycogen to glucose conversion increased	Liver	Blood vessels dilated, secretion of bile increased
Adrenaline and noradrenaline secreted into blood	Adrenal medulla	No effect
Peristalsis reduced, sphincters closed	Large and small intestines	Secretions and peristalsis increased, sphincter relaxed
Smooth muscle wall relaxed, sphincter closed	Bladder	Smooth muscle wall contracted, sphincter relaxed

The parasympathetic nervous system opposes the actions of the sympathetic nervous system by inhibiting activity and conserving energy. For example it constricts the pupils, decreases the heartbeat and has no effect on the adrenal glands. The parasympathetic nervous system also increases activity in the digestive system by stimulating peristalsis and the secretion of saliva.

It is very important to remember that the parasympathetic nervous system only functions effectively when the body is not responding to stress. In other words when it is relaxed. Reflexology calms a person, putting them into a relaxed state in which the parasympathetic nervous system can take over.

How the endocrine system responds to stress

The endocrine system also plays a key role in the body's response to stress. When put under short-term stress such as being physically threatened, our sympathetic nervous system stimulates the adrenal medulla which secretes adrenaline and noradrenaline into the blood stream. These two hormones prepare the body to either fight or flee a situation by causing physiological changes that result in more oxygen and glucose in the blood and a faster circulation of blood to the muscles and heart.

On the other hand, glucocorticoids such as cortisol are secreted by the adrenal cortex to help us deal with long term stress such as the death of a loved one. Glucocorticoids help protect the body from the long term effects of stress, but they also depress the immune system. Through relaxing a person, reflexology encourages the body to cope better with stress.

The Effects Of Reflexology

Holistic relaxation

> 'From the holistic perspective, our suffering comes from forgetting our wholeness. The word 'health' comes from the Anglo Saxon 'häl', whence also came 'heal' and 'whole'. Perhaps the simplest definition of healing is 'to make whole' ... There's an even more profound dimension to the deepest healing – it's also spiritual. The same root that gave us 'heal' and 'whole' gives us 'holy', too.' Dr. Rudolph Ballentine[35]

As mentioned above, reflexology is deeply relaxing and through relaxing the body it reduces the body's need for excess or unnecessary sympathetic and adrenal responses. It also puts the body into a relaxed state so that the parasympathetic nervous system can function effectively.

In addition to relaxing the body, reflexology also relaxes the mind – it is a holistic therapy. The term 'holistic' is derived from the Greek word *holos*, meaning whole, and holistic therapies such as reflexology are based on the idea that health is the result of harmony between the body, mind and spirit. Stresses of any kind, be they physical, psychological, social or environmental, can upset this balance and cause 'dis-ease'.

When a person is unhappy, or under psychological stress (emotional, work or family-related), they can have vague symptoms of ill health such as fatigue, an aching body, tension in the neck and shoulders, a feeling of irritability, disturbed sleep or unhealthy eating habits. This person may not want to go to a doctor because they do not have a specific illness, but if symptoms continue for a long time they can become chronic and cause other illnesses.

This is where reflexology is important. It is natural, non-invasive, drug-free and can help a person to cope better with life's demands. It also gives individuals the opportunity to help themselves and provides a quiet environment in which they can relax and learn to heal themselves.

Improved circulation

'Circulation is life. Stagnation is death.'
Eunice Ingham

It is estimated that our bodies have over 60 billion cells. Every single one of these cells needs oxygen and nutrients to be delivered to it and heat and waste products to be removed from it. If these simple functions do not occur the cell will die.

The importance of good circulation in the body cannot be overstated. Two main substances are circulated in the body – blood via cardiovascular circulation and lymph via lymphatic circulation. The cardiovascular system functions in transporting oxygen, carbon dioxide, nutrients, heat, waste and hormones. It also regulates the body's pH and temperature and the water content of cells. In addition, it helps protect the body against foreign microbes and toxins. The lymphatic system, on the other hand, drains interstitial fluid to prevent tissues from becoming waterlogged, transports dietary lipids and contains specialised tissues and organs that help protect the body against invasion.

Reflexology improves both cardiovascular and lymphatic circulation in three different ways. Firstly, reflexology is deeply relaxing and thus stimulates the parasympathetic nervous system (as discussed above) which encourages the flow of blood to all the organs of the body and lowers blood pressure. Secondly, by massaging the hands and feet which are at the periphery (outer part) of the body, reflexology encourages circulation to the extremities where circulation is often poorer than in the rest of the body. Finally, through the application of pressure to reflexes such as the heart and lymphatic reflexes, reflexology helps stimulate the circulation.

An inspirational story

Reflexology and lupus erythematosus

'Lupus is a chameleon-like disease and difficult to diagnose. I was only diagnosed after I had been severely ill (pleurisy, pneumonia and a large pulmonary embolism) when I was 48 years old. I remained on a daily dose of 15mg of cortisone for several years. Whenever my specialist physician tried to reduce the dose below 15mg my lupus nephritis would flare up.

A friend told me that Natalie had been on a short reflexology course and needed people as case studies. Without any hope I went to Natalie, enjoyed the treatment and decided to go weekly. The next month my doctor remarked that the blood and protein in my urine sample was much less, the following month my urine was clear. I continued my weekly treatments with Natalie and my dose of cortisone was gradually reduced to nil over the following year.

I had no change in medication over this period except the reduction of the cortisone. My kidney function before I began my weekly treatments was 49%, after two years it was 82%. Despite being on 15mg of cortisone daily for several years, when it was gradually withdrawn my adrenal glands came back into action producing the natural cortisone I needed.

I credit reflexology with sending my lupus into remission, improving my kidney function and kick-starting my adrenal glands which had been loafing while I was on artificial cortisone. I still have a monthly treatment to keep my body healthy.'

With special thanks to Dorothy Gray for sharing her inspirational story.

Study tip
Learn your contraindications well – they are often asked in theory, practical and oral exams.

Contraindications And Cautions To Reflexology

'*Contraindication – any situation or condition, especially one of disease, which renders a particular line of treatment unwise or even improper.*'[36]

It is important to know when reflexology cannot help a person and when it should not be used. At times you will have a client who is unwell and you need to know whether or not it is safe for them to receive reflexology.

Although reflexology is generally a safe and non-invasive therapy, there are times when you should either exercise caution or avoid treating a client altogether. The conditions for not giving a treatment are known as *contraindications* and it is vital that you know the contraindications to reflexology and that you respect them.

Some of these conditions, such as gangrene or haemorrhaging, require immediate medical attention and you need to be able to recognise these conditions and know how to refer your client to their GP or a hospital.

Other conditions, such as diabetes, are cautions which require that your client obtain their doctor's permission before receiving reflexology. If they cannot get their doctor's written permission, then they need to sign an informed consent form confirming they are aware of any risks they may be taking. There may be times when your client's doctor may disagree with them receiving reflexology and it is advisable that you respect their wishes. It is important to remember that you, as a reflexologist, are not medically trained and you need to put your client's health and wellbeing first.

Contraindications to reflexology

Acute undiagnosed pain
Any client with severe pain that has not yet been diagnosed needs to be seen by a doctor and should not receive reflexology until they have a proper diagnosis.

Aeroplane flights
Due to the effects of a possible healing crisis, reflexology should not be given within 24 hours of flying.

Contagious or notifiable disease
If a disease is contagious, a reflexologist may be at risk of contracting the disease or of cross-infecting another client.

Deep Vein Thrombosis (DVT)
The formation of a blood clot, or thrombus, in a deep vein of the legs is called a phlebothrombosis or deep vein thrombosis. It is usually characterised by the leg becoming swollen and tender and people at risk of DVT include those who have recently had surgery or prolonged bed rest and pregnant women. Foot reflexology should not be given to a client who has DVT in their legs due to the risk of dislodging the clot.

Diarrhoea and/or vomiting
A person with diarrhoea or vomiting should be under the care of a GP.

Drugs/Alcohol
If a person is under the influence of recreational drugs or alcohol they may not respond normally to reflexology. Wait until the person is sober. If working with a client who is recovering from drug or alcohol dependency, it is recommended that the reflexologist trains in this field first and always works with the supervision and support of medical personnel.

Fever
A fever is an abnormally high temperature and is usually the body's way of dealing with infection. A person with a fever needs to rest and be under the care of a medical practitioner.

Gangrene
Gangrene is the death and decay of tissue due to a lack of blood supply and a person with gangrene needs urgent medical care.

Haemorrhage
A haemorrhage is severe bleeding, either internal or external, and a person who is haemorrhaging needs urgent medical care.

Medical tests or procedures

If a client is due to have a medical test or procedure reflexology should not be done *for the first time* immediately before it. This is because the effects of the reflexology might distort the results of the test or procedure.

Organ transplants

Someone who has had an organ transplant should not receive reflexology as there is a risk that it may affect their medication or that, in trying to return the body to its normal state of homeostasis, reflexology may encourage the body to reject the foreign organ.

Unstable heart conditions

A person with an unstable heart condition should be under medical care and may well be hospitalised. Because reflexology can affect the way the body reacts to certain drugs it is best to wait until the heart condition has been stabilised.

Cautions to Reflexology

AIDS/HIV and Hepatitis

Reflexology is not contraindicated to AIDS/HIV or hepatitis and it can be very beneficial to someone with one of these diseases. However, the reflexologist must be sure to follow the correct hygiene procedures.

Any condition already being treated by a GP or complementary practitioner

If a client has a condition that is already being treated by either a GP or complementary practitioner it is important to gain that their consent to treat their client. This is to ensure your treatment does not interfere with the other practitioner's treatment.

Arthritis

Arthritis is the inflammation of a joint and is generally characterised by pain, swelling and a limited range of movement. There are two main types of arthritis:

Osteoarthritis (wear-and-tear arthritis) – This is a degenerative joint disease caused by ageing, irritation of the joints and general wear and tear. It is a progressive disorder of movable joints, particularly weight-bearing joints such as the knees and hips and is characterised by the deterioration of articular cartilage and the formation of spurs in the joint cavity. It is common in the elderly.

Rheumatoid arthritis – This is an autoimmune disease in which the immune system attacks its own tissues, in this case its own cartilage and joint lining. It is a chronic form of arthritis in which the synovial membrane of the joint becomes inflamed and, if left untreated, thickens and synovial fluid accumulates. The resulting pressure causes pain and tenderness. The membrane then produces an abnormal granulation tissue that adheres to the surface of the articular cartilage and sometimes erodes it completely. The exposed bone ends are then joined by fibrous tissue, which ossifies and renders the joint immovable. Rheumatoid arthritis is thought to be hereditary.

When practising reflexology on a client with arthritis, it is important to adjust one's pressure and avoid relaxation techniques that may be too vigorous, such as the ankle boogie.

Asthma

Asthma is a chronic, inflammatory disorder in which the airways narrow in response to certain stimuli, ranging from pollen and house dust mites to cold air and emotional upsets. It is characterised by periods of coughing, difficulty breathing and wheezing and during an attack the person struggles to exhale. When working with a client who is asthmatic you should know where they keep their asthma pump in case they need it and you should also know how to look after them during an asthma attack. This will be covered in a first aid course.

Cancer

Cancer is the uncontrolled division of body cells and it can affect any tissue in the body. Only a reflexologist trained specifically in cancer care should work with a client who has cancer and should be aware of potential bruising and low platelet counts.

Cellulitis

Cellulitis is a spreading bacterial infection of the skin and a person with cellulitis should be under medical care. Direct pressure to the area should be avoided and if the feet are affected then reflexology should be done on the hands (or vice versa).

Diabetes mellitus

Diabetes mellitus is a disorder in which there is an elevation of glucose in the blood (hypoglycaemia). Symptoms include increased thirst and urination, weight loss in spite of increased appetite, fatigue, nausea, vomiting, frequent infections and blurred vision. Reflexology treatments need to be tailored for diabetic clients as they can have lowered sensitivity (due to peripheral neuropathy), finer skin and be prone to bruising and ulceration on the legs and feet. Short treatments with light pressure are recommended and it is important that the client is regularly monitored by their doctor.

Epilepsy

This refers to a group of disorders of the brain characterised by seizures. Seizures are short, recurrent, periodic attacks of motor, sensory or psychological malfunction and the cause of epilepsy is not always known. However, it can result from a head injury, brain tumour or stroke and seizures are often aggravated by physical or emotional stress or a lack of sleep. Only work with a person who suffers from epilepsy if you know how to look after them during and after an epileptic fit. This is usually covered in a first aid course.

Heart disease and cardiovascular conditions

People with heart disease or cardiovascular conditions often have more than one problem and their bodies can be overburdened with congestion, excess fluid in the tissues and any medication they may be taking. For this reason their doctor may sometimes prefer them not to have any treatment that may interfere with their medication or cause the body to work any harder than it already is. Sometimes, however, doctors are happy for their patients to receive therapies but will need to monitor their progress or perhaps change their medication. Therefore, always ask a client with any heart or cardiovascular condition to obtain their doctor's consent before coming for reflexology. Some of the more common cardiovascular conditions that you may encounter are:

Thrombosis – This is a condition in which a blood clot, or thrombus, is produced. If it is large enough, a blood clot can obstruct the flow of blood to an organ.

Phlebitis – This is inflammation of the walls of a vein. It is characterised by localised pain, redness, tenderness and heat and can often occur as a complication of varicose veins.

Hypertension – Hypertension is abnormally high blood pressure (usually a systolic pressure higher than 140mm Hg or diastolic pressure higher than 90mm Hg). Risk factors include old age, obesity, poor diet, lack of exercise, stress, metabolic defects, genetics and adrenal or kidney disorders.

Hypotension – Hypotension is blood pressure that is low enough to cause symptoms such as dizziness and fainting. Although it is generally healthy, it can cause an insufficient supply of blood to the brain resulting in fainting and dizziness or an insufficient supply of blood to the heart resulting in shortness of breath or chest pain. Hypotension can be caused by a number of factors including heart disease, infection and excess fluid or blood loss.

Kidney infections
Kidney infections are often characterised by impaired kidney function, fluid and urea retention and blood in the urine. Symptoms can sometimes also include fever, shivering and pain. Anyone with a kidney infection must be referred to their doctor.

Nervous/Psychotic conditions
Nervous and psychotic conditions are usually characterised by a loss of contact with reality. Symptoms can include delusions, hallucinations, severe thought or mood disturbances and extremely abnormal behaviour. When treating a client with such a condition it is advisable to have their carer or guardian in the room with you.

Nervous system (dysfunction of)
There are many different disorders of the nervous system but a few that you may encounter are:

Multiple sclerosis – In this disorder patches of myelin and underlying nerve fibres in the eyes, brain and spinal cord are damaged or destroyed. Plaques form on the myelin sheath of the brain and spinal cord and disrupt nerve transmission. This causes weakness, numbness, tremors, loss of vision, pain, fatigue, paralysis, loss of balance and loss of bladder and bowel function. It is thought to be an autoimmune disorder.

Parkinson's disease – This is a progressive disorder which is thought to be due to an imbalance in neurotransmitter activity. Symptoms include involuntary skeletal muscle contractions such as tremor or rigidity, impaired motor performance and slow muscular movements.

Motor neurone disease – This is the degeneration of the motor system. It leads to the progressive weakness and wasting away of muscles and eventual paralysis. Both skeletal and smooth muscles, such as those involved in breathing and swallowing, are affected. However it does not affect the senses. Therefore people with motor neurone disease can still lead intellectually active lives.

A reflexologist needs to have an understanding of the disorder from which their client suffers and should work closely with the carer or guardian.

Neuritis
Neuritis is inflammation of a nerve or group of nerves. It may result from irritation to the nerve produced by injuries, vitamin deficiency or poisons. Reflexology is found to be beneficial to some forms of neuritis but should only be practised in co-operation with the client's doctor.

Sciatica – This is a form of neuritis which is characterised by severe pain along the path of the sciatic nerve. It can be caused by lower back tension, a herniated disc, osteoarthritis or it can result from conditions such as diabetes or pregnancy. It usually only affects one side and symptoms can include pins-and-needles, pain or numbness.

Oedema
Oedema is the excessive accumulation of interstitial fluid in body tissues. It results in swelling and puffiness and can be the result of a local injury, or heart or kidney disease. Oedema in a client needs to be checked by a doctor prior to treatment to ascertain its cause.

Osteoporosis
Osteoporosis is a progressive disease in which bones lose their density and become brittle and prone to fractures. It is common in the elderly and post-menopausal women. Reflexologists need to exercise caution and be aware of the fragility of their client's bones. Deep pressure and rigorous relaxation techniques must be avoided.

Pregnancy
Only a reflexologist trained specifically in pregnancy care should work with a woman who is pregnant.

Prescribed medication
Although reflexology is a gentle and balancing therapy, it does increase the circulation of blood and lymph through the body and promotes the elimination of waste. This means that it may also affect the way in which the body deals with drugs and for this reason it is important that a person on medication is always monitored by their doctor as their body's need for the medication may change. Also, reflexology is a very 'normalising' treatment and at certain times doctors may give their patients drugs that do not normalise the body (for example fertility drugs). At times like this the doctor will not want the normalising effects of reflexology.

Recent operations
If a client has had a recent operation it is necessary to know why they had the operation and what medication they are currently taking. In addition, it is advisable to get their doctor's permission before giving them a treatment.

Study tip
Most contraindications are common sense. To help you remember them, think why they are contraindicated. For example, if you have a bruise on your foot would you want someone to apply pressure to it? If you have a fever or are vomiting would you feel like having someone massage your feet?

Rheumatism

This is a range of disorders which are characterised by aches and pains of the muscles and joints. Reflexologists should avoid pressure on any painful areas and use rigorous relaxation techniques with caution.

Spastic conditions

Spastic conditions are characterised by spasms, which are abnormal, involuntary muscular contractions. Examples of spastic conditions include spastic colon, which is irritable bowel syndrome, and spastic paralysis which is a weakness of the limbs associated with increased reflex activity. Reflexologists need to be aware of any spastic conditions their client may have and tailor their treatment accordingly.

> **Reflexions**
>
> There is much debate over reflexology in pregnancy or cancer care. Reflexology is a safe and gentle complementary therapy and there is no evidence that it can harm an unborn foetus or that it can spread cancer. However, there are certain reflexes and acupoints that should be avoided or worked very lightly in these conditions. Therefore, treatments should only be performed by a therapist who has trained specifically in pregnancy care or cancer care. In addition, any reflexologist who works on someone with either of these conditions should always obtain the permission of the client's doctor or specialist.

Localised contraindications

If a client has a condition that only affects a specific area of the foot or hand, then they can still receive reflexology as long as the affected area is not worked over. A corresponding area can be worked instead. For example, if there is a cut on the big toe then work the thumb. These conditions are called localised contraindications and include:

- After a heavy meal – avoid the reflexes of the digestive system
- Cuts, bruises, abrasions
- Fractures – wait three months for the fracture to heal
- Haematoma
- Localised swelling or inflammation and any undiagnosed lumps or bumps
- Menstruation – avoid deep pressure over the reproductive reflexes as this may encourage a heavier flow
- Scar tissue – wait two years after a major operation or six months for a small scar to heal
- Skin diseases and disorders (skin diseases and disorders specific to the hands and feet are discussed in more detail on pages 62 and 114)
- Sunburn
- Varicose veins – these are abnormally enlarged veins which may be inherited, occur during pregnancy or be caused by an obstruction to the flow of blood. A person with varicose veins is at a higher risk of having a clot in the vein and massaging the foot below the vein may dislodge the clot. Reflexology can be given safely to the hands of a person with varicose veins on their legs.

Study Outline

The history of reflexology

- Reflexology dates back to the ancient cultures of Egypt, China and India.
- The earliest evidence of reflexology was found in Egypt at the tomb of Ankhmahor, Saqqara, in approximately 2330BC.
- In the 1890s Sir Henry Head discovered 'Head zones'.
- In the 1930s Sir Charles Scott Sherrington did pioneering work in neurophysiology.
- Dr William Fitzgerald (1872–1942) founded zone therapy.
- Dr William Fitzgerald worked closely with Dr Edwin Bowers and together they published a number of books on zone therapy and became known as the forefathers of reflexology.
- Eunice Ingham (1889–1974) developed zone therapy into modern reflexology. She was the first person to map the reflexes of the body onto the feet and also discovered the theory of crystal deposits. She was soon known as the mother of modern reflexology.
- In the 1960s Doreen Bayley introduced reflexology to the UK and Hanne Marquardt took it to Germany.

The theory of reflexology

- **Ten longitudinal zones** – The concept of the ten longitudinal zones is that ten pathways of energy flow from the toes and fingertips up through the body and into the head and vice versa. Congestion in a specific zone in the body is reflected in the corresponding zone on the foot or hand.
- **Transverse zones** – There are also transverse zones (body relation lines) on the body and foot – the shoulder line, the diaphragm line, the waistline and the pelvic line. Congestion in a specific zone in the body is reflected in the corresponding zone on the foot or hand.
- **Reflexes** – The hands and feet are 'mini maps' of the body. This means that every structure and organ of the body is reflected in miniature on the hands and feet and can be 'worked' through applying pressure to these reflections.
- **Crystal deposits** – In certain congested reflexes small crystal deposits can be felt. These indicate congestion in the corresponding organ.
- The body's referral areas are as follows:
  Shoulders = Hips
  Arms = Legs
  Elbows = Knees
  Wrists = Ankles
  Hands = Feet

How does reflexology work?

There are many different theories on how reflexology works. These include:
- Pain gate control theory
- Placebo effect theory
- Energy/Electromagnetic theory
- Endorphin/Encephalin release theory
- Autonomic and somatic integration/proprioceptive theory
- Therapeutic relationship theory
- Lactic acid/U-bend theory
- Meridian theory
- Nerve impulse theory

Stress and its effects on the body

- When the body is put into a stressful situation it goes into 'fight or flight' mode. This means that the sympathetic nervous system responds to the situation.
- When the body is relaxed the parasympathetic nervous system counteracts the effects of the sympathetic nervous system and helps the body relax itself and restore its energy.
- Reflexology calms a person, putting them into a relaxed state in which the parasympathetic nervous system can take over.
- During stress the endocrine system releases adrenaline and noradrenaline which help the body to prepare to fight or flee from a situation. Glucocorticoids are released in states of long term stress.

The effects of reflexology

Reflexology has the following effects:
- It is deeply relaxing and reduces the body's need for excess or unnecessary sympathetic and adrenal responses. It also puts the body into a relaxed state so that the parasympathetic nervous system can function effectively.
- It is a holistic therapy working the body, mind and soul of a person.
- It improves both cardiovascular and lymphatic circulation.

Contraindications and cautions to reflexology

Contraindications
- Acute undiagnosed pain
- Aeroplane flights
- Contagious or notifiable disease
- Deep vein thrombosis (DVT)
- Diarrhoea and/or vomiting
- Drugs/Alcohol
- Fever
- Gangrene
- Haemorrhage
- Medical tests or procedures
- Organ transplants
- Unstable heart conditions

Cautions

- AIDS/HIV and Hepatitis
- Any condition already being treated by a GP or complementary practitioner
- Arthritis
- Asthma
- Cancer
- Cellulitis
- Diabetes mellitus
- Epilepsy
- Heart disease and cardiovascular conditions
- Kidney infections
- Nervous/Psychotic conditions
- Nervous system (dysfunction of)
- Neuritis
- Oedema
- Osteoporosis
- Pregnancy
- Prescribed medication
- Recent operations
- Rheumatism
- Spastic conditions

Localised contraindications

- After a heavy meal
- Cuts, bruises, abrasions
- Fractures
- Haematoma
- Localised swelling or inflammation and any undiagnosed lumps or bumps
- Menstruation
- Scar tissue
- Skin diseases
- Sunburn
- Varicose veins

Multiple choice questions

1. **Which of the following are all physical benefits of reflexology?**
   a. Improved blood circulation, reduced muscular pain, improved elimination
   b. Improved elimination, improved sleep patterns, reduction in negative emotions
   c. Balanced sleep patterns, relaxation, elevated moods
   d. Decreased depression, improved lymphatic circulation, reduced elimination.

2. **Who is the mother of reflexology?**
   a. Hanne Marquardt
   b. Doreen Bayley
   c. Eunice Ingham
   d. Renee Tanner.

3. **Which of the following is not a localised contraindication?**
   a. Sunburn
   b. Deep vein thrombosis
   c. Abrasion
   d. Cut.

4. **Which reflexology theory is based on the concept that reflexology works because it is the recipient's expectation that it will work?**
   a. Lactic acid theory
   b. Pain gate control theory
   c. Placebo effect theory
   d. Electromagnetic theory.

5. **Who is the founder of Zone Therapy?**
   a. Dr Shelby Riley
   b. Dr William Fitzgerald
   c. Dr Eunice Ingham
   d. Dr Charles Sherrington.

6. **Which of the following statements is true?**
   a. Reflexology cures all diseases
   b. Reflexology encourages the body to heal itself
   c. Reflexology cures diseases of the circulation only
   d. Reflexology encourages only the nervous system to heal itself.

7. **Which of the following is not a benefit of reflexology?**
   a. Reduced symptoms of stress
   b. Improved sleep patterns
   c. Decreased elimination
   d. Relaxation.

8. **The meridian theory is closely aligned to which of the following?**
   a. Acupuncture
   b. Homeopathy
   c. Alexander technique
   d. Chiropractics.

9. **Who brought reflexology to the UK in the 1960s?**
   a. Renee Tanner
   b. Eunice Ingham
   c. Hanne Marquardt
   d. Doreen Bayley.

10. **Name the referral area to the right shoulder.**
    a. Right knee
    b. Right hip
    c. Left ankle
    d. Left wrist.

2 Foot reflexology

'See to the feet, my friend, and you have seen to the body.'
Outo, Japanese mythology[1]

Foot reflexology is probably the most common form of reflexology and it was on to the feet that Eunice Ingham first mapped the reflexes of the body and where she discovered crystal deposits. In this chapter you will learn about the structure and function of the feet as well as the basic techniques you will need to give a reflexology treatment on the feet.

Student objectives

By the end of this chapter you will be able to:

- Describe the structure of the lower leg and foot, including the bones, muscles, nerves and blood vessels
- Map the body on to the feet
- Read and interpret the feet in preparation for a reflexology treatment
- Perform both relaxation and pressure techniques and give a complete reflexology treatment.

Did you know?
On average, your feet carry you more than five times the circumference of the globe in your lifetime.

The Structure Of The Lower Leg And Foot

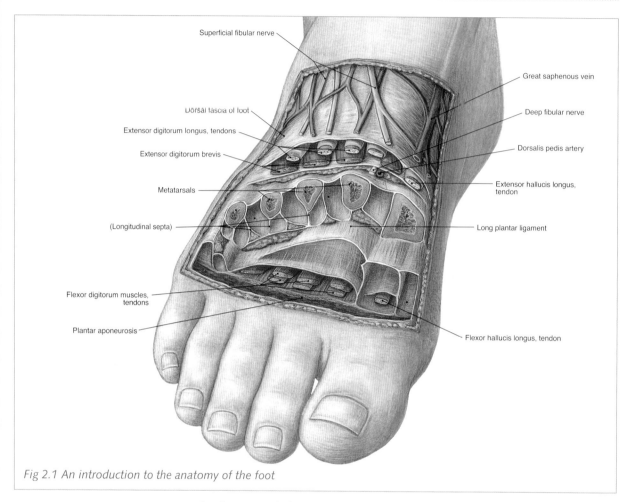

Superficial fibular nerve

Dorsal fascia of foot

Extensor digitorum longus, tendons

Extensor digitorum brevis

Metatarsals

(Longitudinal septa)

Flexor digitorum muscles, tendons

Plantar aponeurosis

Great saphenous vein

Deep fibular nerve

Dorsalis pedis artery

Extensor hallucis longus, tendon

Long plantar ligament

Flexor hallucis longus, tendon

Fig 2.1 An introduction to the anatomy of the foot

The bones of the lower leg and foot

Here is a reminder of some important anatomical terms you will need to know while studying reflexology:

- **Plantar** – the bottom or sole of the foot
- **Dorsum/Dorsal surface** – the top of the foot
- **Medial** – towards the midline of the body (towards the big toe side of the foot)
- **Lateral** – away from the midline of the body (towards the little toe side of the foot)
- **Distal** – further away from a centre of attachment (e.g. the toes are distal to the ankle)
- **Proximal** – closer to a centre of attachment (e.g. the ankle is proximal to the toes)
- **Longitudinal line** – a vertical line (runs from the top to the bottom of the body or vice versa)
- **Transverse line** – a horizontal line (runs from side to side).

Did you know?

One quarter of all the bones in your body are in your feet. If these bones are out of alignment then the rest of your body will be too.

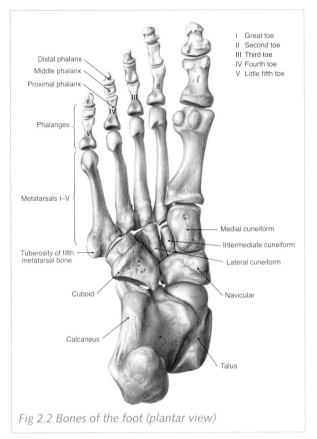

Fig 2.2 Bones of the foot (plantar view)

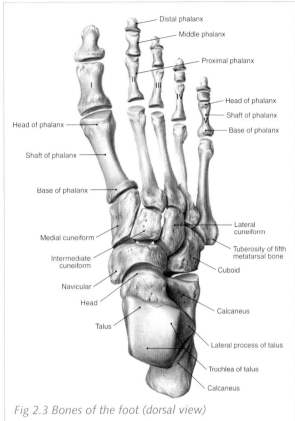

Fig 2.3 Bones of the foot (dorsal view)

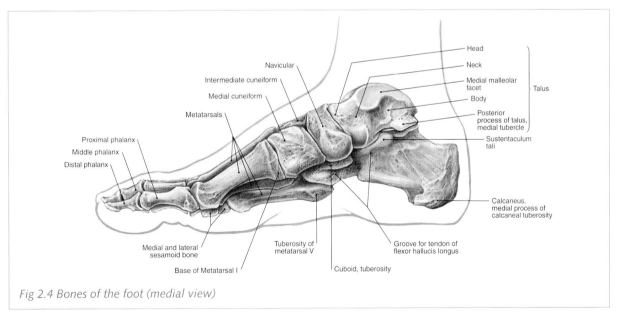

Fig 2.4 Bones of the foot (medial view)

The foot is made up of 26 extremely strong bones that bear the weight of our bodies and enable us to walk, run and jump. These bones fall into three groups, the tarsals, the metatarsals and the phalanges.

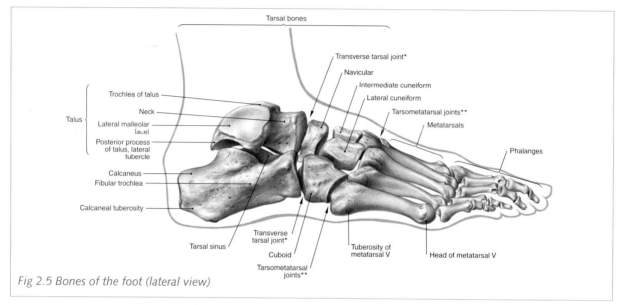

Fig 2.5 Bones of the foot (lateral view)

The lower leg consists of two bones, the larger, stronger tibia which is commonly called the shinbone and the thin fibula which runs parallel to the tibia. The tibia and fibula of the lower leg meet the talus bone of the foot at the ankle joint.

The bones of the foot

Tarsals (7)

The *tarsus*, or back portion, of the foot is made up of seven bones which together are called the tarsals. For ease of learning, the tarsals can be arranged into two rows – the calcaneus and cuboid are the outer strong, solid bones that support the weight of the body while the talus, navicular and the three cuneiforms are the inner bones that give the foot its elasticity. The tarsals are the:

- Talus – this is the ankle bone and it supports the tibia and fibula
- Calcaneus – this forms the heel of the foot
- Cuboid
- Navicular
- Medial cuneiform
- Intermediate cuneiform
- Lateral cuneiform

Metatarsals (5)

Five long bones form the main body and ball of the foot. These are the metatarsals and they are numbered 1 to 5, starting with the medial (big toe) side of the foot.

Phalanges (14)

Fourteen smaller bones work together to form the toes of the foot and these bones are called the phalanges. The big toe is made up of only two phalanges (proximal and distal) while all the other toes are made up of three phalanges (proximal, middle and distal). The big toe is sometimes called the *hallux*.

Did you know?

The word 'navicular' means boat-shaped and the navicular bone in your foot is so-called because it is shaped like a boat. Similarly, the word 'cuneiform' means wedge-shaped and this perfectly describes the shape of the three cuneiform bones in your foot. Finally, the cuboid bone is shaped like a cube.

The Arches of the Foot

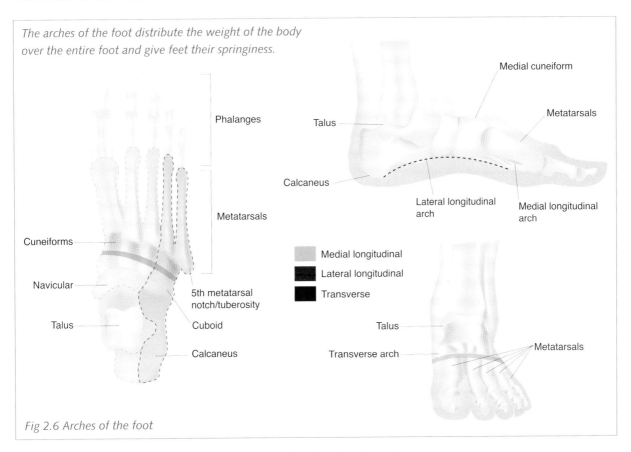

The arches of the foot distribute the weight of the body over the entire foot and give feet their springiness.

Medial cuneiform

Metatarsals

Talus

Calcaneus

Lateral longitudinal arch

Medial longitudinal arch

Phalanges

Metatarsals

Cuneiforms

Navicular

5th metatarsal notch/tuberosity

Talus

Cuboid

Calcaneus

Medial longitudinal

Lateral longitudinal

Transverse

Talus

Transverse arch

Metatarsals

Fig 2.6 Arches of the foot

The bones of the foot are arranged into three arches that distribute the weight of the body over the entire foot and also give the foot its 'springiness' and movement. These arches are the:

Medial longitudinal arch – runs longitudinally down the medial length of the foot. It consists of the calcaneus, navicular, all three cuneiforms and the medial first three metatarsals.

Lateral longitudinal arch – runs longitudinally down the lateral length of the foot. It consists of the calcaneus, cuboid and the lateral two metatarsals.

Transverse arch – runs transversely across the foot and is formed by the cuboid, all three cuneiforms and the bases of the five metatarsals.

The muscles of the lower leg and foot

The muscles that move the feet generally originate in the tibia and fibula of the leg, cross the ankle joint and insert into the foot. They can be divided into anterior, posterior and lateral compartments.

Study tip

A reminder of some anatomical terminology:

Anterior – at the front

Aponeurosis – a sheet-like tendon that attaches muscles to bone, to skin or to another muscle

Evert – turning the sole of the foot outwards

Hallux – big toe

Interosseous membrane – membrane between bones

Invert – turning the sole of the foot inwards

Malleolus – ankle bone

Phalange – toe or finger

Posterior – at the back

Anterior muscles

The anterior compartment of the leg contains the muscles that dorsiflex the ankle joint and extend the toes. Its tendons are held firmly to the ankle by the transverse ligament of the ankle (superior extensor retinaculum) and the cruciate ligament of the ankle (inferior extensor retinaculum).

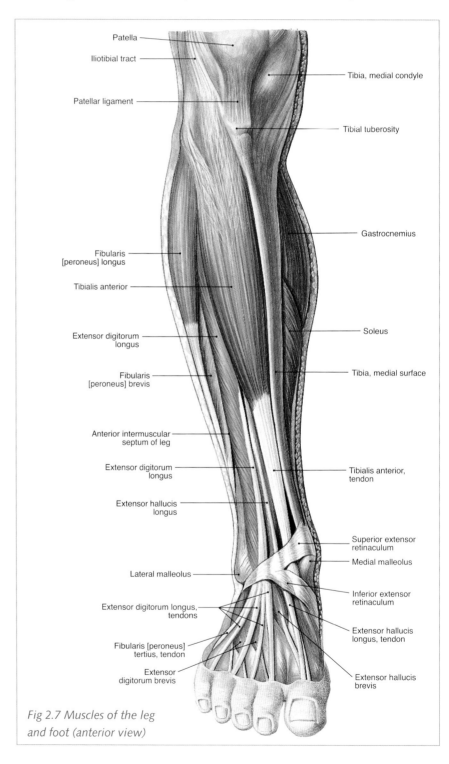

Fig 2.7 Muscles of the leg and foot (anterior view)

Posterior muscles

The posterior compartment of the leg contains the muscles that plantar flex the foot and flex the toes.

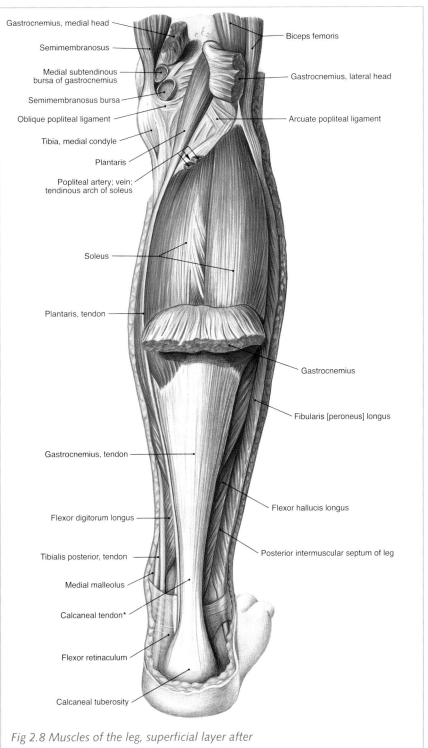

Gastrocnemius, medial head

Semimembranosus

Medial subtendinous bursa of gastrocnemius

Semimembranosus bursa

Oblique popliteal ligament

Tibia, medial condyle

Plantaris

Popliteal artery; vein; tendinous arch of soleus

Soleus

Plantaris, tendon

Gastrocnemius, tendon

Flexor digitorum longus

Tibialis posterior, tendon

Medial malleolus

Calcaneal tendon*

Flexor retinaculum

Calcaneal tuberosity

Biceps femoris

Gastrocnemius, lateral head

Arcuate popliteal ligament

Gastrocnemius

Fibularis [peroneus] longus

Flexor hallucis longus

Posterior intermuscular septum of leg

Fig 2.8 Muscles of the leg, superficial layer after partial removal of the gastrocnemius muscle

Did you know?

The Achilles tendon (calcaneal tendon) is the strongest tendon in the body. It is made up of the tendons of the gastrocnemius, soleus and plantaris muscles.

ANTERIOR MUSCLES OF THE LOWER LEG AND FOOT

Name	Origin	Insertion	Basic actions
Tibialis anterior	Tibia and interosseous membrane	Medial cuneiform and metatarsal 1	Dorsiflexes ankle joint and inverts foot.
Extensor hallucis longus	Fibula and interosseous membrane	Hallux (big toe)	Dorsiflexes ankle joint, inverts foot and extends big toe.
Extensor digitorum longus	Tibia, fibula and interosseous membrane	Phalanges 2–5 (4 outer toes)	Dorsiflexes ankle joint, everts foot and extends toes 2–5.
Peroneus (fibularis) tertius	Extensor digitorum longus muscle	Metatarsal 5	Helps dorsiflex ankle joint and evert foot.

Study tip

If you hold the foot in your hand so that you are looking at its sole and gently dorsiflex the foot by pushing the toes backwards, you will see and feel a tight tendon that runs longitudinally from the heel to between the big toe and the second toe. This is the flexor hallucis longus tendon. Take note of it as it will be a helpful guideline when you are finding the reflexes on the feet. Also be careful not to press it too hard during a treatment as it can be very sensitive.

POSTERIOR MUSCLES OF THE LOWER LEG AND FOOT

Name	Origin	Insertion	Basic actions
Gastrocnemius	Femur and knee capsule	Heel via the Achilles tendon	Plantar flexes ankle joint and aids flexion of knee. Is a postural muscle.
Soleus	Tibia and fibula	Heel via the Achilles tendon	Plantar flexes ankle joint.
Flexor hallucis longus	Fibula and interosseous membrane	Hallux (big toe)	Flexes big toe. Helps plantar flex ankle joint. Helps invert foot and stabilise the inside of the ankle.
Flexor digitorum longus	Tibia	Phalanges 2–5 (4 outer toes)	Flexes the joints of the lateral 4 toes. Helps plantar flex ankle joint and invert foot.
Tibialis posterior	Tibia and fibula and interosseous membrane	Tarsals and metatarsals 2–4	Plantar flexes ankle joint and inverts foot.

Lateral Muscles

The lateral compartment of the leg contains the muscles that plantar flex the ankle joint and evert the foot.

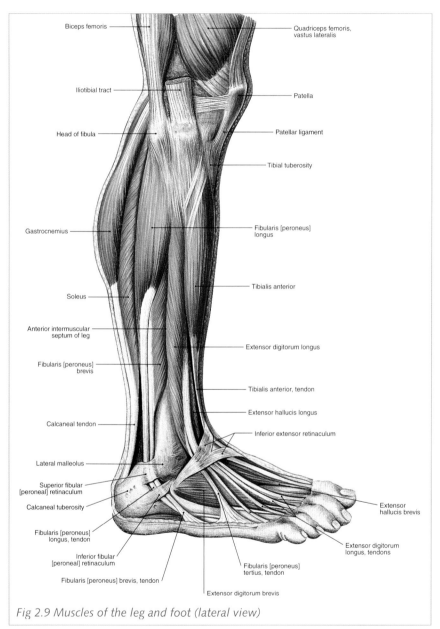

Biceps femoris
Quadriceps femoris, vastus lateralis
Iliotibial tract
Patella
Head of fibula
Patellar ligament
Tibial tuberosity
Gastrocnemius
Fibularis [peroneus] longus
Tibialis anterior
Soleus
Anterior intermuscular septum of leg
Extensor digitorum longus
Fibularis [peroneus] brevis
Tibialis anterior, tendon
Extensor hallucis longus
Calcaneal tendon
Inferior extensor retinaculum
Lateral malleolus
Superior fibular [peroneal] retinaculum
Calcaneal tuberosity
Extensor hallucis brevis
Fibularis [peroneus] longus, tendon
Inferior fibular [peroneal] retinaculum
Extensor digitorum longus, tendons
Fibularis [peroneus] brevis, tendon
Fibularis [peroneus] tertius, tendon
Extensor digitorum brevis

Fig 2.9 Muscles of the leg and foot (lateral view)

LATERAL MUSCLES OF THE LOWER LEG AND FOOT			
Name	**Origin**	**Insertion**	**Basic actions**
Peroneus (fibularis) longus	Fibula	Metatarsal 1, cuneiform 1	Helps plantar flex ankle joint and evert foot.
Peroneus (fibularis) brevis	Fibula	Metatarsal 5	Helps plantar flex ankle joint and evert foot.

Muscles on the dorsum of the foot

The muscles that extend the toes are located on the top/dorsum of the foot.
Note: Not all the muscles on the dorsum of the foot are discussed here.

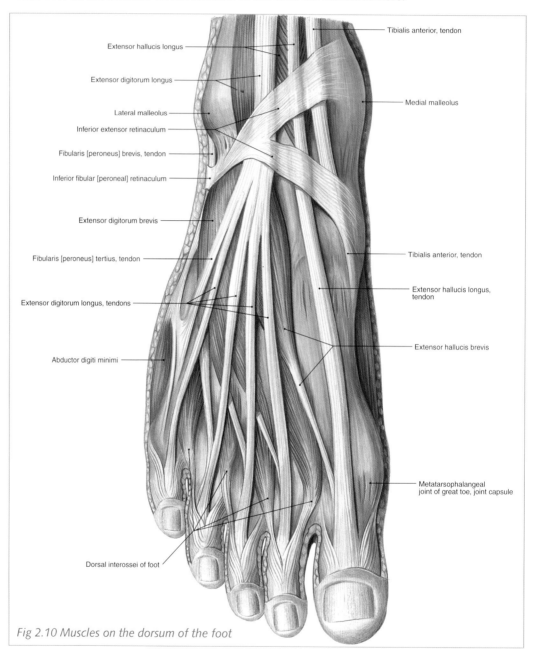

Fig 2.10 Muscles on the dorsum of the foot

MUSCLES ON THE DORSUM OF THE FOOT			
Name	**Origin**	**Insertion**	**Basic actions**
Extensor digitorum brevis	Calcaneus	Phalanges/toes 2–4	Extends toes.
Extensor hallucis brevis	Calcaneus	Hallux (big toe)	Extends the big toe.

Muscles on the sole of the foot

The muscles that flex the toes are located on the sole/plantar aspect of the foot. **Note:** Not all the muscles on the sole of the foot are discussed here.

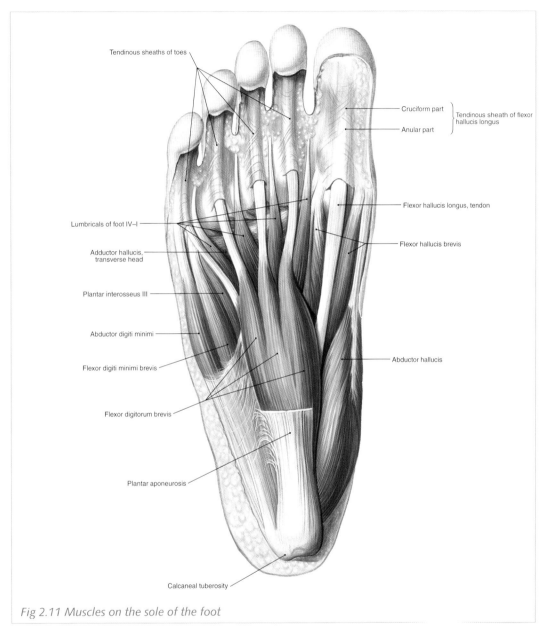

Fig 2.11 Muscles on the sole of the foot

MUSCLES ON THE SOLE OF THE FOOT			
Name	**Origin**	**Insertion**	**Basic actions**
Abductor hallucis	Calcaneus, plantar aponeurosis and flexor retinaculum	Hallux (big toe).	Abducts and flexes big toe.
Flexor digitorum brevis	Calcaneus, plantar aponeurosis	Phalanges 2–5	Flexes toes.

The nerves of the lower leg and foot

Anterior (femoral and saphenous nerves)

On the front of the leg is the large femoral nerve. This nerve arises from the lumbar plexus of the spinal column and it branches into the saphenous nerve which innervates the medial aspect of the thigh and lower leg.

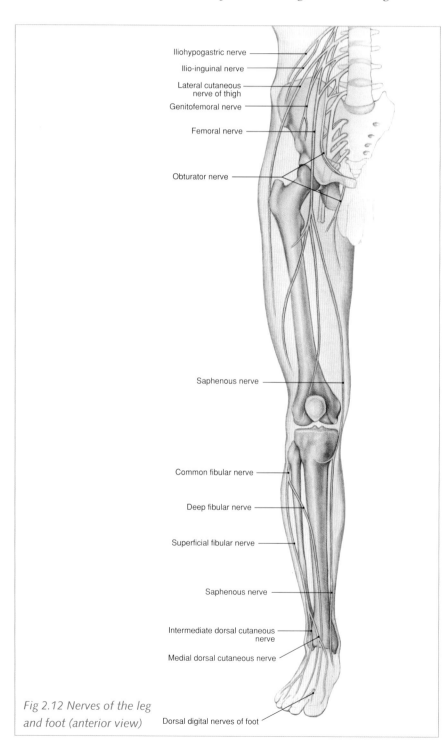

Iliohypogastric nerve

Ilio-inguinal nerve

Lateral cutaneous nerve of thigh

Genitofemoral nerve

Femoral nerve

Obturator nerve

Saphenous nerve

Common fibular nerve

Deep fibular nerve

Superficial fibular nerve

Saphenous nerve

Intermediate dorsal cutaneous nerve

Medial dorsal cutaneous nerve

Dorsal digital nerves of foot

Fig 2.12 Nerves of the leg and foot (anterior view)

Posterior (sciatic and tibial nerves)

The sciatic nerve is a large nerve consisting of two nerves, the tibial and common peroneal (fibular) nerves, bound together by a sheath of connective tissue. The sciatic nerve arises from the sacral plexus of the spinal column and descends down the back of the thigh. It then splits into the tibial and common peroneal (fibular) nerves. The tibial nerve descends down the back of the lower leg and branches into the sural, medial and lateral plantar nerves.

Lateral (common peroneal/fibular nerve)

The common peroneal (fibular) nerve which arises from the sciatic nerve descends down the lateral side of the leg and has both superficial and deep branches.

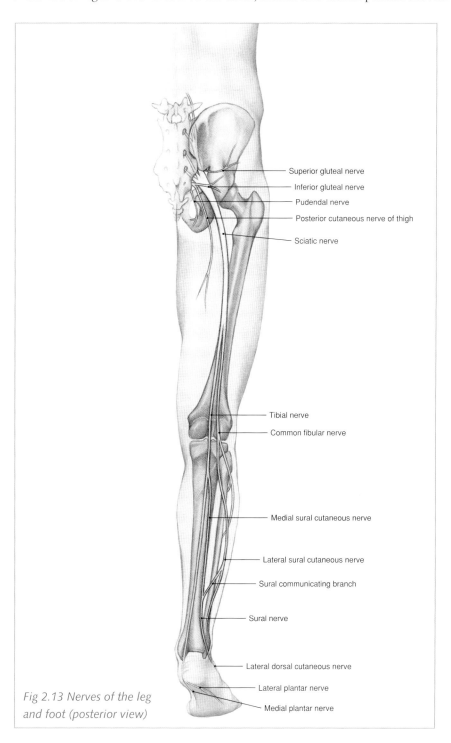

Fig 2.13 Nerves of the leg and foot (posterior view)

Labels:
- Superior gluteal nerve
- Inferior gluteal nerve
- Pudendal nerve
- Posterior cutaneous nerve of thigh
- Sciatic nerve
- Tibial nerve
- Common fibular nerve
- Medial sural cutaneous nerve
- Lateral sural cutaneous nerve
- Sural communicating branch
- Sural nerve
- Lateral dorsal cutaneous nerve
- Lateral plantar nerve
- Medial plantar nerve

Did you know?
The sciatic nerve is the largest nerve in the body.

The blood vessels of the lower leg and foot

Arteries

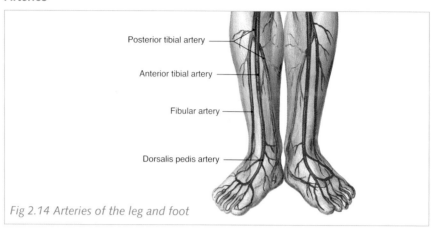

Fig 2.14 Arteries of the leg and foot

The lower leg is supplied with blood by the external iliac artery which becomes the femoral artery once it enters the thigh. As the femoral artery descends through the leg it becomes the popliteal artery which then divides into the anterior and posterior tibial arteries.

The anterior tibial artery continues over the top of the foot as the dorsalis pedis artery.

The posterior tibial gives off the peroneal branch and then becomes the plantar artery (medial and lateral plantar) supplying the sole of the foot.

Together with the dorsalis pedis, the plantar artery and its branches form the plantar arch from which the digital arteries arise.

Veins

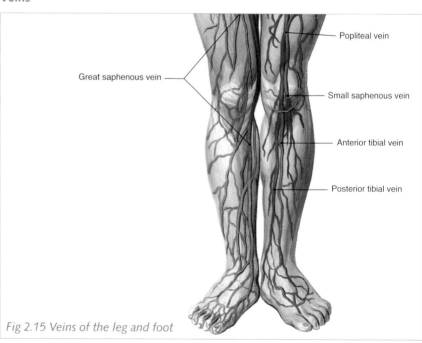

Fig 2.15 Veins of the leg and foot

Veins of the lower limb are divided into two groups – superficial and deep veins:

- Superficial veins are the great saphenous and small saphenous veins:
  - Great saphenous vein – the longest vein in the body and runs up the inner thigh, beginning at the dorsal venous arch and emptying into the femoral vein in the groin.
  - Small saphenous vein – begins behind the ankle joint and ascends up the back of the leg where it joins the popliteal vein behind the knee.
- The deep veins follow the course of the arteries and have the same names: anterior tibial, posterior tibial, popliteal, femoral, external iliac, internal iliac and common iliac veins.

Mapping The Body Onto The Feet

In Chapter 1 you learned the basic concepts behind reflexology. These are:

- the body can be divided into longitudinal and transverse zones and any congestion in a zone in the body can be worked on the corresponding zone on the hand or foot.
- the hands and feet are maps or mirrors of all the organs and structures in the body and any congestion in the body can be worked in the corresponding reflex on the hand or foot.

We will now look at these basic concepts in relation to the feet.

The ten longitudinal zones of the feet

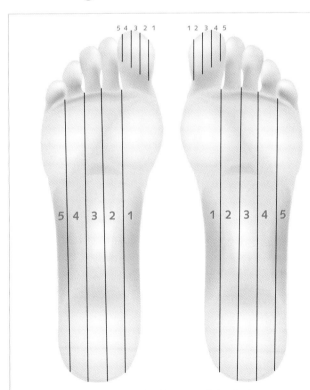

Study tip
Learn the following diagrams by heart as it is essential to know where to locate the zones or reflexes.

To remember the longitudinal zones of the foot simply count your toes and always start with the big toe as zone 1 and finish with the little toe as zone 5.

Remember that your big toe itself contains five zones because all the zones of the body merge in your head.

Fig 2.16 The ten longitudinal zones of the feet

The transverse zones/body relation lines of the feet

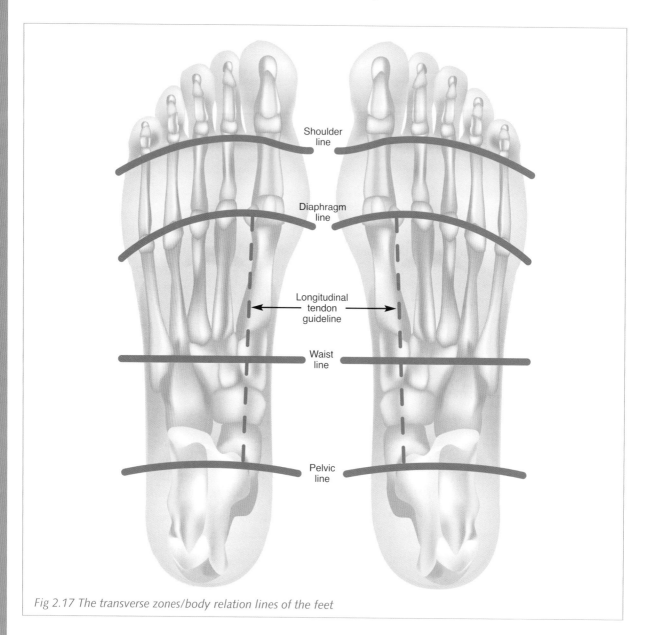

Shoulder line

Diaphragm line

Longitudinal tendon guideline

Waist line

Pelvic line

Fig 2.17 The transverse zones/body relation lines of the feet

The transverse lines can be easily located:

- The shoulder line is found at the base of the toes.
- The diaphragm line lies just below the metatarsal pad or ball of the foot where the colour and texture of the skin changes.
- The waistline can be located by feeling along the lateral edge of the foot until you feel a bone protruding outwards. This is the fifth metatarsal bone and by drawing a line directly across the foot from this protuberance you will find the waistline.
- Finally, the pelvic line lies at the beginning of the heel, once again where there is a change in the colour and texture of the skin.

The reflexes of the feet

Note: As you read more about reflexology, you will discover that there are different versions of the foot and hand charts and that the location of some reflexes differs from chart to chart and book to book. One reason for this is that some books give 'anatomical' reflexes while others show 'energetic' reflexes. Neither of these is better than the other. The charts in this book are based on the anatomical location of the reflexes and any energetic reflexes noted have been termed 'helper' reflexes.

> *'When we take a broad overview of the many different applications of reflexology around the world ... we see therapists working with feet, hands, ears, face, and other body parts, manipulating reflexes with many different energy forms... .What do they all have in common? They communicate with a reflexion of the whole in a part through the exchange of some kind of energy or another. The existence of many locations for a particular reflex, which used to be a strong argument for the critics of reflexology, now turns into a magnificent strength for our profession.'* Peter Lund Frandsen[2]

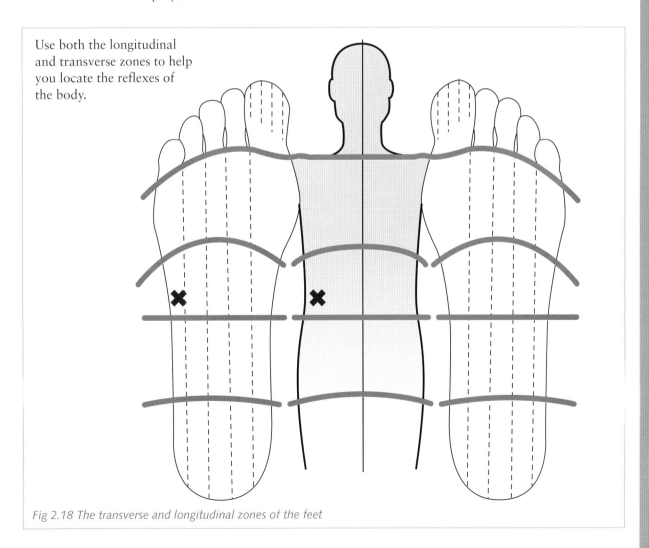

Use both the longitudinal and transverse zones to help you locate the reflexes of the body.

Fig 2.18 The transverse and longitudinal zones of the feet

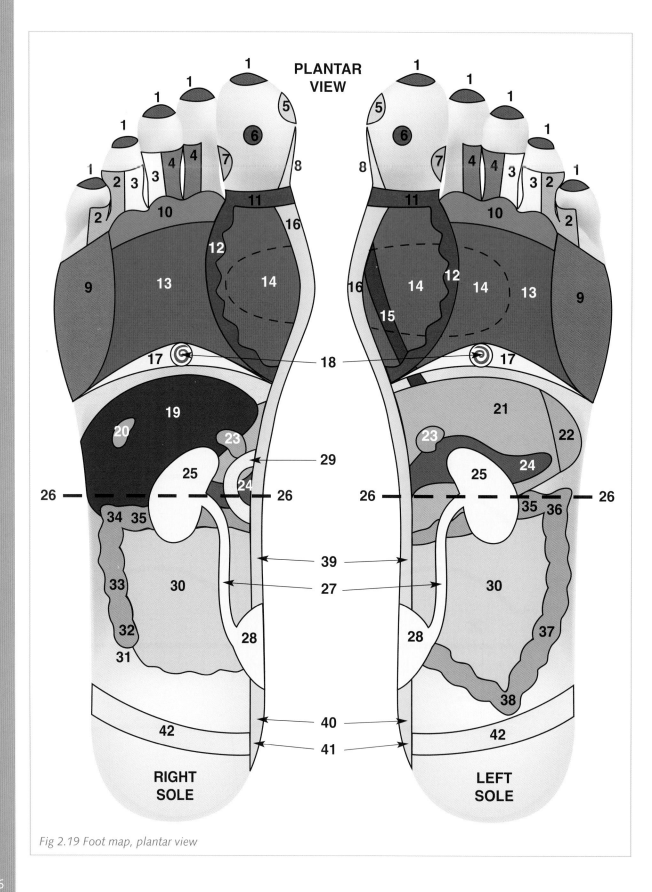

Fig 2.19 Foot map, plantar view

Key to foot maps

1. Brain/Sinuses
2. Outer ear
3. Inner ear
4. Eye
5. Pineal/Hypothalamus
6. Pituitary
7. Side of neck
8. Cervical spine
9. Shoulder/Arm
10. Helper to eye, inner ear and Eustachian tube
11. Neck/Thyroid/Parathyroid/Tonsils
12. Bronchial/Thyroid helper
13. Chest/Lung
14. Heart
15. Oesophagus
16. Thoracic spine
17. Diaphragm
18. Solar plexus
19. Liver
20. Gallbladder
21. Stomach
22. Spleen
23. Adrenals
24. Pancreas
25. Kidney

26. Waist line
27. Ureter
28. Bladder
29. Duodenum
30. Small intestine
31. Appendix
32. Ileocaecal valve
33. Ascending colon
34. Hepatic flexure
35. Transverse colon
36. Splenic flexure
37. Descending colon
38. Sigmoid colon
39. Lumbar spine
40. Sacrum
41. Coccyx
42. Sciatic nerve
43. Upper jaw/Teeth/Gums
44. Lower jaw/Teeth/Gums
45. Neck/Throat/Tonsils/Thyroid/Parathyroid
51. Fallopian tubes/Vas deferens/Lymphatics
52. Lymphatics of groin
53. Nose
54. Spine
56. Uterus/Prostate
57. Chronic area – reproductive/rectum

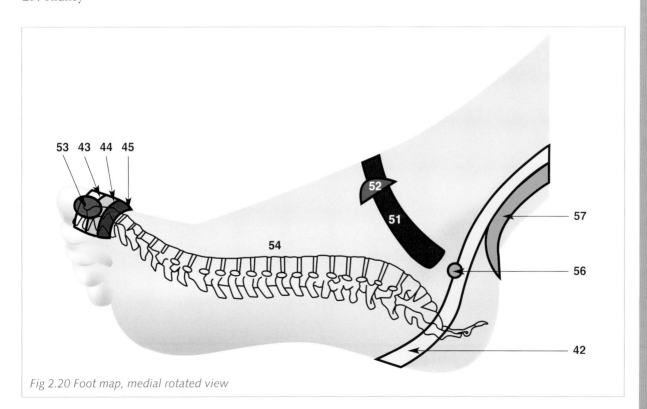

Fig 2.20 Foot map, medial rotated view

Key to foot maps

43. Upper jaw/Teeth/Gums
44. Lower jaw/Teeth/Gums
45. Neck/Throat/Tonsils/Thyroid/ Parathyroid
46. Vocal cords
47. Inner ear helper

48. Lymphatics of chest
49. Chest/Breast/Mammary glands
50. Mid-back
51. Fallopian tubes/Vas deferens/Lymphatics
52. Lymphatics of groin

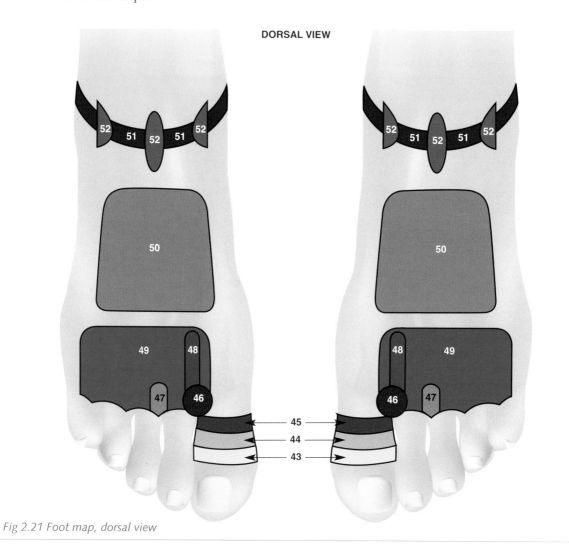

DORSAL VIEW

Fig 2.21 Foot map, dorsal view

Referral areas

The referral area for the foot is the hand. Therefore, if for some reason you are unable to work a client's foot or part of the foot work their hand as follows:

- Foot – hand
- Ankle – wrist
- Big toe – thumb
- Smaller toes – fingers

Key to foot maps

9. Shoulder/Arm
28. Bladder
42. Sciatic nerve
43. Upper jaw/Teeth/Gums
44. Lower jaw/Teeth/Gums
45. Neck/Throat/Tonsils/Thyroid/Parathyroid
46. Vocal cords
47. Inner ear helper
48. Lymphatics of chest

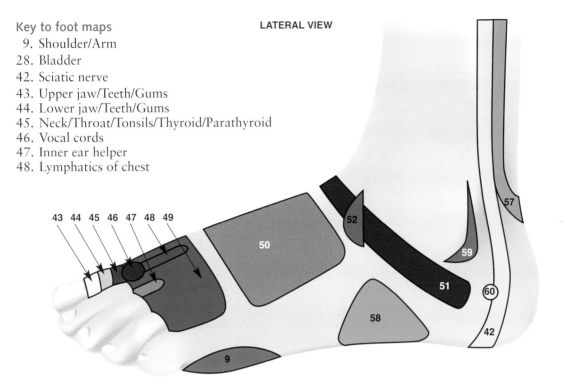

Fig 2.22 Foot map, lateral view

49. Chest/Breast/Mammary glands
50. Mid-back
51. Fallopian tubes/Vas deferens/Lymphatics
52. Lymphatics of groin
53. Nose
55. Penis/Vagina
56. Uterus/Prostate
57. Chronic area – reproductive/rectum
58. Leg/Knee/Hip/Lower back helper
59. Hips
60. Ovaries/Testes

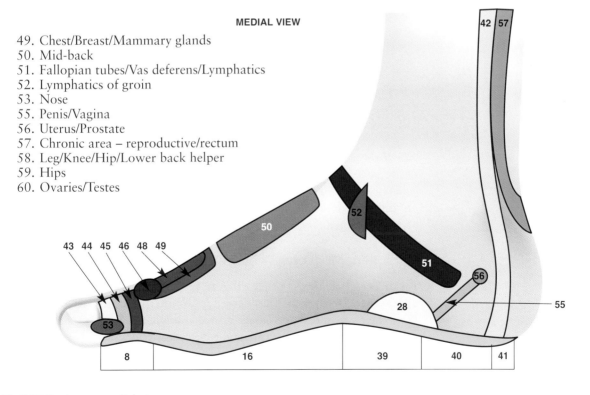

Fig 2.23 Foot map, medial view

Foot reflexology

Reading And Interpreting The Feet

Your feet are more than simply structures upon which you walk. They are a mirror of your body and soul, revealing your health, energy and even your emotions. By looking closely at a person's feet you will find that every detail is telling you something about that person – a mole, a bunion, even a verruca is telling you what is going on inside your client.

Before every reflexology treatment spend a few minutes assessing your client's feet and listen to what they are telling you:

- Get a general overview of the feet.
- Look for any local contraindications.
- Look at the colour of the feet.
- Smell them.
- Feel their temperature.
- Feel for excess moisture or dryness.
- Feel the tone of the feet.
- Look and feel for changes in skin texture.
- Look and feel for any structural foot disorders.
- Move the feet to check for mobility and flexibility.
- Examine the nails.

Please note

The following tables give suggestions of what different foot conditions may reflect – these are only suggestions and should not be used to diagnose your client's condition. Rather, use these suggestions as a basis from which you can chat to your client about their health.

For example, if a client has a verruca on her chest reflex, do not say to her that she has a problem with her lungs. Only a medically qualified professional can make such a diagnosis. Instead, question her about her current health and medical history regarding her chest. Does she smoke? Does she suffer from frequent coughs? Is she asthmatic? As a child did she have frequent chest infections or perhaps bronchitis? If her answer to all of these is no, then look at a deeper level – an emotional level. Has she suffered any emotional trauma? The verruca on her chest reflex is showing that there is an energy blockage that can be caused by a number of different things from the physical to the emotional. It is not showing a specific disease.

Get a general overview of your client's feet

Before even touching your client's feet, have a look at their general appearance. Do they look well cared for or are they neglected and dirty? Does their size and shape reflect that of your client's body? Are they equal in size? Does their skin texture and tone reflect your client's age? How do they fall when your client is lying down relaxed – are the medial malleoli (ankle bones) symmetrical or asymmetrical? Are there blemishes such as scars, freckles or moles?

DESCRIPTION OF FOOT	HOW CAN THIS RELATE TO YOUR CLIENT'S HEALTH?
General care	The way in which your client cares for their feet can reflect how much they care for themselves and how much time they have to look after themselves. It can also give clues about their self-esteem and emotional state.
Size and shape	The feet should be equal in size and shape and should be proportional to the size and shape of your client's body. A marked difference in the feet can reflect an imbalance in the right and left sides of the body.
Age of the foot	The skin texture and tone should resemble the age of your client. It is not uncommon for an elderly person to have thin or fragile skin, a loss of elasticity, pigmentation, poor muscle tone and brittle bones. However, if you find these conditions in a young person's feet they are indicative of an imbalance and poor health.
How do the feet fall?	When your client is lying down in a relaxed position, the medial malleoli should be symmetrical and the feet should lie symmetrically. If they do not fall symmetrically then ask your client if they have any problems with their hips or lower spine. If you notice that their ankle bones are falling inwards towards one another then look at your client's arches as they may be suffering from pes planus which can lead to lower back ache and digestive problems (see page 67).
Blemishes (scars, freckles, moles)	Even blemishes on the feet reveal something about your client's health. If they have a scar always ask them how they got it as recent scarring is a local contraindication. Freckles and moles often indicate hereditary weaknesses so take note of the zone, reflex and meridian on which they lie. Be aware that a hereditary weakness only indicates that your client may be prone to imbalances in a certain organ, it does not necessarily mean that they have an imbalance with that organ. For example, your client may have a mole or freckle on their bladder reflex but have no problems at all with their bladder. However, their mother and grandmother may have suffered from bladder problems or frequent urinary tract infections. This indicates that if your client is healthy and looks after themselves they should have no problems but if they become run down and do not look after themselves they may start to develop urinary or renal problems.

Look for any local contraindications

It is important to be aware of any local contraindications before you touch your client's feet. Local contraindications are localised areas that are contraindicated to reflexology. This means that to avoid cross-infection or hurting your client, you must not touch these areas. Local contraindications include:

- Cuts, bruises, abrasions
- Fractures
- Haematoma
- Localised swelling or inflammation and any
- undiagnosed lumps or bumps
- Scar tissue
- Skin diseases
- Sunburn
- Varicose veins.

Common skin diseases and disorders that affect the foot and are local contraindications include eczema, tinea pedis and verrucae.

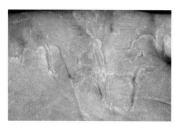

Eczema

Eczema

Eczema is an inflammatory condition that is characterised by itchiness, redness and blistering. It can be either dry or weeping and can lead to scaly and thickened skin. There are many different causes of eczema and a client with chronic eczema should be referred to a medical professional. Avoid the affected area during a reflexology treatment and rather treat the corresponding reflexes on your client's hands.

Reflexions

Eczema is a difficult disorder to treat because it is so closely linked to one's lifestyle, stress levels and diet. All these aspects need to be taken into consideration as part of the treatment and your client will need to make lifestyle changes, especially to their diet, in order to see results. In Chinese medicine, the lungs and the skin are closely linked. It is said that 'the lungs rule the exterior of the body'[3] and it is not uncommon for a person with eczema to have a history of asthma or vice versa. In fact, physicians once called asthma 'eczema on the inside'[4].

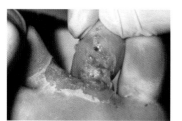

Tinea pedis (Athlete's foot)

Tinea pedis (Athlete's foot)

Athlete's foot is a common fungal infection found between the toes. Its symptoms include scaling, with or without redness and itching. Fungal infections are highly contagious and more common in elderly people, diabetic patients and those who use public facilities such as swimming pools or gym showers. They develop in warm, damp parts of the feet (often between the toes) and spread rapidly.

You may come across clients who have fungal foot infections and you should observe high standards of hygiene to avoid cross-infection. During a treatment cover or avoid the infected areas and work the corresponding reflexes on your client's hands instead. After the treatment, always dispose of any paper towels, cotton wool or rubber gloves used to treat the condition and wash thoroughly all linen and any areas the feet may have come into contact with. Finally, remember to always wash your hands well.

Reflexions

Fungal infections can indicate an imbalance in the lymphatic or digestive systems so pay extra attention to these reflexes during a treatment. You may suggest that your client take a probiotic supplement. Also advise them to use an anti-fungal foot powder, keep their feet covered in public areas and suggest they visit a chiropodist or doctor if the infection does not clear up.

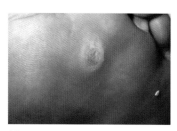

Verruca

Verrucae (Plantar warts)

Verrucae are warts which grow into the sole of the foot. They appear as firm, rough growths and because they are located on the sole of the foot, they can be painful due to the weight of the body on them.

Verrucae are thought to be caused by viruses which need a 'host' cell in which to survive and because they are contagious, you should not touch them during a treatment. Instead, work the corresponding reflexes on your client's hand and suggest they see a chiropodist.

Reflexions
Take note of the reflexes on which the verrucae are found. For example, they are quite common on the lung reflexes of chronic smokers.

Look at the colour of the feet

Your client's feet should be a healthy colour that corresponds to their natural skin tone. If, however, their feet are unusually pale, blue, red or yellow then you need to take note.

DESCRIPTION OF FOOT	HOW CAN THIS RELATE TO YOUR CLIENT'S HEALTH?
Pale/Bluish feet	Pale or bluish feet often suggest poor circulation.
Red or shiny areas	Red or shiny areas can suggest local inflammation. To avoid hurting your client, you should ask them if they have injured the area or have gout or arthritis. If there is no physical cause for the red and shiny area then be aware that it could reflect a reflex that is unusually congested.
Yellowish feet	Feet that have a yellow hue to them often reflect an overworked liver. There are many things that can cause the liver to work extra hard so ask your client about any medication they may be taking, their alcohol consumption and their general diet. Remember that Indian or Mediterranean people often have a natural yellow undertone.

Smell the feet

Smelling your client's feet can give you an insight into their health. Healthy feet should not have a strong or offensive odour.

DESCRIPTION OF FOOT	HOW CAN THIS RELATE TO YOUR CLIENT'S HEALTH?
Offensive odour	If your client's feet have a particularly strong and offensive odour, firstly check there are no local foot infections. If there are none then you need to consider your client's foot hygiene, as wearing dirty or synthetic socks or plastic shoes can make the feet smell worse than usual. In addition, look at how well their body is eliminating its waste. A person who suffers from chronic constipation can often have offensive smelling feet.
Sweet odour	A diabetic person's feet often have an unusually sweet odour.

Feel the temperature of the feet

Run your hands over your client's feet and take note of the temperature. Both feet should be warm and there should be no localised hot or cold areas.

DESCRIPTION OF FOOT	HOW CAN THIS RELATE TO YOUR CLIENT'S HEALTH?
Cold feet	Unusually cold feet can suggest poor circulation.
Localised hot or cold areas	Small areas that are extremely hot or cold suggest a congested reflex. Look at the reflex affected.

Feel for excess moisture or dryness

Run your hands over your client's feet and feel for excess moisture or dryness.

DESCRIPTION OF FOOT	HOW CAN THIS RELATE TO YOUR CLIENT'S HEALTH?
Damp or moist, sweaty feet	Damp, sweaty feet can indicate a number of imbalances but most commonly they show that the person is either feeling nervous or under a lot of stress. On a more serious note, chronically sweaty feet can indicate a hormonal imbalance.
Damp or moist with flaking skin between the toes	If your client's feet have dampness with flaking skin between the toes this could be a fungal infection such as tinea pedis.
Very dry skin (sometimes with flaking), dehydrated	Feet that are covered with dry and flaking skin generally reflect poor health and nutrition.

Feel the tone of the feet

Hold the feet and gently squeeze and press them to determine their muscle tone. Healthy feet should be firm yet pliable but sometimes you will find they are unusually tight or soft and almost lifeless. The muscle tone of the feet reflects the general muscle tone of your client's body and also reveals a great deal about their energy levels and emotional state.

DESCRIPTION OF FOOT	HOW CAN THIS RELATE TO YOUR CLIENT'S HEALTH?
Tight, hard feet	Feet that are tight and hard often reflect a body that is tight, hard and 'wound-up'. Common in people who are suffering with muscle tension caused by stress and anxiety.
Flaccid or soft, 'empty' feet	You will sometimes find that a person's feet are unusually soft and feel almost 'empty' – as if you could just push your thumbs right through them. Feet such as these are common in people who are exhausted and run down or who are recovering from a chronic illness.
Localised tight or soft areas	If only a specific area of the foot is noticeably tight or soft compared to the rest of the foot then look at the zone, reflex and meridian of the area and relate it to your client's health.

Look and feel for changes in skin texture

Using your eyes and your hands, ascertain the texture of your client's feet. Healthy feet are firm and smooth and should be free of any hard skin, roughness, cracks or puffiness and swelling. Extreme changes in skin texture can lead to calluses, corns or heel fissures.

Calluses

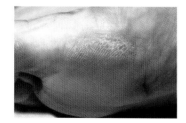

Callus

Calluses are thick, protective layers of skin that form in response to repeated pressure and friction. They are usually caused by ill-fitting shoes or uneven weight distribution and are common on the tops and cushions of the toes, especially toes 4 and 5 which sometimes appear to have a 'knife-edge'. Calluses can also occur on the ball or heel of the foot. Refer your client to a chiropodist if their calluses become painful or cause a burning sensation.

Reflexions
Calluses on the neck or shoulder reflex are common in people who suffer from tension in these areas.

Corns
Corns are cone-shaped areas of thickened skin that have no root. They form in response to repeated pressure and friction and are most commonly found on the joints of the toes. Occasionally, they do also occur on the sole of the foot. If corns are left to grow unmanaged they exert pressure on nerve endings and cause stabbing pains. Corns should be treated by a chiropodist.

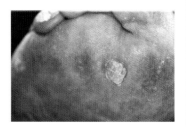

Corn

Heel fissures
Heel fissures develop when the skin covering the heel of the foot is left to dry, thicken and eventually crack. These cracks can bleed or become infected and heel fissures can be very painful if not looked after. Heel fissures tend to occur more in people who wear ill-fitting shoes or flat open shoes that constantly slap the back of the foot (such as flip-flops). Heel fissures are also common in pregnant women.

DESCRIPTION OF FOOT	HOW CAN THIS RELATE TO YOUR CLIENT'S HEALTH?
General hard, rough skin	If your client's feet are covered in hard, rough skin they may be wearing the wrong sized shoe, generally neglect their feet or simply walk barefoot all the time – discuss such habits with them.
General dry, flaky skin	Feet that are covered with dry and flaking skin tend to reflect poor health and nutrition.
Thin, fragile skin	Thin, fragile skin is normal on a elderly person but can indicate poor health on a younger person.
Localised flaking and wrinkling of skin	If the skin flakes or wrinkles in a specific area then you need to look at what zone and reflex is affected. For example, wrinkles over the digestive reflex are commonly found in people with sluggish digestive systems.
Calluses	If your client has a callus always look at the zone and reflex where it is found. In addition, discuss their posture and footwear with them.
Corns	If your client has a corn always look at the zone and reflex where it is found. In addition, discuss their posture and footwear with them.
Heel fissures or cracked heels	The heel of your client represents the lower back and hips and people with heel fissures often suffer with lower back ache, hip problems or from reproductive disorders.
Generalised puffiness and swelling, oedematous	If your client's foot is puffy and swollen always check that they have not injured it as this could be causing the swelling. If the entire foot is puffy and swollen this could indicate a problem with fluid retention or oedema and if the case is severe it is important that you refer your client to a doctor as the fluid retention could be indicative of an underlying condition. If the fluid retention is not severe then look at your client's circulation and lymphatic drainage.
Localised puffiness and swelling	If a specific area of the foot is puffy then look at the zone, reflex and meridian affected. Often a person with reproductive or hip disorders has puffy ankles.

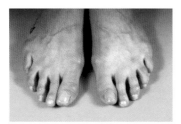

Bunions

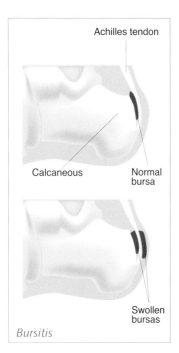

Achilles tendon

Calcaneous

Normal bursa

Swollen bursas

Bursitis

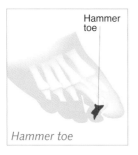

Hammer toe

Hammer toe

Look and feel for any structural foot disorders

Look carefully at the shape and structure of your client's feet and gently run your hands over them feeling for any unusual bumps or growths and you will discover a lot about your client's body.

Many structural disorders of the feet are thought to be either genetic or caused by poor posture and ill-fitting shoes. They do, however, also reveal imbalances in your client's health. These disorders include bunions, bursitis, hammer toes, hallux valgus, heel spurs, high arches, flat feet, plantar digital neuritis, plantar fasciitis and club foot.

When giving a reflexology treatment to a person with any structural foot disorders do not apply pressure to areas of inflammation. Instead, work around these areas and work the corresponding hand reflexes if necessary. Always be aware of which zones, reflexes and meridians are affected by the pressures or deformities of the feet and relate these to the client's health.

It is also important to advise your client on possible postural changes or improvements and ensure that they wear correctly fitting shoes. If necessary refer them to a podiatrist who can supply them with arch supports.

Bunion
A bunion is a painful, swelling of the joint between the big toe and the first metatarsal (metatarsophalangeal joint). A bursa, and bursitis, often develops at this joint and the big toe can become laterally displaced. This displacement is known as hallux valgus. It is thought that bunions can be hereditary or caused by ill-fitting shoes.

Unfortunately, once a bunion has developed, reflexology cannot change it. However, treatments can help with skeletal pain, especially back pain, which often results from a bunion. Reflexology can also improve blood circulation and energy flow in a client suffering from this condition. Moreover, homecare advice such as suggesting the client changes their shoes and walking habits can help to prevent the condition from worsening.

Bursitis
Bursitis is the inflammation of a bursa. It is characterised by inflammation, pain and limited movement and is usually caused by overuse or irritation from unusual use. Bursitis may also be caused by injury, gout, arthritis or some infections. During a reflexology treatment, do not apply any pressure to the inflamed area.

Hallux valgus
Hallux valgus is the lateral displacement of the big toe in which it moves inwards towards the other toes. It usually accompanies a bunion.

Hammer toes
Hammer toes are painful, rigid toes that are fixed in a contracted position and cannot be straightened. Usually the second, third and fourth toes are affected. Hammer toes often accompany other foot disorders such as bunions or high arches and can also lead to corns and nail problems. The most common cause of hammer toes is poorly fitting shoes.

Heel spur

Heel spurs are bony growths under the heel of the foot and are usually caused by excessive pulling on the heel bone by tendons. They are not always painful, but can cause pain and difficulty in standing or walking, especially if the tissues surrounding the spur are inflamed.

Pes cavus (High arches)

Pes cavus is the opposite of pes planus and is characterised by unusually high arches in the feet. These high arches result in stiffness of the foot and limited movement and can cause pain, calluses and claw foot. High arches are generally inherited or can be caused by chronic illness, especially neurological illnesses. A client with pes cavus should be referred to a podiatrist who can advise them on correctly fitting shoes and give them arch supports.

Pes planus (Flat foot or dropped arches)

Pes planus, commonly called flat foot, is a condition in which the arches of the feet drop, the ankles lean in towards one another and the foot spreads. Because the arches support the foot and absorb shock when the body is in motion, pes planus often results in fatigue, pain and backache. Pes planus is sometimes hereditary but can also be the result of joint overload or weakness, nutritional deficiencies in children or chronic illness. Foot exercises that help strengthen the arch should be recommended.

Plantar digital neuritis

Plantar digital neuritis is the inflammation of a nerve in the foot. It usually affects the fourth toe and is characterised by pain, tenderness and a loss of function. Avoid the area when giving a reflexology treatment.

Plantar fasciitis

Plantar fasciitis is the inflammation of the plantar fascia at its point of attachment to the calcaneus bone. It is characterised by pain and tenderness of the heel. During a reflexology treatment do not work on the inflamed area, but stretch and knead the calf muscles as they tend to shorten with this condition.

Talipes equinovarus (Clubfoot)

Clubfoot, or talipes equinovarus, is a birth defect in which the foot is twisted out of shape. Two types of clubfoot exist – positional and true. Positional clubfoot is caused when the foot has been held in an unusual position in utero and it can often be corrected through physical therapy after birth. True clubfoot, on the other hand, is usually only corrected through surgery because either the bones of the leg or foot or the muscles of the calf are underdeveloped.

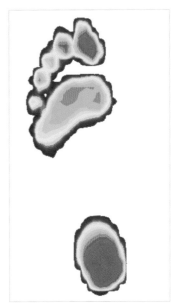

Pedogram showing pes cavus

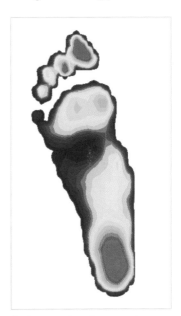

Pedogram showing pes planus

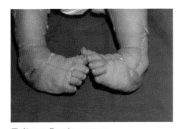

Talipes Equinovarus

DESCRIPTION OF FOOT	HOW CAN THIS RELATE TO YOUR CLIENT'S HEALTH?
Toes	Any disorders affecting the toes can indicate congestion or imbalances in the head. This can include headaches or problems with the eyes, ears, nose, mouth, teeth, neck and throat. Also be aware of which zone and meridian the affected toe represents. In addition to this, always look at your client's posture and their footwear.
Ball of the foot	The ball of the foot represents your client's thoracic area and any disorders in this area will reflect congestion in the thoracic area (neck, shoulders, lungs, heart, thymus gland and chronic thyroid helper). Bunions lie on the reflex for the thoracic spine. Thus, they can often indicate chronic tension between the shoulder blades or thyroid/energy imbalances.
Arches	The medial longitudinal arch of the foot represents the spine and it should be neither too high nor too low, flexible and free from problems. In addition, both arches should be the same. If one arch is different from the other you will often find that there will be an imbalance in the muscles along the spine. Stiff and inflexible arches represent a stiff and inflexible spine while high arches (pes cavus) indicate back pain, especially of the thoracic area. Flat feet, on the other hand, reveal lower back ache and often digestive disorders as well. Remember that all the nerves feeding every organ in the body come off the spine so problems with the spine can lead to problems in other areas as well.
Heel	The heel of the foot represents the pelvis of the body. This includes the lower back, hips, reproductive and urinary organs.

Move the feet to check for mobility and flexibility

Taking one foot at a time, gently rotate the foot at the ankle joint and move it from side-to-side and back and forth. Do this very gently to avoid hurting your client, especially if they are elderly or suffer from any bone or joint problems. The foot should be mobile and flexible and move easily.

Any problems with the mobility and flexibility of the foot usually represent bone and joint problems such as general stiffness or arthritis. Inflexibility can also reflect a rigid or inflexible personality.

Arthritis
Arthritis is the inflammation of a joint. There are two main types of arthritis and both can affect the feet. They are osteoarthritis and rheumatoid arthritis and are discussed in more detail on page 30.

When treating a client with either form of arthritis, it is important not to apply pressure to any areas of inflammation. Always avoid these areas and work the corresponding reflexes on the hands. Pay particular attention to the reflexes of the adrenal glands, skeletal and circulatory systems as well as reflexes for any areas affected by arthritis. For example, if your client suffers with arthritis in the hips then make sure you spend time working the hip reflex on the foot.

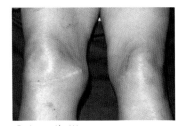

Osteoarthritis

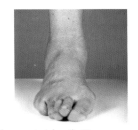

Rheumatoid arthritis

Reflexions
Working the reflex for the adrenal glands will help your client's body cope with pain and inflammation. Thus, this reflex should always be worked in cases of arthritis, gout or any other disorders characterised by pain and inflammation.

Gout

Gout is the build-up of uric acid and its salts in the blood and joints and it often occurs in the big toe. Crystals accumulate in, irritate and erode the cartilage of joints. Eventually, the bones can fuse, leading to an immovable joint. Symptoms include inflammation, swelling, pain, tenderness and a loss of mobility. Gout occurs primarily in middle-aged and older males and is suspected to be caused by diet, an abnormal gene or environmental factors such as stress. During a reflexology treatment do not apply pressure to the affected area which will usually be inflamed and painful. Do, however, focus on the reflexes for the circulatory system as well as the organs of elimination and the adrenal glands.

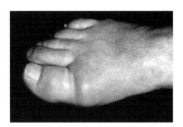

Gout

Hallux rigidus

Hallux rigidus is the stiffening of the joint between the hallux (the big toe) and the metatarsals. It is usually caused by damage to the nerves, injury or arthritic inflammation.

DESCRIPTION OF FOOT	HOW CAN THIS RELATE TO YOUR CLIENT'S HEALTH?
Rigid and inflexible feet	Rigid and inflexible feet indicate rigid and inflexible joints and imbalances in the skeletal system. They can also represent a rigid and inflexible personality.

Examine the nails

Finally, have a good look at your client's toe and finger nails. The nails can be affected by many skin conditions and can also be indicators of internal imbalances, nutritional deficiencies, neglect or stress and anxiety. It is important to be able to recognise diseases and disorders of the nails in order to avoid cross-infection. The toes and fingers represent the head, and disorders of the nails can often be linked to disorders of the head such as headaches. Nail problems also indicate imbalances in the meridians. Refer to page 225 for more information on meridian therapy.

During a treatment do not touch the affected nails, as this could be painful for the client and the nails may also be infectious. Rather, treat the same reflex area on the client's hand. Advise the client not to cut their nails too short or down the sides and to keep the area very clean to prevent further infection. Also suggest that the client does not pull stockings or socks on too tightly as this could also damage the nails. If the condition is very painful, recommend that they visit a chiropodist.

Agnail (Hang nail)

Hang nail is characterised by dry, split cuticles. It is often caused by poor manicure or pedicure techniques, the use of detergents or soaking the hands in water for long periods. Although a harmless disorder, it can become infected.

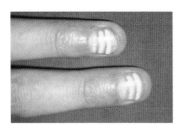

Beau's lines

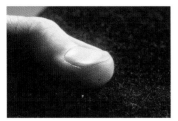

Koilonychias (spoon nail)

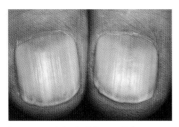

Leuconychia (white nails)

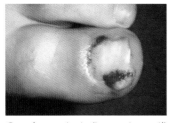

Onychocryptosis (ingrowing nail)

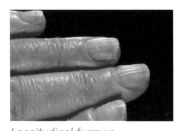

Longitudinal furrows

Anonychia
Anonychia is the congenital absence of a nail.

Beau's Lines
Beau's lines are transverse (horizontal) ridges or grooves on the nail plate. They can reflect a temporary retardation of growth due to ill health, a very high fever or a zinc deficiency in the body.

Egg Shell Nails (Soft, thin nails)
Eggshell nails are unusually soft, thin, white nails that are curved over the free edge. They can be the result of poor diet, ill health, medication or some nervous disorders.

Koilonychias (Spoon nail)
Koilonychias is the term given to spoon-shaped, concave nails resulting from abnormal growth. Spoon nails can be congenital, due to a lack of minerals or as a result of illness. The nails are also thin, soft and hollowed.

Leuconychia (White nails Or white spots)
Leuconychia is the term given to white spots or streaks on the nail or to nails that are white or colourless. Leuconychia is often the result of trauma to the nail or air bubbles. It can also be an indication of poor health. The white spots will grow out with the nail.

Longitudinal furrows
Longitudinal (vertical) ridges can occur on the nail as a result of uneven nail tissue growth. To some extent they are normal in adults and increase with age. However, severe ridges can result from injury to the nail matrix through poor manicure or pedicure techniques or from the excess use of detergents and other harsh chemicals. They can also be caused by conditions such as psoriasis and poor circulation.

Onychauxis (Thick nails)
Onychauxis is an unusual thickness of the nail caused by trauma to the nail matrix, fungal infection or neglect. It can also be hereditary.

Onychocryptosis (Ingrowing nail)
Onychocryptosis is an ingrowing nail – a condition in which the sides of the nail penetrate the skin. It is characterised by red, shiny skin around the nail and can be very sensitive and painful if touched. Ingrowing nails are most common on the big toe and can be caused by ill fitting shoes or improper nail cutting.

Onycholysis (Separation of the nail from the nail bed)
Onycholysis is the separation of the nail from the nail bed. It usually begins to loosen at the free edge and continues up to the lunula, but does not fall off. It can be caused by illness, trauma, infection, certain drugs or abuse of the nails.

Onychomycosis (Fungal infection of the nail)
Onychomycosis is a fungal infection of the toe nails in which the nails become thickened, yellow and chalky and give off a distinct odour. Onychomycosis is contagious and should be treated as soon as possible. (See tinea ungium.)

Onychophagy (Nail biting)
Nail biting is common in people who suffer from stress or anxiety. It can result in an exposed nail bed which is inflamed and sore. Onychophagy is the term given to nails that have become deformed through excess nail biting.

Onychoptosis (Nail shedding)
Onychoptosis is a condition in which parts of the nail shed. It usually occurs during ill health or as a reaction to some drugs. It can also be caused by trauma to the nail.

Onychorrhexis (Brittle nails)
Onychorrhexis is the term given to dry, brittle, splitting nails that also have longitudinal ridges. It is common in old age or people with arthritis or anaemia. It can also be caused by poor manicure or pedicure techniques and excess soaking of the hands in water or detergents.

Paronychia (Bacterial infection of the cuticle and nail wall)
Paronychia is a bacterial infection of the skin surrounding the nails. The tissues become red, swollen and painful. It is a common infection that can be the result of injury, nail biting or poor manicure or pedicure techniques.

Pterygium (Overgrowth of cuticle)
This is the condition in which the cuticle becomes overgrown and grows forward, sticking to the nail plate. The cuticle can become dry and split and it is usually a result of neglect or poor nail care.

Severely bruised nail
Bruised nails are a result of physical damage or trauma to the nail bed. A clot of blood forms under the nail plate and, in some cases, a severely bruised nail can fall off.

Tinea ungium (Ringworm of the nail)
Tinea ungium is ringworm of the nail. It is a fungal infection characterised by thickened and deformed nails. Infected nails may separate from the nail bed, crumble or flake off.

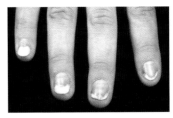

Onycholysis (separation of the nail from the nail bed)

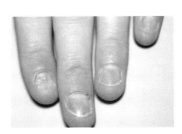

Onychophagy (nail biting)

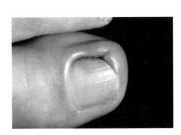

Paronychia (bacterial infection of the cuticle and nail wall)

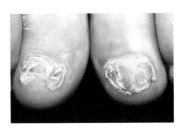

Tinea ungium (ringworm)

Case Studies: Reading The Feet

Marion

Marion is 71 years old. As a baby she had chronic whooping cough and from the age of 10 she has suffered with back problems. Four years ago she broke her right leg and had to have surgery to both her knee and hip. Since then she has had chronic problems with her hips and knees and can no longer walk without a stick. Marion has also had an underactive thyroid for the last 32 years, is diabetic and suffers from advanced arthritis in both knees. In addition, although she went through menopause many years ago, she still has gynaecological bleeding almost every day, has hot flushes and has recently been diagnosed with fibroids. Marion's feet are red, swollen and very warm to touch. The right foot is notably warmer than the left.

Photo 1 is a lateral view of Marion's feet and reveals the following:

- Her lower back reflex (on the dorsum of her foot) is swollen and puffy. Marion was in a car accident 5 years ago and cracked a lumbar vertebrae. Since then she has suffered with lower back problems. Her hip reflex (the ankle) is swollen and puffy and she suffers with chronic hip problems.
- Her ovary reflex (below the ankle) is very congested, swollen and puffy and has a build-up of hard, dry skin on it. Although Marion had six children with no problems, she has had gynaecological bleeding every day since menopause, still experiences hot flushes and has uterine fibroids.
- Her knee reflex (slightly below and in front of the ankle) is puffy and swollen. Marion has arthritis in both knees and has also had problems with her right knee since she broke her leg.
- The dry, rough skin on her pelvic reflex (the heel) emphasises her gynaecological, lower back and hip problems.

Photo 2 shows a build-up of hard, dry skin on Marion's brain reflex (tip of the big toe). Marion suffers from weekly headaches.

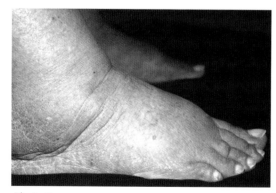

Photo 1

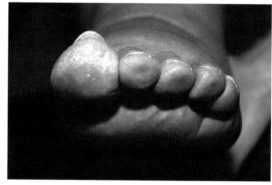

Photo 2

In **photos 3** and **4** the skin over Marion's digestive reflex (area between the ball of her foot and the heel) and pelvic reflex (the heel) is loose and saggy. She says she has no problems with her digestive system itself, however, she does suffer with flatulence and bloating. In addition, the pancreas is part of

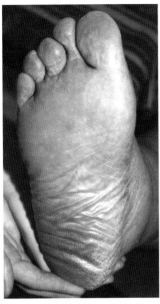

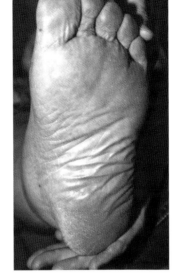

Photo 3

Photo 4

the digestive system and lies in the area where the skin is loose. As we know, Marion is diabetic.

The loose skin over her pelvic area reminds us of her gynaecological problems. The dry, hard skin over her heel also emphasises her lower back and gynaecological problems. We can see in photos 3 and 4 that the skin over Marion's thyroid reflex (neck of the big toe) is loose and saggy. This reflects the thyroid imbalance that she has had for many years.

Finally, there is discolouration and a slight build-up of dry skin on Marion's chest reflexes (ball of the foot) and the area is slightly swollen. Marion says she had very bad bronchitis one month ago.

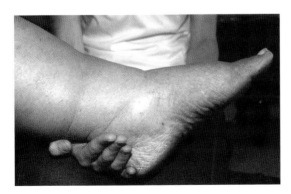

Photo 5

Photo 5 shows how flat Marion's arch is. Flat, or dropped arches reflect both digestive disorders and lower back problems. Marion suffers with flatulence and bloating as well as chronic lower back ache.

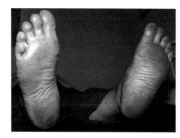

Julie

Julie is Marion's 50 year old daughter. She was a very healthy child and teenager and had two children while still quite young. However, she later developed both uterine fibroids and ovarian cysts and after numerous procedures had a total hysterectomy at the age of 42. Since then she feels she has not been herself and her health has not been good. Julie suffers from stress and tension and a few years ago she suffered with severe depression. Like her mother, she also has an underactive thyroid and chronic lower back pain. She has degeneration of the lumbar vertebrae.

The top photo on the left shows both of Julie's feet and the first thing we notice is their overall dryness and that the right foot is worse than the left. Interestingly, she feels most of her problems, especially her back ache, are on the right side of her body. Looking at the next two photos we can see the following:

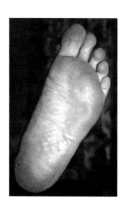

- A callus on her occipital reflex (on the base of the big toe, just above the neck of the toe). Julie suffers from chronic headaches that develop from her neck and move up the back of her head into the occipital region.
- Loose, saggy skin over her thyroid reflexes (the neck of the big toe). Like her mother, Julie has an underactive thyroid gland. Note that there is also a deep horizontal wrinkle over the thyroid helper reflexes (which lie in zone one, just beneath the ball of the foot).
- A build-up of dry skin and puffiness over her chest reflexes (the balls of her feet). A year ago Julie was hospitalised with bronchial pneumonia and a slightly enlarged heart.
- Zones 3–5 of Julie's liver reflex (on the right foot only, below the ball of the foot, extending across all zones) are markedly swollen. Although she has no liver problems she does take medication and supplements, both of which affect the liver.
- The skin over Julie's digestive reflexes (the area between the ball of the foot and the heel) is loose and saggy. Again, she has no problems here but does suffer from bloating.
- Although it is not easy to see from the photo, Julie's bladder reflex (on the arch of the foot, close to the heel) is dry and callused. She finds that since having had her hysterectomy she needs constantly to relieve her bladder and also struggles with minor incontinence when she sneezes.
- Finally, Julie's heels are dry, callused and splitting and this reflects both her gynaecological problems (cysts and fibroids and menopausal hot flushes) and the lower back pain.

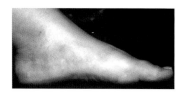

Julie has a fungal infection of the toenails called onychomycosis. This is clearly seen in the bottom photo where you can see the yellow discolouration and chalky/granular texture of the nails. The toenails are reflexes for the head and Julie does suffer with headaches. You will also learn in Chapter 5 that two major meridians run through the big toe. These are the spleen/pancreas meridian and the liver meridian. The spleen/pancreas meridian also runs through the pelvis and an imbalance in this meridian is sometimes exhibited as cysts, fibroids and menstrual problems. Julie has a history of cysts and fibroids.

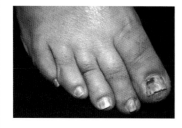

Reflexology Techniques

Reflexology is more than a simple foot massage. It is a deeply relaxing experience in which a person can release not only physical tension, but also emotional and spiritual unease. It is vital that you, as a therapist, are always properly prepared for your client and that you work on them with positive intentions. This chapter introduces the basic techniques that make up a reflexology treatment. **Note:** The techniques described below are demonstrated in the accompanying DVD.

Preparation

Positioning your client

One of the main aims of a reflexology treatment is to relax the client. It is therefore important that they are comfortable throughout the treatment. Reflexology is usually carried out with the client either lying on a massage couch or a specially designed reflexology chair. You should always:

- support your client's head and back with cushions to ensure they are comfortable. You must be able to see their face so that you can monitor any reactions they may express. Therefore your client should be in a semi-reclining position.
- place a support under their knees to ease pressure off their lower back.
- cover your client with a towel or blanket to keep them warm and give them a feeling of security.

Positioning yourself

You should sit comfortably with both feet flat on the floor, an upright upper body and relaxed shoulders. Ideally, the client's feet will be at the same height as your solar plexus so that you can examine and move the feet easily without having to bend or hunch over them. It is also recommended that you use a chair or stool that has wheels so that you can move easily around the client's feet. This will enable you to work the feet comfortably from different positions without strain.

Cleaning the feet

Before working on your client's feet it is very important that you clean them first. There are a number of different antiseptic products you can use and once you have cleaned the feet make sure you dispose of any cotton wool or wipes you have used. Remember to always use a new wipe for each foot to avoid cross-contamination and always wash your hands before and after every treatment.

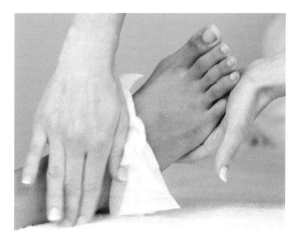

Cleaning the feet

Choosing a medium

It is not essential use a medium when performing a reflexology treatment. In fact, many reflexologists choose not to use a medium because they find it makes their thumbs and fingers slip and so prevents them from working deeply. The following mediums are available:

- Talc, liquid talc and corn starch – these dry out the tissue and are helpful if your client has sweaty feet or you have sweaty hands. Be aware, however, that they should be used sparingly as airborne particles can cause respiratory problems and their use is not recommended for clients who are asthmatic or have a dust allergy.
- Cream or lotion – many reflexologists enjoy working with creams, especially when performing relaxation techniques.

It is not advisable to use oil during a treatment as it makes the feet too slippery to work on properly.

> **Reflexions**
> Unusually damp or sweaty feet are a sign that there is an imbalance in the body. They can indicate that your client is feeling nervous or stressed. They can also suggest a hormonal imbalance.

Holding the feet

Reflexology should be an enjoyable experience for both the giver and receiver and at the end of the treatment you should be as relaxed and balanced as your client. However, this is not always the case for many therapists – especially those new to reflexology. It is not uncommon for students to find that their hands and thumbs ache and their necks and shoulders become sore and tense. Discomforts such as these can indicate that:

- Your posture is incorrect. Always ensure both feet are flat on the floor and the client's feet are approximately in line with your solar plexus. If possible, use a stool or chair on wheels so that you can move around the feet rather than twisting your body around the feet.
- You are not holding the feet properly. Focus on learning to hold and support the feet properly and you will develop good techniques that will be easy and enjoyable to perform.

The first rule of reflexology is to always use both your hands during a treatment. Either both hands are working the same reflexes on either foot at the same time, or one hand works a reflex while the other hand supports the foot. Your working hand is usually referred to as the 'working hand' while the other hand is called the 'support hand'. Both hands are always close together and your working hand is always pushing into or working through the feet into the support hand. Never have a lazy hand!

In the standard support grip, always:

- Keep your support hand as close to your working hand as possible.
- Take the foot in the support hand with your four fingers on top of the foot and the thumb beneath the foot. The web of your hand between your fingers and thumb will be touching the side of the foot.

Study tip
Make sure you learn the following vocabulary well:

Working hand – the hand that is applying pressure and working a reflex
Support hand – this hand is always close to the working hand and supports or holds the foot
Leverage – the pressure provided by the rest of your working hand, and sometimes the support hand, in opposition to your working thumb or finger.

Place the fingers of the working hand on top of the support hand so that if you inadvertently squeeze these fingers the pressure will go into your support hand and not directly into the client's foot.

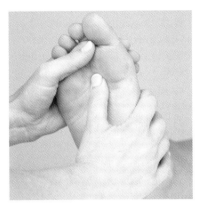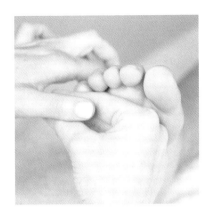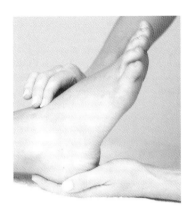

Working and supporting the feet

It is important that you are aware of the functions of the support hand. It:

- Supports the foot being worked on and keeps it still
- Acts as a barrier to the working hand's fingers and so protects the foot from unnecessary pressure or pinching
- Provides an area off which the working hand's fingers can 'lever'
- Helps spread or open up the foot to make deeper reflexes more accessible
- Reassures the client by giving a sense of continual contact.

Use both your hands during a treatment – your working hand pushes through your client's foot into your support hand while your support hand pulls your client's foot into your working hand.

In addition, pressure is gained through what is called leverage. Leverage is the pressure provided by the rest of your working hand, and sometimes your support hand, in opposition to your working thumb or finger. To understand this concept better, place the thumb of your working hand onto your forearm and press it as hard as you can into your arm without letting the rest of that hand touch the forearm. See what little pressure you get. Now, place the thumb of your working hand onto your forearm and wrap the rest of your working hand around your forearm so that your fingers are working in opposition to your thumb. Now, press as hard as you can and you will see how much more pressure you get from doing this and how much easier it is on your thumb.

Finally, throughout your treatment, always keep the foot bent slightly towards you so that the longitudinal tendon is not exposed as this would cause discomfort. A relaxed foot also allows for deeper penetration without unnecessary discomfort.

Relaxation techniques

Reflexology is a holistic therapy which treats the whole person – mind, body and soul. Relaxation is an integral part of reflexology and it is important to spend the first few minutes of every treatment using relaxation techniques prior to working specific reflexes with the deeper pressure techniques. When your client is relaxed, their body will balance and heal itself naturally. Relaxation techniques also loosen up stiff muscles, ligaments and tendons and improve circulation to the body as a whole and to the reflexes to which they are applied. Finally, they give your client time to unwind before you begin working specific reflexes.

While doing the relaxation techniques, take note of the flexibility of the joints, the springiness and resilience of the tissues, the texture of the skin and the presence of any congestion or crystalline deposits. Also have a look at the nails and the general structure of the feet. Use this time to start building up a picture of your client's health and balance.

Relaxation techniques can also be interspersed throughout the treatment when you feel you need to pay extra attention to a particular area or if a client has a reaction during the treatment. You can also use the same relaxation techniques at the end of your treatment to ensure the body is completely balanced and to close off the treatment.

Greeting the feet/Palming/First contact and solar plexus breathing

The way in which you first touch your client's feet will set the tone for the entire treatment so take your time and gently, but firmly, welcome your client's feet. You can spend as long as you like on this technique as it is very good for stress and will help your client to slow down and unwind in preparation for their treatment. Try to work with your client's breathing and also remember to breathe deeply and slowly yourself. You will work both feet at the same time in this technique, your right hand on their left foot and your left hand on their right foot.

Note
Use the following techniques in any order. Remember that you don't have to use every technique in every treatment. Be aware of any contra-indications, especially arthritic joints, pregnancy and diabetes and tailor the techniques accordingly.

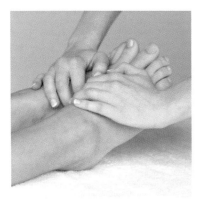

Greeting the feet

1. Begin by placing your hands on top of the feet and take a few deep breaths.

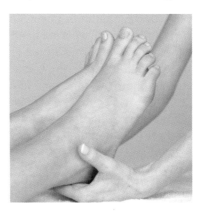

2. Slide your hands to the heels and gently pull them towards you. As you pull, lean backwards slightly so that the movement pulls the heels backwards.

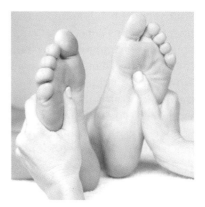

3. Slide your hands up the soles of the feet and place your thumbs on the solar plexuses.

Practical tip: Moving your own body

When giving a treatment try to keep your own body as relaxed and fluid as possible to prevent straining or tensing your muscles. Remember that you never need to use your own strength to achieve deep pressure. Instead, use the weight of your body. When you press into a point and want more depth and pressure simply lean forwards into the point and when you want to lessen the pressure simply lean back. You now have a choice – just follow your instincts and do what feels right for your client:

- Ask them to take a deep breath and as they breathe in lean your body forwards so that your thumbs press into the solar plexus. As they breathe out lean back to release the pressure on the solar plexus. Repeat three times.

- Or, if your client is very stressed and their solar plexus feels tight and tender, spend some time unwinding the solar plexus by moving your thumbs in an anticlockwise direction.

- Or, simply lean into the solar plexus and maintain pressure on it while your client continues to breathe deeply. Hold the solar plexus until you feel your client begin to relax – this can take up to a minute.

Effleurage/Stroking

There are few things more relaxing than the flowing, warming movements of effleurage. This is a simple, almost instinctive, technique that encourages deep relaxation and also promotes circulation throughout the whole body.

As well as using effleurage to begin and end your treatment, use it when you change techniques or move to different areas of the foot. It is a good technique to use if your client becomes too sensitive or uncomfortable for deep pressure techniques or if they have an emotional reaction during a treatment. Finally, effleurage should always be used for any circulatory and lymphatic conditions. The technique itself is a natural movement:

- With your fingers together let your hands mould the contours of the feet, ankles and lower legs as you stroke them.
- Keep your entire hand in contact with the skin and use more pressure as you stroke up towards the heart and less as you come down to the toes.
- Establish a rhythm in sync with both yours and your client's breathing.

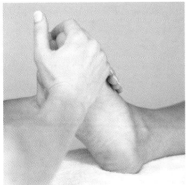
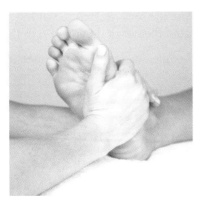
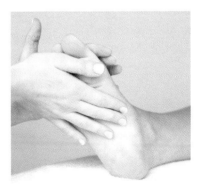

Effleuraging the feet

Side to side/back and forth slapping

Slapping or creating friction on the sides of the feet is another technique that encourages circulation and promotes the flow of energy. It is a great technique to use for any circulatory disorders as well as fatigue. In addition, it releases tension in the spine and also helps with disorders of the nervous system. However, it is a vigorous technique that creates a lot of movement in the pelvic area and it is, therefore, contraindicated during pregnancy.

Side friction/back and forth slapping is carried out on one foot at a time:

- Place the palms of your hands on either sides of the foot with your hands straight and your fingertips pointing upwards as if in a prayer position.
- Vigorously rub your hands up and down the foot to move it from side to side.

Note: the heel remains in contact with the couch so that it can act as a pivot.

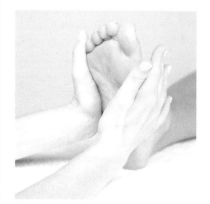 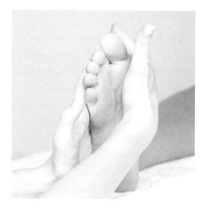 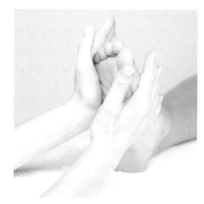

Side to side/Back and forth slapping

Foot squeezing

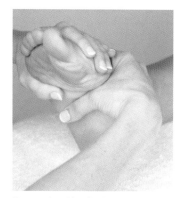

Foot squeezing is a firm, fast technique that is extremely beneficial for circulatory disorders. The secret behind this technique is in its speed and firmness – it should feel as if you are trying to squeeze and pump the blood out of the foot. Foot squeezing is carried out on one foot at a time:

- Begin by placing your hands on either side of the foot, as close to the ankle as possible. Wrap your hands around the foot with your fingers on the top of the foot and your thumbs on the bottom.
- Squeeze your hands into the foot and at the same time twist them both inwards.
- Release the pressure and repeat the movement working up the foot to the toes and then back down again to the ankle.

Squeezing the foot

Ankle boogie/Ankle loosening/Hook in ankles

The ankle boogie is another very powerful technique that releases tension in the hips and spine. However, it is contraindicated in pregnancy and is also not advisable for elderly, frail or arthritic clients because it is such a vigorous technique. The ankle boogie is performed on one foot at a time:

- Place the heels of your hands on either side of the foot, just below the ankle bones. Ensure your palms are facing upwards.
- Rapidly move the hands back and forth so that as your right hand goes backwards your left one comes forwards and vice versa.

- This should be a fast, strong movement that causes the foot to 'flap' from side to side.

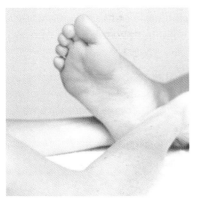 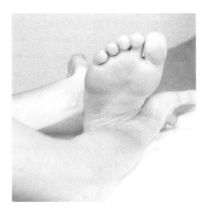 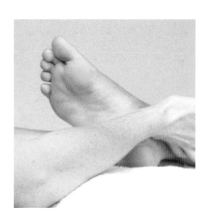

Ankle boogie

Ankle stretch and rotation/circumduction

Working the ankles helps to release any tension in the pelvic area, including the hips and sacral spine, and encourages circulation to the reproductive organs. In stretching and rotating the ankles the calf muscles are also stretched and this helps with any disorders of the ankles or wrists (remember the wrists are referral areas to the ankles). When stretching the ankles it is best to work one foot at a time:

- Support the heel of the foot with one hand and place the palm of your working hand on the ball of your client's foot.
- In time with your client's breath, lean forwards into your working hand and push into the ball of the foot to encourage dorsiflexion. Your support hand will gently pull the heel towards you. Hold the stretch and then release.
- Now, keeping the support hand under the heel, place the palm of your working hand on the top of the foot and lean backwards, pulling the foot towards you and encouraging plantarflexion. Your support hand will gently guide the heel backwards. Hold the stretch and release.
- Take care not to overstretch the ankles, especially with elderly, frail or arthritic clients.

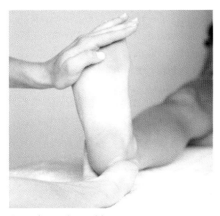 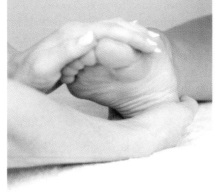

Stretching the ankle

Ankle rotation is also done on one foot at a time. If you are working on your client's right foot, then use your right hand as your support hand and your left hand as your working hand. If you are working on your client's left foot, use your left hand as the support hand and your right hand as the working hand. This means that you will be holding the lateral edge of the foot when rotating it (see photos below).

- Support the heel of the foot with one hand and hold the lateral edge of the foot with your working hand. Try to hold the foot just below the toes so that the webbing between your thumb and fingers is in contact with the edge of the ball of the foot.
- Slowly rotate the foot in large, smooth circles. Rotate it both clockwise and anticlockwise several times.
- If the foot does not move smoothly it is an indication of tension in the pelvic area, especially the hips and sacral spine.

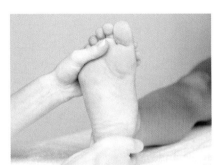 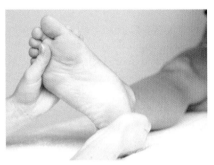

Rotating the ankles

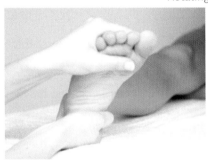 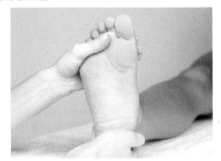

Lower leg massage
The entire lower leg, especially the calf muscle, can be massaged with deep, flowing techniques such as effleurage and kneading. The fingers or knuckles may be used. Massage to this area not only stimulates the flow of blood to the feet, it also stimulates 'helper' reflexes to the reproductive area and therefore benefits women trying to become pregnant. The back of the lower leg along the Achilles tendon is, in fact, sometimes called the 'chronic reproductive' reflex. Deep work to this area must, however, be avoided if a client is already pregnant as acupoints are located here.

Spinal twist/Foot wringing
Anyone suffering with stiffness or tension in the back will love this technique. It is a strong technique that releases tension and helps relieve backache. However, because it is such a strong technique it should not be used on anyone who has arthritis in the foot.

Work one foot at a time:

- Place both your hands together, palms down, on the medial edge of the foot with your fingers on the top of the foot and your thumbs on the bottom. The webbing between your fingers and thumbs should be in contact with the medial edge of your client's foot (their spinal reflex).
- The hand closest to your client's ankle will be the support hand and the hand nearer the toes will be the working hand.
- Keep your support hand very still and firm and with your working hand slowly and strongly 'twist' the spinal reflex in both directions. It should feel as if you are wringing water out of a wet towel.
- Repeat this movement up the length of the spine and back down again.

Sometimes you will hear a cracking sound when performing the spinal twist. Do not be alarmed by this, it is simply an indication that tension is being worked out of the spine.

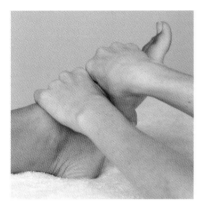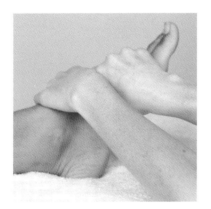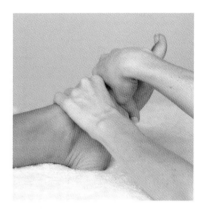

The spinal twist

Shoulder sandwich

Everybody seems to love receiving this technique. It is a warming, relaxing technique that releases tension in the neck, shoulders and thoracic spine and that also helps with respiratory and stress-related disorders. The shoulder sandwich is done on one foot at a time:

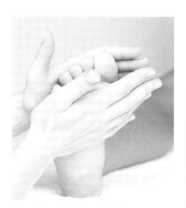

- Place the palms of your hands on either side of the lateral edge of the foot, directly over the shoulder reflex. The foot should be 'sandwiched' between your two palms with your fingers facing towards the big toe. It may help to move your chair around so that you are sitting close to the small toe of the foot and facing your body towards the big toe.
- Slowly and firmly move your hands in large circular movements. Move one hand ahead of the other – it is the same movement you would use to roll dough into a ball.
- Repeat in the other direction.

The shoulder sandwich

Metatarsal manipulation/Chest or lung relaxation

Working or manipulating the metatarsals opens up the chest, deepening breathing and helping to relieve tension. It is a beneficial technique for any respiratory or stress-related disorders and it also helps release stiffness in the shoulders and thoracic spine. Work one foot at a time:

- Support the top of the foot with a flat palm and place the fist of your working hand on the ball of the foot.
- As your client breathes in, lean into your fist and push inwards.
- As they breathe out, release the pressure by moving your body backwards.
- Repeat this a few times and then use the knuckles of your working hand to knead the ball of the foot and release any tension there.

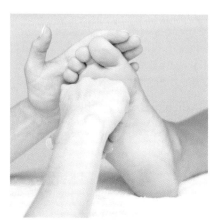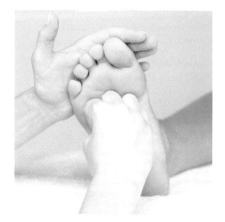

Knuckling the foot

Practical tip: Breathing

'*If the autonomic nervous system is the gearbox that moves us into one state of readiness or another, breathing is the gearshift, the lever we grasp to shift from one of those states to the next.*' Otto Schmidt, biophysicist[5]

Have you noticed that when you are stressed you often do not breathe properly and if you stop for a minute and take a few deep breaths you feel you can cope better with a situation? Breathing is integral to relaxation and stress-relief and should be an integral part of every reflexology treatment. To make it part of your treatments do the following:

- Encourage your client to focus on their own breath, to 'listen' to it and 'feel' it. This will help them to relax and unwind and take their mind off any stressful events or situations they may be thinking about.
- Let your client's breathing establish the 'rhythm of the treatment by applying and releasing pressure in sync with their breaths and letting your movements flow in time with their breathing.
- Finally, remember to breathe yourself. When first learning reflexology students often concentrate so much on their techniques that they forget to breathe themselves. This stiffens the body and as a result the movements do not flow so well. Relax, make an effort to breathe deeply and, ideally, follow your client's breathing so that a rhythm develops between your client, your movements and you.

Intercostal sliding

Intercostal sliding is a technique that helps to relax the chest muscles, open up the thoracic cage and encourage deep breathing. In doing this it helps with breathing difficulties, respiratory problems and stress-related conditions. Work one foot at a time:

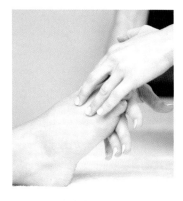

Intercostal sliding

- Place the back of your support hand on the sole of the foot and the tips of your working fingers on the top of the foot between the toes.
- Slowly and deeply slide your fingers down the dorsum of the foot, between the metatarsals. Picture the metatarsals as the ribs and the spaces between them as the intercostals muscles.
- Repeat the movement a number of times.

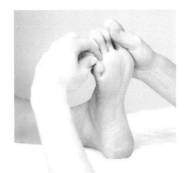

Stretching the toes individually

Toe stretching and rotation/Toe circumduction

The toes are the reflexes for the neck and in working them you release tension and stiffness in the neck and shoulders. This technique also helps relieve sinusitis and is very good for conditions of the nervous system. It is, however, contraindicated if there is any arthritis in the toes. This technique takes a bit of time as each toe needs to be worked on individually:

- Begin by taking a toe between your fingers and thumb and pull it to create a good stretch. At times you may hear a clicking sound – don't worry, this simply indicates you are releasing tension in the neck area.
- Still maintaining the toe stretch, rotate the toe slowly in both directions a few times.
- Release the toe and move onto the next one.
- Once you have stretched and rotated each toe, open your fingers and slide them between the toes so that the toes are opened. Maintaining this position, move your fingers to encourage movement between the toes.
- If your client is suffering from neck tension, you may not be able to slide all your fingers between their toes. Don't force your fingers, simply let them go as far as they can and spend some extra time working on the neck and shoulder reflexes to help relax these areas.

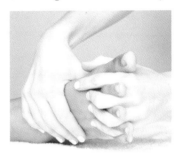

Rotating the toes together

Hacking and pummelling

Hacking and pummeling are two vigorous techniques that can be used to waken up and energise your client. They boost the circulation of the blood, encourage the elimination of waste and generally boost the flow of energy through the body. However, because they are so vigorous, they are not recommended for diabetic or pregnant clients. Diabetic clients often suffer with poor peripheral circulation and this technique may bruise their feet while it is too strong a technique for a pregnant woman. Hacking and pummelling are both done the same way, with one slight difference – if hacking, use the edges of your fingers and if pummelling, use the edge of a closed fist.

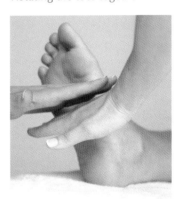

Hacking

- The lateral edge of the hand is always used so begin by placing one hand slightly above the other with your palms facing downwards, your thumbs closer to your body and your small fingers closer to the sole of the foot.
- Rhythmically beat the sole of the foot by striking it with the lateral edge of your fingers or fists, one hand at a time.
- Continue with this movement for as long as you think is necessary and ensure you develop a rhythm.

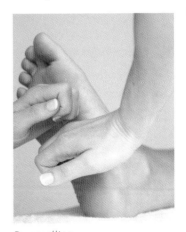

Pummelling

Zone walking/Zone clearing

Zone walking is one of the most important and therapeutic techniques you will learn as it is extremely calming and very balancing. It is recommended for any stress-related condition or energetic imbalance and can also be used to calm a client who suddenly becomes upset or reacts negatively during a treatment. Zone walking is done with both the thumb-walk or finger-walk technique. These are pressure techniques and are described on page 87. Work on one foot at a time:

- Hold the heel of the foot in your support hand and, starting with zone one, thumb-walk from the heel up the sole of the foot to the tip of the big toe. Ensure you only walk in zone one and remember to move your support hand up as your working thumb moves up so that by the time you are walking the big toe your support hand is behind the toes.
- Once you have finished walking zone one, return your thumb to the heel and thumb-walk zone two, three, four and five. NB, for ease of learning you are recommended to work from zone one to zone five. This is not essential however and if you wish you can also work from zone five to zone one instead.

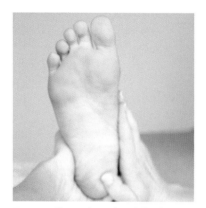
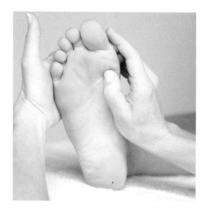
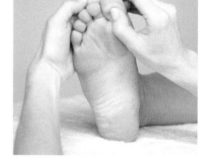

Zone walking the sole of the foot

Having thumb-walked all five zones on the sole of the foot, use your fingers to finger-walk down the five zones on the dorsum of the foot.

While walking each zone be aware of any congestion you may feel beneath your fingers and thumb. You can always stop and work out that congestion or make a note of it and return to it later in the treatment.

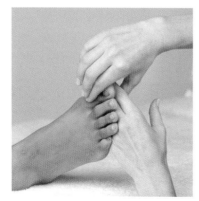
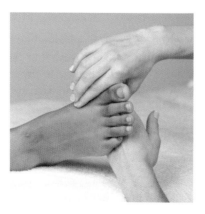
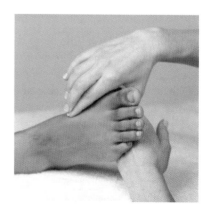

Zone walking the top of the foot

Pressure techniques

Pressure techniques form the basis of your reflexology treatment and, although it takes a while to master them, if you are doing them correctly they should always feel comfortable and easy. When performing a treatment, ensure that your own body is relaxed so that you do not injure yourself while trying to help someone else.

Practical tip: Pressure

The saying 'no pain, no gain' does not apply to reflexology and although some people enjoy deep pressure it should not be the focus of your treatment. In fact, some reflexologists do not use any pressure at all yet they still have outstanding results.

If, however, you want to use deep pressure in your treatments it is important that you do so without hurting yourself in the process. There are four steps to working deeply – each has been discussed in more detail in the previous pages:

- Use your support hand to draw the foot towards your working hand.
- Use the fingers of your working hand in opposition to your thumb to gain leverage.
- Move your body in towards the foot to gain more pressure and move it backwards to reduce the pressure.
- Work with your client's breath – the more relaxed they are the more their body will 'accept' the pressure.

Thumb-walking/Caterpillar crawl

Thumb-walking forms the basis of almost every reflexology treatment. Unfortunately, it is also the technique that damages the reflexologist's thumbs most often because it is done incorrectly. Take time to learn how to perform the technique properly from the start to avoid any injuries. To begin with, you need to find the correct hand position for thumb walking:

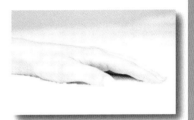

Finding the correct position for thumb walking

- Place your hand on a table, with your palm facing downwards and completely relaxed.
- You will notice that your thumb does not lie down flat. Instead, it rests on its edge – this is the edge of your thumb that you will use when thumb-walking. It is called the working edge of the thumb.

Now, learn thumb-walking on your own hand before practising it on someone's feet:

- Start at the bottom of the hand, near the wrist and aim to work in a straight line up towards your fingers.
- Place the working edge of your thumb on your opposite hand and wrap your working fingers around your hand to provide leverage.
- Begin by bending the top/distal joint of your thumb so that the working edge pushes into the flesh of your opposite hand.
- Now release the pressure by straightening the joint and moving upwards by a millimeter.
- Bend the joint and apply pressure again. Continue these tiny movements up to the fingertips.

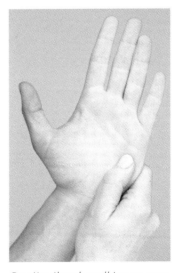

Practise thumb-walking on your own hand

- The focused, tiny movements should remind you of a caterpillar crawling along a surface.

Finally, you can practise on someone's feet. Try walking longitudinally up the foot from the heel to the toes and then walk transversely from one side of the foot to the other. Note that zone walking is a relaxation technique that uses thumb-walking. Please refer to page 86 for more information on zone walking.

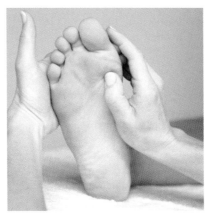

Thumb-walking up the sole of the foot

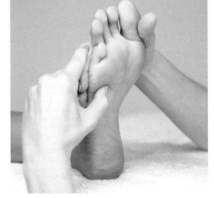

Transverse thumb-walking across the foot

Practical tip: The rules of thumb-walking

Thumb-walking forms the bulk of most treatments so try to be aware of the following:

- All movements should be very small. Imagine the foot has hundreds of tiny squares on it, like graph paper. Each one of those squares should be worked. If your thumb-walking consists of large, sliding movements you will miss many important reflexes of the feet.
- Do not over-extend your top/distal thumb joint when straightening it. To avoid over-extending this joint, remember to not completely straighten it during thumb-walking. Instead, always have it bent slightly.
- While walking the feet let your thumbs be your eyes and ears and listen to what the feet have to tell you. With practice you can feel areas of tension, emptiness, hardness, crystals and changes in temperature. All of these are signals of imbalances or congestion in specific areas.

Thumb-rotation

Thumb-rotation is a similar movement to thumb-walking, but there are two fundamental differences – the tip and not the medial edge of the thumb comes into contact with the foot, and the movement involves a rotation on each point. Begin by learning the technique on your opposite hand again:

- Place the tip of your working thumb on your opposite hand and wrap your working fingers around your hand to provide leverage.
- Begin by bending the top/distal joint of your thumb so that the tip pushes into the flesh of your opposite hand and then rotate this tip in a circular motion.
- Now release the pressure by straightening the joint and moving upwards by a millimeter.

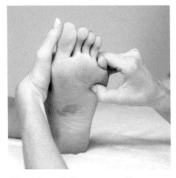

Thumb-rotating across the diaphragm line

Foot reflexology

- Bend the joint and apply pressure again. Continue these tiny movements up to the fingertips.
- Once you have mastered thumb-rotation on your own hand you can practise it on someone's feet.

Finger-walking

Reflexologists usually work the sole of the foot with their thumbs and the top, or dorsum, of the foot with their fingers. Your index finger will be your working finger and it often helps to strengthen or support this finger by placing your middle finger on top of your index finger:

- Place your support hand under the foot and your working finger on the top of the foot.
- Bend your finger so that the tip pushes into the top of the foot.
- Then straighten the finger and move it a millimeter forwards. Bend the joint again.
- Repeat this process as you move along the foot.

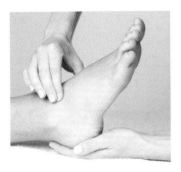

Finger-walking the Fallopian tubes/vas deferens

Finger-rotation

Finger-rotation is similar to thumb-rotation, except that the finger is used. Once again, use your index finger as the working finger and support it with your middle finger:

- Place your support hand under the foot and your working finger on the top of the foot.
- Bend your finger so that the tip pushes into the top of the foot. Now rotate the finger in a small circular movement.
- Then straighten the finger and move it a millimeter forwards. Bend the joint again.
- Repeat this process as you move along the foot.

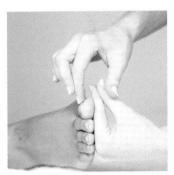

Finger-rotating across the face reflex

Thumb-hook/Hook-in, back-up/Bumblebee action

The thumb-hook is probably the deepest and strongest of all the techniques you will learn and it must be used with care, both for you and your client. As it is such a powerful technique it can hurt your client if performed on a very tender point and it can also hurt your thumb if done incorrectly. Do not use this technique too often. Instead, save it for specific reflexes that require the most accuracy and very deep stimulation.

Begin by locating the exact reflex you wish to work on and place the tip of your thumb on the reflex. When you are sure you are exactly on the reflex, bend the top/proximal joint of the thumb to a 90° angle, apply deep pressure and simultaneously swing your hand so your wrist comes upwards. When you first bend the joint your thumbnail will be facing the ceiling but when you have swung your hand around the thumbnail will be facing the floor. Now pull upwards so that the tip of the thumb hooks in and backs up into the flesh. Hold this position and maintain the pressure for as long as necessary (10–60 seconds). To avoid damaging your thumb while performing this technique ensure you use your support hand to draw the reflex into your working thumb. Also make sure your proximal thumb joint is at a 90° angle and that the thumb is not straight.

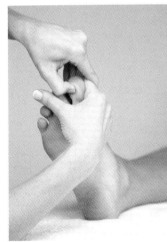

Thumb-hooking the pituitary reflex

Knuckling

Reflexology techniques are not only performed with the tips of the thumbs and fingers. You can also use your knuckles and you will find they are powerful tools that give a lot of depth and pressure to a treatment while at the same time letting you rest your thumbs and fingers. There are two ways you can use your knuckles:

- Work a specific reflex with the knuckle of one finger instead of the thumb.
- Work an entire region with knuckles of all four of your fingers at the same time.

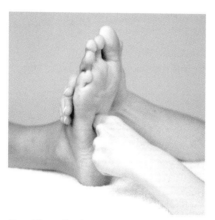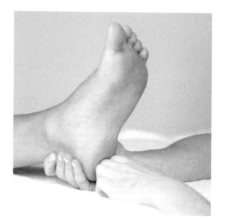

Knuckling the feet

Practical tip: Avoiding injury

As a reflexologist your hands are your source of income and if you overuse them or use them incorrectly you may injure them and have to stop working. Here are a few tips to prolong the life of your hands:

- Do not only use your thumb during a treatment. Make an effort to constantly change between your thumb, fingers and knuckles.
- Always ensure your thumbs or fingers are pointing in the direction that your hand is travelling. In other words, do not work backwards. For example, if you are working from the toes down towards the heels your elbow should be up and the tip of your thumb pointing downwards. Do not have the tip of your thumb pointing up to the toes while you are working downwards to the heel.
- Move your arms, wrists and elbows to ensure you are always comfortable. For example, when working vertical lines from the heels to the toes, drop your wrist and elbow and work upwards. When working vertical lines from the toes down to the heels, elevate your arms. Finally, when working horizontal lines elevate your elbow out to the side.
- Always ensure you are comfortable, your back is straight, your shoulders are dropped and you have both feet on the floor. If you are not comfortable then change your position as you will not be able to give a good treatment and you may injure yourself.
- Most importantly, if a technique feels uncomfortable or hurts you in any way, do not do it and use another technique.

Interpreting reflex points

So how do you know when a reflex is congested or needs extra work? The answer is quite straightforward – there should be a consistency in the feet in terms of texture, colour and temperature. Any area that is different from the rest of the foot requires attention.

Always begin a treatment by reading the feet as discussed on page 60. Any inconsistencies, imbalances or notable conditions should draw your attention to areas and reflexes on the feet that need some extra work.

After reading the feet you can begin your reflexology treatment with some relaxation techniques. While performing these techniques take note of what you feel on the feet and also how easily they can be manipulated. This will tell you which reflexes need to be re-worked.

Finally, as you do your treatment, you or your client will feel certain sensations that indicate imbalances or congestion. It is important that your client gives you feedback and lets you know how the treatment feels.

Important

Clients often want to know which reflexes are sensitive on them and what it means. You need to answer their questions carefully as they may not understand the concept of energy imbalances and instead interpret what you say as a diagnosis. For example, if you say 'that is your liver reflex' a client may think they have a problem with their liver when in fact it is just an imbalance in the energy of that area. If you are at all concerned about your client's health, refer them to a doctor and do not try to diagnose their condition yourself.

Sensitive or painful reflexes

Sensitive areas generally reflect an imbalance in a reflex and you will need to spend some extra time working these reflexes. There are a number of different ways you can work sensitive reflexes:

- **Holding** – Simply hold the reflex and apply as little or as much pressure as you feel necessary.
- **Pin-pointing** – Use your thumb or knuckle to apply pressure to the point, pushing inwards and upwards while using your support hand to pull the foot into your thumb or knuckle. Be careful not to hurt your client, especially if the reflex is painful.
- **Rotating** – If the reflex is very painful then spend a few minutes 'unwinding' it. Place your thumb on the reflex and gently and slowly unwind it in an anti-clockwise direction. Start with tiny circles that slowly spiral outwards until you are making large circles over the entire transverse zone in which the reflex lies. Imagine you are taking any excess energy out of the reflex and spreading it through the foot to rebalance the energy.
- **Rocking** – Hold the reflex with a bent thumb and rock back and forth several times.
- **Pinch 'n' Rotate** – Pinch the reflex between your thumb and index finger and using a deep pressure, rotate both digits several times.

Note:

- The ovaries/testes and uterus/prostate reflexes are often worked by holding/pinching these reflexes between the thumb and index finger and then rotating the entire foot into these digits instead of rotating the digits themselves.
- The reflexes for the lymphatics are also worked through a pinching action. This time, however, the webbing between the toes is pinched between the thumb and index finger.

Tight reflexes

Reflexes can sometimes feel very tight and they usually represent an excess of energy. They can be worked by:

- Simply holding your thumb gently over the reflex and applying minimal pressure until you feel the tension beneath beginning to give.
- Unwinding the reflex as described above.

Empty reflexes

Sometimes you will feel as if you could push your thumbs right through a reflex. They feel so soft that you could describe them as empty. Reflexes such as these usually indicate a lack of energy and should be worked by:

- **Winding up the reflex.** To wind up a reflex place your thumb over it and rotate it in a clockwise direction. Start with large circles that gather the energy from the rest of the foot and then slowly decrease these circles so they become small and focused on the reflex. This will draw the energy into the reflex.
- **Pumping the reflex.** You can also place your thumb on the reflex and use a pumping action to apply and release pressure on the area. This helps to stimulate the point.

Crystal deposits

It is not unusual to feel crystal deposits, especially in the shoulder reflex. These deposits feel like small grains of sand and need to be broken down by deep rubbing and pushing. Spend a few minutes on these deposits until you can no longer feel them.

Adapting techniques

Every person is different and you will need to change your techniques to suit each client. Always check they are happy with your pressure and be aware that if you are treating an elderly client, a young child, a pregnant woman, a diabetic or someone who is very ill they may not be able to cope with what other people might consider normal pressure – so use a lighter pressure. Also, if you are treating someone who is very stressed and wound up use slower and gentler techniques to relax them. You will learn more about how to adapt your techniques for specific conditions in Chapter 7.

Study Outline

The Structure of the Lower Leg and Foot

- The bones of the lower leg are the tibia and fibula.
- The foot is composed of 7 tarsal bones (the talus, calcaneus, cuboid, navicular, medial cuneiform, intermediate cuneiform and lateral cuneiform); 5 metatarsals and 14 phalanges.
- There are three arches in the foot:
  - **Medial longitudinal arch** – consists of the calcaneus, navicular, all three cuneiforms and the medial first three metatarsals.
  - **Lateral longitudinal arch** – consists of the calcaneus, cuboid and the lateral two metatarsals.
  - **Transverse arch** – consists of the cuboid, all three cuneiforms and the bases of the five metatarsals.
- The anterior muscles of the lower leg dorsiflex the ankle joint and extend the toes. These include the:
  - Tibialis anterior
  - Extensor hallucis longus
  - Extensor digitorum longus
  - Peroneus tertius
- The posterior muscles of the lower leg plantar flex the foot and flex the toes. These include the:
  - Gastrocnemius
  - Soleus
  - Flexor hallucis longus
  - Flexor digitorum longus
  - Tibialis posterior
- The lateral muscles of the lower leg plantar flex the ankle joint and evert the foot. These include the:
  - Peroneus (fibularis) longus
  - Peroneus (fibularis) brevis
- The muscles on the dorsum of the foot extend the toes. They include the:
  - Extensor digitorum brevis
  - Extensor hallucis brevis
- The muscles on the sole of the foot flex the toes. They include the:
  - Abductor hallucis
  - Flexor digitorum brevis
- The nerves of the lower leg and foot include the:
  - Femoral nerve
  - Saphenous nerve
  - Sciatic nerve
  - Tibial nerve
  - Common peroneal nerve

- The arteries of the lower leg and foot are the:
  - Popliteal artery
  - Anterior tibial artery
  - Dorsalis pedis artery
  - Posterior tibial artery
  - Peroneal artery
  - Medial plantar artery
  - Lateral plantar artery
  - Digital arteries

- The veins of the lower leg and foot are the:
  - Dorsal venous arch
  - Great saphenous vein
  - Small saphenous vein
  - Popliteal vein
  - Anterior tibial vein
  - Posterior tibial vein

Mapping the body onto the feet

To revise this section please study the diagrams on pages 56–59 of this chapter.

Reading and interpreting the feet
- Get a general overview of the feet.
- Look for any local contraindications.
- Look at the colour of the feet.
- Smell the feet.
- Feel the temperature of the feet.
- Feel for excess moisture or dryness.
- Feel the tone of the feet.
- Look and feel for changes in skin texture.
- Look and feel for any structural foot disorders.
- Move the feet to check for mobility and flexibility.
- Examine the toenails.

Relaxation techniques in a nutshell

Greeting the feet
Working both feet at a time, place both hands on the top of the foot, slide them down to the heels, gently pull the heels and then slide your thumbs to the solar plexus. Work the solar plexus in sync with your client's breathing.

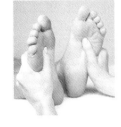

Effleurage
Use long, stroking movements to massage the feet.

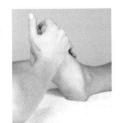

Side to side
Place your palms on either side of the foot in a prayer position and rub them up and down.

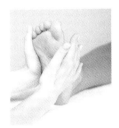

Foot squeezing
Place your hands on either side of the foot and squeeze and twist your hands inwards in a pumping action. Move the hands up and down the feet.

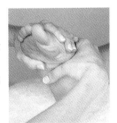

Ankle boogie
Place the heels of your hands on either side of the ankle and move them back and forth so the foot flaps from side to side.

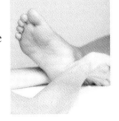

Ankle stretch and rotation
Support the heel of the foot with one hand and use the other to dorsiflex and plantar flex the foot and rotate the ankle in both directions.

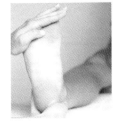

Lower leg massage
Work one leg at a time and use your hands, fingers or knuckles to deeply effleurage and knead the calf muscle.

Spinal twist
Place both hands on the arch of the foot and, keeping one hand still, use the other to twist the arch up and down.

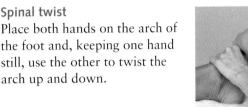

Shoulder sandwich
Sandwich the lateral edge of the foot between your two hands and move them in a circular motion.

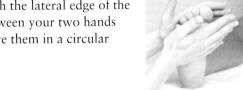

Metatarsal manipulation
Support the dorsum of the foot with one hand and use your knuckles to push into the ball of the foot in time with your client's breathing.

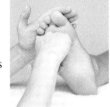

Intercostal sliding
Support the sole of the foot with one hand and use the fingers of your other hand to slide down between the metatarsals.

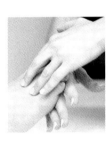

Toe stretching and rotation
Working one toe at a time, pull it and rotate it in both directions.

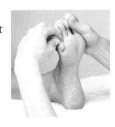

Once you have done this slide your fingers through the gaps between the toes to create movement in this area.

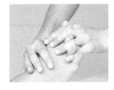

Hacking

Using flat hands, beat the sole of the foot with the lateral edge of your fingers.

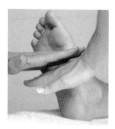

Finger-rotation

Using the tip of the index finger, apply small circular movements to a point on the foot before releasing the pressure and moving it forwards a fraction.

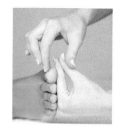

Pummelling

Using a closed fist, beat the sole of the foot with the lateral edge of your fist.

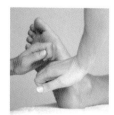

Thumb-hook

Push the tip of your thumb into a reflex and at the same time swing your hand upwards to hook your thumb deeply into the reflex.

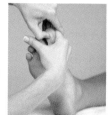

Zone walking

Using the thumb-walking technique, walk up and down each of the five zones of the foot.

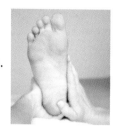

Knuckling

Use either one or all of your knuckles to work a reflex.

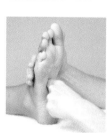

Pressure techniques in a nutshell

Thumb-walking

Using the lateral edge of the thumb, bend and straighten the thumb so that it moves along the foot in a tiny crawling movement.

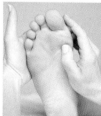

Thumb-rotation

Using the tip of the thumb, apply pressure to the foot and then rotate the thumb before releasing the pressure and moving along in tiny movements.

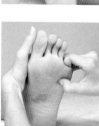

Finger-walking

Using the tip of your index finger to apply pressure, bend and straighten the finger so that it moves along the dorsum of the foot with tiny, crawling movements.

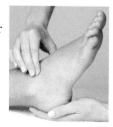

Multiple choice questions

1. **Which of the following are all tarsals?**
   a. Calcaneus, radius, talus, cuboid
   b. Hamate, capitate, ulna, sacrum
   c. Cuneiform, navicular, calcaneus, cuboid
   d. Radius, ulna, capitate, cuboid.

2. **A client presents with tinea pedis. What would you do?**
   a. Give them a full treatment, working all areas of the foot
   b. Give them a full treatment, working the hand instead of the infected foot
   c. Give them a full treatment, spending extra time working the areas of tinea pedis
   d. Do not give them any treatment at all and advise them to seek medical advice.

3. **Which of the following techniques would you use if you wished to work a point very deeply?**
   a. Effleurage
   b. Thumb-hook
   c. Zone-walking
   d. Foot squeezing.

4. **Which of the following techniques would you use if you wished to relax your client?**
   a. Effleurage
   b. Thumb-hook
   c. Thumb-rotation
   d. Finger-rotation.

5. **While looking at your client's feet you notice their toenails are thickened, yellow and have a granular texture as well as a strong smell. What could this be?**
   a. Eczema
   b. Onychophagy
   c. Dermatitis
   d. Onychomycosis.

6. **Which of the following techniques is contraindicated in pregnancy?**
   a. Zone-walking
   b. Spinal twist
   c. Ankle boogie
   d. Thumb-rotation.

7. **Which of the following techniques would be most beneficial for a client suffering with asthma?**
   a. Spinal twist
   b. Intercostal sliding
   c. Toe stretching
   d. Ankle boogie.

8. **Which arch in the foot is composed of the cuboid, all three cuneiforms and the bases of the five metatarsals?**
   a. Transverse arch
   b. Medial longitudinal arch
   c. Lateral longitudinal arch
   d. Intermediate longitudinal arch.

9. **What is the action of the gastrocnemius muscle?**
   a. Everts the foot
   b. Inverts the foot
   c. Plantar flexes the ankle joint
   d. Dorsiflexes the ankle joint.

10. **What do yellow feet indicate?**
    a. Diabetes
    b. Osteoporosis
    c. A kidney imbalance
    d. A liver imbalance.

3 Hand reflexology

Although foot reflexology is more popular, it is hand reflexology that has the most powerful effects on the emotions. Perhaps this is because we communicate so much with our hands and are able to express emotions such as love, tenderness and even anger with them.

When you first learn hand reflexology you may find it more difficult than foot reflexology because the hands are so much smaller and it is more difficult to locate the reflexes. Don't give up, however, because hand reflexology is an easy and accessible therapy. It can be used in public places such as exhibitions, airports or shopping malls where people do not want to take off their shoes and socks. It is also popular with people who have contraindications on their feet, are ticklish on their feet or are simply shy about their feet. It can be used quickly in first aid situations and, finally, you can always show your clients how to work reflexes on their own hands.

Student objectives

By the end of this chapter you will be able to:

- Describe the structure of the forearm and hand, including the bones, muscles, nerves and blood vessels
- Map the body onto the hands
- Read and interpret the hands in preparation for a reflexology treatment
- Perform a complete reflexology treatment on the hands.

The Structure Of The Forearm And Hand

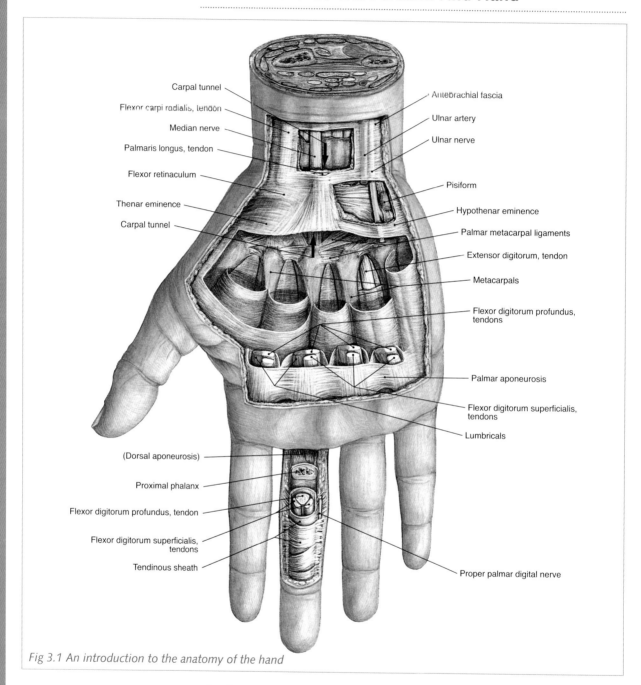

Carpal tunnel

Flexor carpi radialis, tendon

Median nerve

Palmaris longus, tendon

Flexor retinaculum

Thenar eminence

Carpal tunnel

Antebrachial fascia

Ulnar artery

Ulnar nerve

Pisiform

Hypothenar eminence

Palmar metacarpal ligaments

Extensor digitorum, tendon

Metacarpals

Flexor digitorum profundus, tendons

Palmar aponeurosis

Flexor digitorum superficialis, tendons

Lumbricals

(Dorsal aponeurosis)

Proximal phalanx

Flexor digitorum profundus, tendon

Flexor digitorum superficialis, tendons

Tendinous sheath

Proper palmar digital nerve

Fig 3.1 An introduction to the anatomy of the hand

The bones of the forearm and hand

The forearm consists of two bones – the ulna and radius. The hand itself is made up of 27 bones that fall into three regions – the carpals, metacarpals and phalanges.

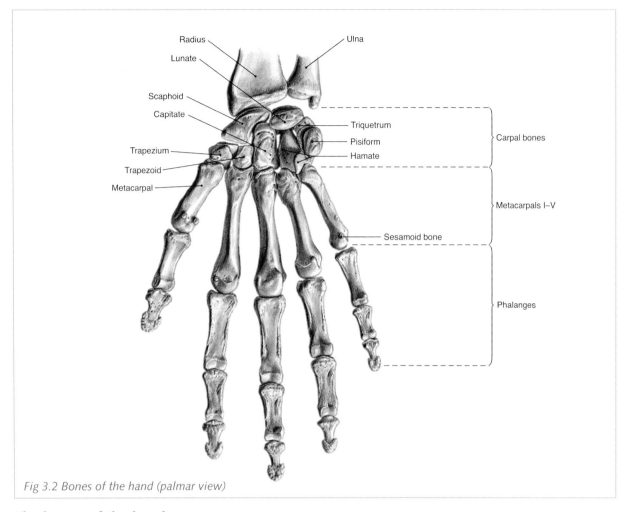

Fig 3.2 Bones of the hand (palmar view)

The bones of the hand

Carpals (8)
The wrist, or carpus, consists of eight small bones arranged in two irregular rows of four bones each. They are bound together by ligaments. The carpals are the:

- Trapezium
- Trapezoid
- Capitate
- Hamate
- Scaphoid
- Lunate
- Triquetrum
- Pisiform

Metacarpals (5)
Five metacarpals form the palm of the hand. They are numbered 1 to 5, starting with the thumb side of the hand.

Phalanges (14)
Fourteen phalanges make up the fingers. Each finger has a proximal, middle and distal phalange. The thumb has only proximal and distal phalanges. The thumb is sometimes called the *pollex*.

The muscles of the forearm and hand

Some of the muscles located on the upper arm move the forearm. They originate on the scapula or humerus, pass over the elbow joint and insert into the radius and ulna.

MUSCLES THAT MOVE THE FOREARM			
Name	Origin	Insertion	Basic actions
Biceps brachii	Scapula	Radius and bicipital aponeurosis	Flexes the elbow joint, supinates the forearm and aids flexion of the shoulder.
Brachialis	Humerus	Ulna	Flexes elbow joint.
Brachio-radialis	Humerus	Radius	Flexes elbow joint.
Triceps brachii	Scapula and humerus	Ulna	Extends elbow joint.
Pronator teres	Humerus and ulna	Radius	Pronates forearm and hand.
Supinator	Humerus and ulna	Radius	Supinates forearm and hand.

The muscles of the forearm move the wrist and can be divided into anterior and posterior compartments. The tendons of these muscles are held close to the bones by strong fibrous bands called retinacula. The flexor retinaculum (transverse carpal ligament) is found on the palmar surface of the carpal bones while the extensor retinaculum (dorsal carpal ligament) is found over the dorsal surface of the carpal bones.

Note: Only those muscles relevant to reflexology are discussed here. There are many other muscles of the forearm and hand that are not mentioned.

Anterior muscles
The anterior muscles of the forearm originate on the humerus (the bone of the upper arm) and insert on the carpals, metacarpals and phalanges. They flex the wrist or fingers.

Muscles of the arm

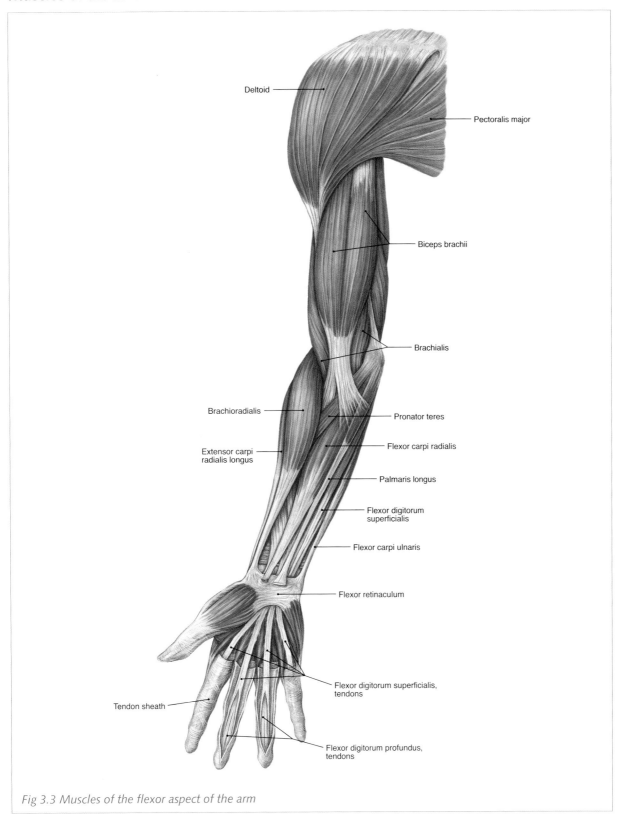

Deltoid

Pectoralis major

Biceps brachii

Brachialis

Brachioradialis

Pronator teres

Flexor carpi radialis

Extensor carpi
radialis longus

Palmaris longus

Flexor digitorum
superficialis

Flexor carpi ulnaris

Flexor retinaculum

Flexor digitorum superficialis,
tendons

Tendon sheath

Flexor digitorum profundus,
tendons

Fig 3.3 Muscles of the flexor aspect of the arm

Muscles of the arm

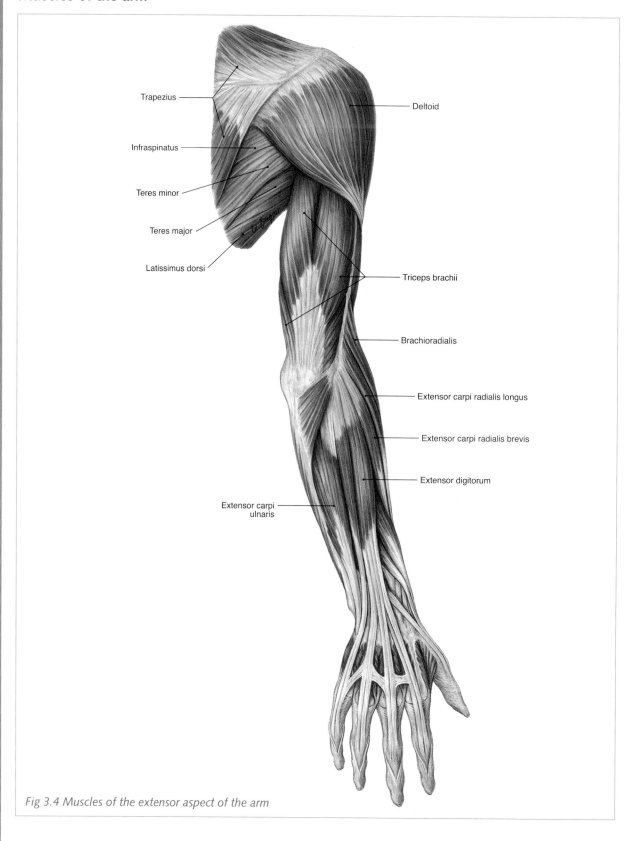

Trapezius

Infraspinatus

Teres minor

Teres major

Latissimus dorsi

Deltoid

Triceps brachii

Brachioradialis

Extensor carpi radialis longus

Extensor carpi radialis brevis

Extensor digitorum

Extensor carpi ulnaris

Fig 3.4 Muscles of the extensor aspect of the arm

ANTERIOR MUSCLES OF THE FOREARM AND HAND

Name	Origin	Insertion	Basic actions
Flexor carpi radialis	Humerus	Metacarpals 2 and 3	Flexes and abducts wrist.
Flexor carpi ulnaris	Humerus and ulna	Carpals and metacarpals	Flexes and adducts wrist.
Flexor digitorum superficialis	Humerus, ulna and radius	Middle phalanges	Flexes middle phalanges of each finger.

Posterior muscles

The posterior muscles of the forearm originate on the humerus and insert on the metacarpals and phalanges. They extend the wrist or fingers.

POSTERIOR MUSCLES OF THE FOREARM AND HAND

Name	Origin	Insertion	Basic actions
Extensor carpi radialis longus	Humerus	Metacarpal 2	Extends and abducts wrist.
Extensor carpi radialis brevis	Humerus	Metacarpal 3	Extends and abducts wrist.
Extensor digitorum	Humerus	Phalanges of the four fingers	Extends fingers.
Extensor carpi ulnaris	Humerus and ulna	Metacarpal 5	Extends and adducts wrist.

Muscles of the thenar and hypothenar eminences

The thenar eminence is a raised area of firm tissue found on the radial side of the palm of the hand, beneath the thumb. It is composed of the muscles that move the thumb, namely the abductor pollicis brevis, flexor pollicis brevis, opponens pollicis and adductor pollicis. Not all of these muscles are discussed here. Take note of the thenar eminence as it can become a problem area if you are thumb-walking incorrectly.

The hypothenar eminence is an area of soft tissue found on the ulnar side of the palm, beneath the little finger. It is composed of the muscles that move the little finger. Namely, the palmaris brevis, abductor digiti minimi, flexor digiti minimi brevis and opponens digiti minimi. These are not discussed here.

Muscles of the arm

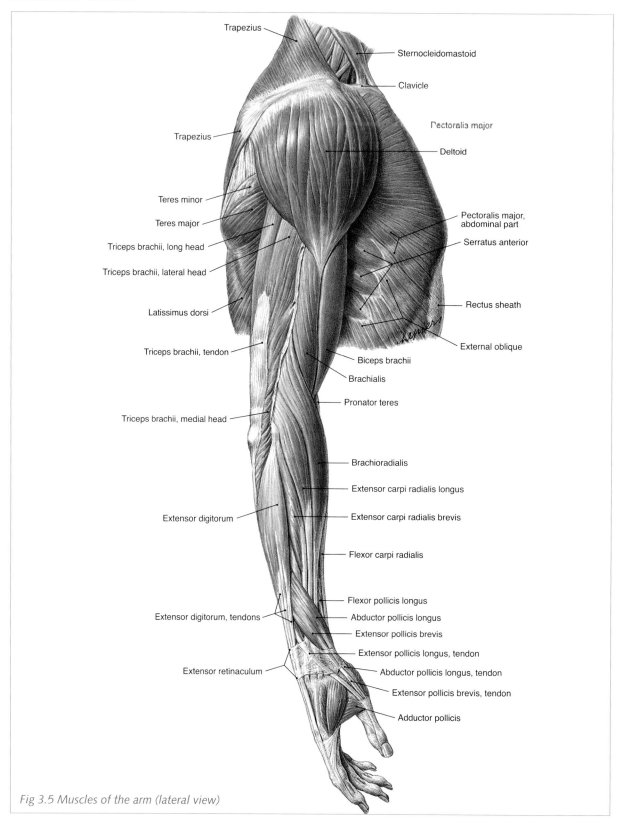

Trapezius

Sternocleidomastoid

Clavicle

Pectoralis major

Trapezius

Deltoid

Teres minor

Teres major

Pectoralis major,
abdominal part

Triceps brachii, long head

Serratus anterior

Triceps brachii, lateral head

Latissimus dorsi

Rectus sheath

Triceps brachii, tendon

External oblique

Biceps brachii

Brachialis

Pronator teres

Triceps brachii, medial head

Brachioradialis

Extensor carpi radialis longus

Extensor carpi radialis brevis

Extensor digitorum

Flexor carpi radialis

Flexor pollicis longus

Extensor digitorum, tendons

Abductor pollicis longus

Extensor pollicis brevis

Extensor pollicis longus, tendon

Extensor retinaculum

Abductor pollicis longus, tendon

Extensor pollicis brevis, tendon

Adductor pollicis

Fig 3.5 Muscles of the arm (lateral view)

MUSCLES THAT MOVE THE THUMB			
Name	Origin	**Insertion**	**Basic actions**
Abductor pollicis brevis	Flexor retinaculum and scaphoid	Thumb	Abducts the thumb.
Flexor pollicis brevis	Flexor retinaculum and capitate, trapezium, trapezoid and metacarpal 1	Thumb	Flexes the thumb.

The nerves of the forearm and hand

The forearm and hand are innervated by three main nerves which emerge from the brachial plexus:

- **Radial nerve** – supplies the muscles on the posterior aspect of the arm and forearm. At the elbow (cubital fossa) it divides into the deep and superficial radial nerves.
- **Median nerve** – supplies the muscles on the anterior aspect of the forearm and divides into common palmar digital nerves which innervate some of the muscles of the hand.
- **Ulnar nerve** – supplies some of the muscles of the forearm and most of the muscles of the hand. It has dorsal, palmar, deep and superficial branches and also divides into common palmar digital nerves in the hand.

The skin of the arm and hand is also innervated by cutaneous nerves.

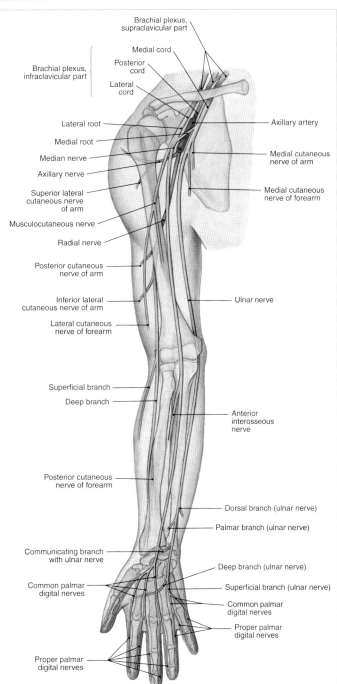

Fig 3.6 Nerves of the upper limb – overview

The blood vessels of the arm and hand

Arteries

The arms are supplied with blood by the subclavian arteries which become the axillary arteries at the armpits and the brachial arteries in the arms. Once in the forearm, the brachial artery splits into the radial and ulnar arteries which feed the superficial and deep palmar arches of the palm. These in turn supply the digital arteries of the fingers and thumb.

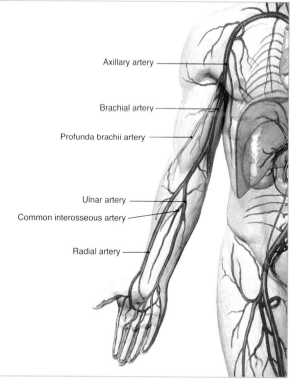

Axillary artery

Brachial artery

Profunda brachii artery

Ulnar artery

Common interosseous artery

Radial artery

Fig 3.7 Arteries of the arm and hand

Veins

The veins of the arm and hand are divided into two groups – superficial veins and deep veins. The superficial veins are the cephalic, median cubital, basilic and median antebrachial veins. The cephalic vein drains the lateral (radial) aspect of the arm, beginning at the back of the hand and emptying into the axillary vein.

At the elbow the cephalic gives off a branch called the median cubital vein which slants upwards to join the basilic vein.

The basilic vein begins at the back of the hand and drains the medial (ulnar) aspect of the arm, emptying into the axillary vein.

The median antebrachial veins begin at the palm of the hand and ascend on the medial (ulnar) aspect of the forearm and end in the median cubital veins at the elbow.

The deep veins follow the course of the arteries and have the same names – dorsal metacarpal, palmar venous arch, ulnar, radial, brachial, axillary and subclavian veins.

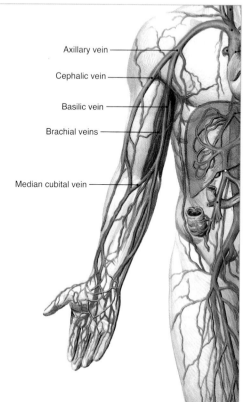

Axillary vein

Cephalic vein

Basilic vein

Brachial veins

Median cubital vein

Fig 3.8 Veins of the arm and hand

Mapping The Body Onto The Hands

At this stage, you should have a good understanding of how reflexology
works and also how to locate the zones and reflexes of the body on the feet.
Now it is time to apply this knowledge to the hands.

The ten longitudinal zones of the hands

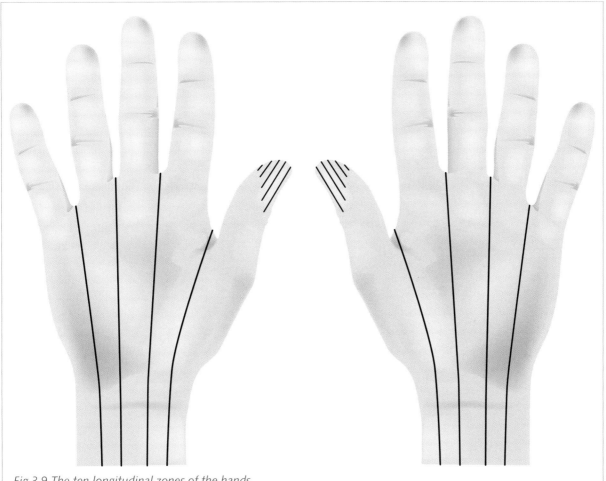

Fig 3.9 The ten longitudinal zones of the hands

Fig 3.10 The reflexes of the hands – palmar view

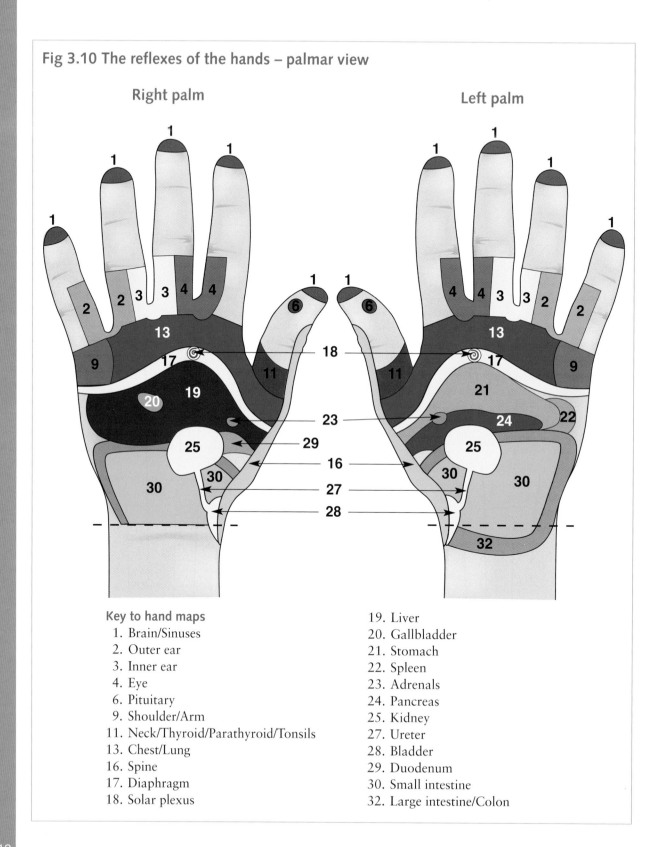

Right palm   Left palm

Key to hand maps
1. Brain/Sinuses
2. Outer ear
3. Inner ear
4. Eye
6. Pituitary
9. Shoulder/Arm
11. Neck/Thyroid/Parathyroid/Tonsils
13. Chest/Lung
16. Spine
17. Diaphragm
18. Solar plexus
19. Liver
20. Gallbladder
21. Stomach
22. Spleen
23. Adrenals
24. Pancreas
25. Kidney
27. Ureter
28. Bladder
29. Duodenum
30. Small intestine
32. Large intestine/Colon

Fig 3.11 The reflexes of the hands – dorsal view

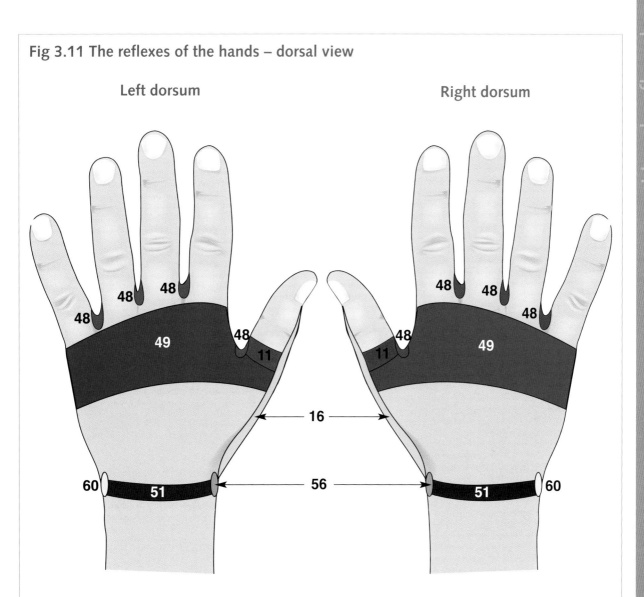

Left dorsum

Right dorsum

Key to hand maps
11. Neck
16. Spine
48. Lymphatics of upper body
49. Chest, breast, mammary glands
51. Fallopian tubes/Vas deferens/Lymphatics of lower body
56. Uterus/Prostate
60. Ovaries/Testes

The transverse zones/body relation lines of the hands

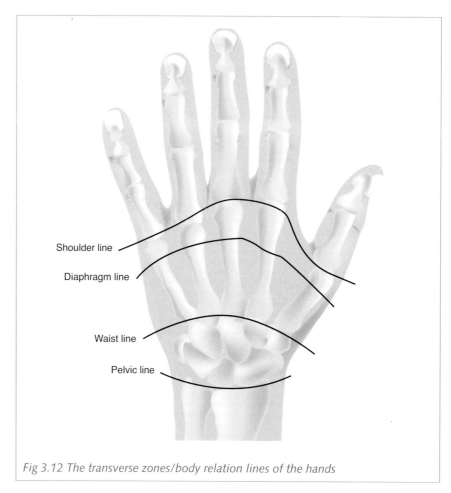

Shoulder line

Diaphragm line

Waist line

Pelvic line

Fig 3.12 The transverse zones/body relation lines of the hands

Locating the transverse zones on the hands is a little more difficult than finding them on the feet. However, there are specific markers to help you:

- **Shoulder line** – The shoulder line is located where the fingers and thumb join the ball of the hand.
- **Diaphragm line** – Hold your hands with your palms facing towards you and bend all your fingers towards you. You will see that the ball of your palm also bends towards you at a natural crease. Your diaphragm line falls on this crease. Take note that in zone 1 it lies very close to your shoulder line.
- **Waist line** – The waistline is more difficult to locate. Feel down the medial edge of your hand between your diaphragm line and your wrist (pelvic line) and you will feel a slight protrusion approximately half way down. Now feel down the lateral edge of your hand between your diaphragm line and your wrist (pelvic line) and again you will feel a slight protrusion approximately half way down. These protrusions indicate where the waistline should be placed.
- **Pelvic line** – The pelvic line is located on the wrist, where the hand meets the arm.

Reading And Interpreting The Hands

Before performing a reflexology treatment on someone's hands, spend a few minutes reading and interpreting them in the same way as you would the feet. You will find that the hands are not as easy to read as the feet, but you can still pick up a great deal of information from them:

- Get a general overview of the hands.
- Look for any local contraindications.
- Look at the colour of the hands.
- Feel the temperature of the hands.
- Feel for excess moisture or dryness.
- Look and feel for changes in skin texture.
- Look and feel for any structural hand disorders.
- Examine the fingernails.

Get a general overview of your client's hands

Look at a person's hands and you will get an insight into their character and health. Dr Rudolph Ballentine, a highly experienced medical doctor and psychiatrist who has written many books on holistic health, said the following: 'The shape of the hand is what strikes us first. I am still astonished by the dramatic differences among the many hands that are extended to me when I meet new people. Some are damp, small, and nearly formless, seemingly hesitant to declare themselves. Others are large, square, and almost wooden, suggesting the angular construction of a table or a homemade chair. And then there are those that are hot and oily, full of fire and determination. To grasp such a hand is to feel invaded by the insistent intention and impatience of its owner.'[1]

DESCRIPTION OF HAND	HOW CAN THIS RELATE TO YOUR CLIENT'S HEALTH?
General care	The way in which your client cares for their hands can often reflect how much they care for themselves and how much time they have to look after themselves. It can also give clues to one's self esteem and emotional states.
Size and shape	The hands should be equal in size and shape and should be proportional to the size and shape of your client's body. A marked difference between the two hands can reflect an imbalance in the right and left sides of the body.
Age of the hands	The skin texture and tone of the hands should resemble the age of your client. It is not uncommon for an elderly person to have thin or fragile skin, a loss of elasticity, pigmentation, poor muscle tone and brittle bones. However, if you find these conditions in a young person's hands they are indicative of an imbalance and poor health.
Blemishes (scars, moles)	If your client has a scar always ask them how and when they got it as recent scarring is a local contraindication. Moles often indicate hereditary weaknesses so take note of the zone, reflex and meridian on which they lie. Take note that freckles are common on the hands and are not usually included in a hand reading.

Look for any local contraindications

It is always important to be aware of any local contraindications before you touch your client's hands. Local contraindications are localised areas that are contraindicated to reflexology. This means that in order to avoid either cross-infection or hurting your client, you must not touch these areas. Local contraindications include:

- Cuts, bruises, abrasions
- Fractures
- Haematoma
- Localised swelling or inflammation and any undiagnosed lumps or bumps
- Scar tissue
- Skin diseases
- Sunburn.

Skin diseases and disorders that affect the hand specifically include skin cancers, candidiasis, dermatitis, eczema, tinea corporis, psoriasis and warts.

Skin cancers

There are three main types of skin cancer and long-term sun damage generally plays a role in their development. These cancers are:

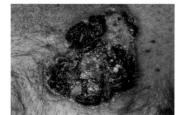

Basal cell carcinoma

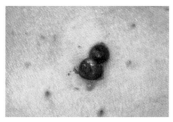

Melanoma

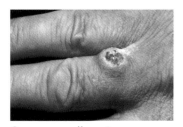

Squamous cell carcinoma

- **Basal cell carcinoma (rodent ulcers)** – This is the most common form of skin cancer and it can appear in many forms. For example, it may appear as raised bumps that break open and form scabs; or as a flat pale or red patch; or it may be an enlarged papule with a thickened, pearly border. Basal cell carcinomas may also be mistaken for sores that constantly bleed, scab and heal. Basal cell carcinomas rarely metastasise (spread to distant parts of the body). However, they can invade surrounding tissues and this can be serious if the carcinomas are located close to the brain, eyes or mouth.
- **Melanoma** – This is a cancer that originates in the melanocytes of the skin. It can develop in sun-exposed areas or on moles and it can metastasise. Melanomas vary in appearance and signs to watch for include moles or freckles that are growing, changing in colour or changing in shape, moles that bleed or break open, or irregular black or gray lumps that appear on the skin.
- **Squamous cell carcinoma (prickle-cell cancer)** – This usually occurs on sun-exposed areas in fair-skinned people. Occasionally, it may develop in areas that are not exposed to the sun, for example, the mouth. It is characterised by a thick, scaly, warty appearance and if left untreated it can develop into an open sore that grows into the underlying tissue. In addition to prolonged sun exposure, causes of squamous cell carcinoma include certain chemicals, chronic sores, burns and scars. Squamous cell carcinomas do occasionally metastasise.

Candidiasis

Candidiasis, also called candidosis, is a fungal infection caused by the yeast *Candida*. This yeast is normally found in the mouth, digestive tract and vagina but it can infect other areas of the body if it is allowed to grow unchecked. Pregnant women, obese people, people taking antibiotics and diabetics are more prone to candidiasis. Different forms of candidiasis that affect the hands include:

- **Infections in the skin folds between the fingers** – this is characterised by a bright red rash with a softening and sometimes breaking down of the skin. The rash may itch or burn and small pustules may appear.
- **Candidal paronychia** – this is candidiasis of the nail bed and is characterised by redness and swelling that may lead to the nail turning white or yellow and separating from the nail bed.

Tinea corporis (Body ringworm)

Tinea corporis is commonly called ringworm and is a fungal infection. It appears as round patches that have pink scaly borders and clear centres. It is often very itchy and be aware that it is very contagious.

Dermatitis and Eczema

Dermatitis is a broad term for inflammation of the upper layers of the skin and it includes a variety of symptoms that usually involve itching, blistering, redness and swelling. Severe symptoms include oozing, scabbing and scaling. Dermatitis can be caused by allergens, irritants, dryness, scratching or fungi.

- **Contact dermatitis** is an itchy rash that is confined to a specific area and it is the result of direct contact with a substance. It can be caused by cosmetics, metals such as nickel, certain plants such as poison ivy, drugs in some creams and certain chemicals used in the manufacture of clothing.
- **Eczema** is a form of dermatitis that can be caused by either internal or external factors. It is characterised by itchiness, redness and blistering. It can be either dry or weeping and can cause scaly and thickened skin.

Psoriasis

Psoriasis is a chronic disorder characterised by raised, red patches that have silvery scales. These patches are caused by unusually rapid cell growth, but the reason for this rapid cell growth is unknown. Some people with psoriasis will also have deformed, thickened nails. Psoriasis often runs in families and can be aggravated by sunburn, injury or stress. It is sometimes improved through gentle exposure to the sun.

Warts

Warts are small, firm growths that have a rough surface. They are caused by a virus and can grow in clusters or as an isolated growth. Warts on the body are generally painless.

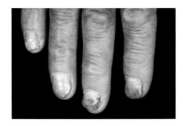
Candidiasis

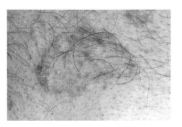
Tinea corporis (body ringworm)

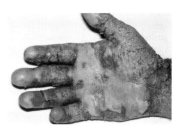
Contact dermatitis

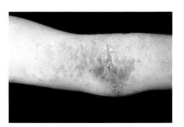
Eczema

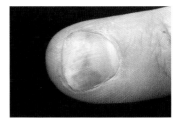
Psoriasis

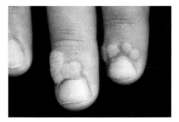
Warts

Look at the colour of the hands

Like the feet, the hands should be a healthy pinkish colour which indicates good circulation and metabolism. In general, the palm of the hand reflects the state of the internal organs whilst the fingers and fingernails usually relate to the circulation.

DESCRIPTION OF HANDS	HOW CAN THIS RELATE TO YOUR CLIENT'S HEALTH?
Red palms	Unusually red palms indicate an imbalance in the internal organs of the body and sometimes constipation.
Blue thenar eminence	If the thenar eminence of the hand is unusually blue there may be an imbalance in the stomach and you should discuss your client's diet.
Pale or blue fingertips	This reflects poor circulation.

Feel the temperature of the hands

Run your hands over your client's hands and note the temperature. Both hands should be warm and there should be no localised hot or cold areas.

DESCRIPTION OF HANDS	HOW CAN THIS RELATE TO YOUR CLIENT'S HEALTH?
Cold hands	Unusually cold hands can suggest poor circulation and are common in smokers, people who drink a lot of tea or coffee or who do not exercise.
Localised hot or cold areas	Small areas that are extremely hot or cold suggest a congested reflex. Look at the reflex affected.

Feel for excess moisture or dryness

Run your hands over your client's hands and feel for excess moisture or dryness.

DESCRIPTION OF HANDS	HOW CAN THIS RELATE TO YOUR CLIENT'S HEALTH?
Damp or moist, sweaty hands	Damp, sweaty hands usually indicate that your client is nervous. This is not uncommon, especially in the first few treatments. However, if your client continually suffers with excessive sweating then you need to look at their endocrine function.
Very dry skin (sometimes with flaking), dehydrated	Hands that are covered with dry and flaking skin generally reflect poor health and nutrition and a lack of bodily fluids.
Generalised puffiness and swelling, water retention or oedematous hands	Some water retention is not unusual in overweight clients and pregnant women. However, if your client has unusually swollen and puffy hands or they have pitting oedema then refer them to their doctor. To test for pitting oedema press into the skin above your client's wrist for the count of five. If your finger leaves an impression in their skin that does not go away after approximately 30 seconds then they need to be seen by their doctor.

Look and feel for changes in skin texture

In general, the texture of the hands should be smooth and soft. However, calluses (thick, protective layers of skin) and build-ups of dry skin are not uncommon. Make a note of the zone, reflex and meridian where there are textural changes and relate this to your client's health. Once you have got an overview of the skin on the hands, take a close look at the fingers. The fingers represent the reflexes of the head and skin changes on them can reveal a great deal about a person.

DESCRIPTION OF HANDS	HOW CAN THIS RELATE TO YOUR CLIENT'S HEALTH?
Heavy vertical ridges or lines on the fingers	Deep lines running longitudinally up the fingers indicate fatigue and exhaustion and are present in people who have used up all their energy.
Transverse lines across the fingers	Transverse lines going across the fingers usually indicate that there is an energy blockage manifesting in the head. These lines often point to problems of the head and neck such as headaches, eye, ear, nose or throat disorders, breathing problems, neck strain or anxiety.

Look and feel for any disorders of the hands

There are many disorders that can affect the shape and structure of the hands and you should be aware of the impact these disorders can have on a person's life, especially if their hands are distorted. They may feel embarrassed by the shape of their hands or they may struggle with things that one often takes for granted such as holding a cup. This is when hand reflexology can have a positive effect.

Abnormal bending of the fingers

Injuries and disorders such as rheumatoid arthritis can cause the fingers to bend abnormally so that they cannot be straightened. It is important that you, as a reflexologist, do not try to straighten these fingers as you will simply cause pain to your client. Abnormal bending of the fingers includes:

- **Mallet finger** – the tip of the finger does not straighten.
- **Swan-neck deformity** – the finger bends in three places: the joint at the base of the finger flexes, the middle joint extends and the top joint flexes.
- **Boutonnière deformity** – the middle joint bends inward toward the palm and the top joint bends outward away from the palm.

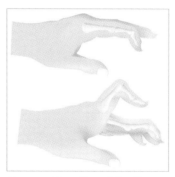

Abnormal bending of the fingers

Arthritis

Arthritis can affect any joints of the body and it commonly affects the hands. For more information on arthritis please turn to page 30.

Carpal tunnel syndrome

This is the compression of the median nerve as it passes through the wrist. It is often caused by repetitive, forceful use of the wrist when it is in the wrong position and is also common in pregnancy, diabetes, rheumatoid arthritis and people who have an underactive thyroid gland. Carpal tunnel syndrome is characterised by numbness and tingling of the thumb and first three fingers and the thumb also tends to be weak. The little finger is often symptom-free. Look at Figure 3.1 on page 100 and you will see where the median nerve passes through the carpal tunnel at the top of the hand.

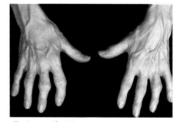

Osteoarthritis

Cubital tunnel syndrome (Ulnar nerve palsy)

Cubital tunnel syndrome is compression of the ulnar nerve at the elbow. It can be caused by an abnormal bone growth, or repeatedly leaning on or bending the elbow for prolonged periods. It is common in some sports people. Cubital tunnel syndrome is characterised by pain and numbness at the elbow and a tingling sensation in, and a weakening of, the ring and little

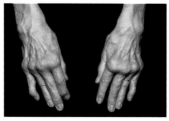

Rheumatoid arthritis

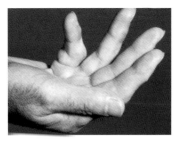

Dupuytren's contracture

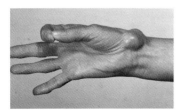

Ganglion cyst

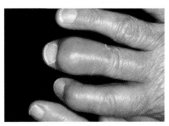

Gout

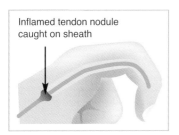

Inflamed tendon nodule caught on sheath

Trigger finger

finger. The ability to pinch the thumb and index finger together can sometimes be affected and if cubital tunnel syndrome becomes chronic and severe, the hand can become deformed.

Dupuytren's contracture
In Dupuytren's contracture the fascia inside the palms progressively shrinks and causes the fingers to curl inwards. Eventually the hands take on a clawlike shape. Dupuytren's contracture is often inherited but can also occur in diabetics, alcoholics and epileptics.

Ganglia (Ganglion cysts)
A ganglion cyst is a fluid-filled growth that usually develops near joints or tendon sheaths on the hand or foot. The cause of ganglion cysts is unknown. They can be removed by surgery, but they can also disappear over time.

Gout
Although gout is most commonly found in the big toe, it can also affect the wrist or fingers. Please turn to page 69 for more information on gout.

Trigger finger (Flexor digital tenosynovitis)
Trigger finger occurs when a finger locks in a bent (flexed) position. In trigger finger, a tendon that flexes a finger becomes inflamed and swollen. When the finger flexes, the tendon is able to move out of its surrounding sheath, however it is unable to go back into it and so the finger remains in a flexed position. It can result from repetitive use of the hands or from inflammatory conditions such as arthritis.

Examine the fingernails

Finally, have a good look at your client's fingernails. As with the toenails, they can be affected by many nail conditions and are also indicators of internal imbalances, nutritional deficiencies, neglect or stress and anxiety. It is important to be able to recognise diseases and disorders of the nails in order to avoid cross-infection. These are covered in detail on pages 69–71. In addition to the disorders covered on these pages, the fingernails are often used to help diagnose other disorders. This table only gives suggestions and symptoms of certain disorders and is not intended as a diagnostic tool.

DISORDER	HOW CAN THIS BE SEEN IN THE FINGERNAILS?
Lack of iron/anaemia	Spoon-shaped, concave or blanching nails can point to a lack of iron.
Lack of oxygen or respiratory disorders	Blue or purple nails, or nails that curve unusually (Hippocratic nails) can be signs of respiratory disorders.
Thyroid imbalances	Thyroid imbalances can show themselves in nails that have no moon in the base, nails that are unusually soft and prone to infection, nails that are very ridged or have fanning lines on them and Hippocratic nails.
Skin disorders	Skin disorders are sometimes accompanied by pitted nails.
Problems with the lumbar spine	Hippocratic nails (extremely arched or curved nails) can suggest lumbar problems.
Vitamin A deficiency	Extremely thin, egg shell like nails that are almost transparent and pale blue can indicate a deficiency of vitamin A.

Case Study: Reading The Hands

Martin is a 37 year old man who has for the last few years been under extreme stress in all aspects of his life. He has had a very ill child, changed both homes and jobs a number of times, struggled financially and separated from his partner. Although he has tried to look after his health his stress levels have taken a toll on his body.

Photo 1 is of Martin's little finger on his left hand and its condition is typical of all his other fingers. Looking at this finger both vertical and transverse ridges can be seen. The deep vertical ridges reflect Martin's fatigue and exhaustion. In addition to the extreme stress he is under, Martin also suffers with insomnia and is exhausted on all levels – physical, emotional and spiritual. The transverse ridges going across his finger reflect the chronic neck tension that he suffers from, as well as the fact that he wears glasses. In addition, transverse ridges indicate extreme anxiety. These ridges can also indicate headaches and breathing problems. Although Martin is not aware of having these, they often accompany stress.

In **photo 2**, Martin's left palm, the following can be seen:

* Calluses are present on the shoulder reflex and the shoulder line. Martin does suffer with chronic neck and shoulder tension.
* Discolouration of the chest reflex. Due to his extreme levels of stress, Martin has actually developed a heart condition which is reflected in the discolouration of his chest reflex.
* Discolouration and wrinkling of the skin in zones 1–3, particularly over the reflexes for the digestive system. The digestive system is one area of the body that is always affected by stress and Martin needs to take special care with his diet during this time.

Both longitudinal ridges and white spots are evident on Martin's fingernails as shown in **photo 3**. These reflect Martin's poor diet, chronic stress and high levels of anxiety.

Photo 4 is of Martin's right palm and once again callusing on the shoulder line is evident. There is also a small callus that has developed over the adrenal reflex. This reflects the prolonged stress Martin has been under.

Photo 5 shows the tip of Martin's right thumb. Deep ridges and cracks have developed over this area which is the reflex for the brain. Once again, this indicates chronic stress, anxiety and a severe lack of homeostasis.

Because Martin's condition is so chronic and severe, I recommended that he go for counselling as well as visit his doctor for a thorough check-up.

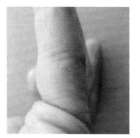

1. Left hand little finger

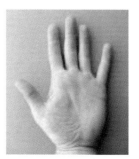

2. Left hand palm

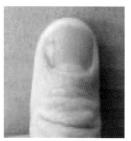

3. Left thumb nail

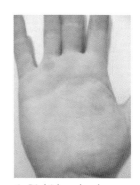

4. Right hand palm

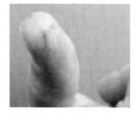

5. Right thumb end

Reflexology Techniques

In Chapter 2 you learned how to perform the basic reflexology techniques on the feet. These techniques are exactly the same as you will use on the hands. To revise these techniques, please turn to page 75. On the following pages you will see how to apply these techniques to the hands.

Preparation

Positioning your client and yourself
Your client needs to be comfortable during their treatment so put them into a position in which they can relax. You have two options:

- They can lie on a massage couch with their arms stretched out next to them. Place your chair next to their right hand and work this hand until you have completed it then move your chair to the other side of the couch and work the left hand.
- They can sit across a desk or table from you with their hands stretched out in front of them. Sit opposite them and work their hands.

Be aware that when giving a hand reflexology treatment clients can sometimes feel as if their personal space is being invaded. To avoid this try to work in as professional an environment as possible and have your client either lying on a massage couch or seated across a desk from you. If you cannot work in such an environment and need to place your client's hands in your lap, ensure you put a pillow on your lap first.

Hygiene
Before your client sits or lies down, ask them to wash their hands with soap and water. Do the same.

Choosing a medium
The medium you use on the hands is up to you. Some reflexologists choose not to use any medium at all, while others prefer to use cream or lotion. If you or your client has particularly sweaty hands you may choose to use talc, corn starch or liquid talc. These should be used with caution and are not recommended if your client has respiratory problems or dust allergies.

Holding the hands

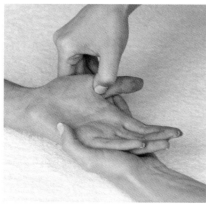

Working reflexes on the palm

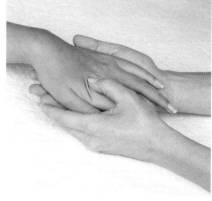

Working reflexes on the top of the hand

As with the feet, always use both your hands during a hand reflexology treatment. One hand is the working hand and the other the support hand. Place your support hand underneath your client's hand and use your working hand to apply pressure to the reflexes.

Relaxation techniques

Always begin and end every treatment with a relaxing hand massage. Feel free to use any relaxing massage techniques you may already know as well as those listed below.

Greeting the hands/First contact and solar plexus breathing

Your first contact with your client's hands sets the tone for the entire treatment so focus on touching your client with confidence, warmth and care. You can either work both hands together or one at a time. Hold their hand between your hands and ask them to take a few deep, relaxing breaths in and out. Breathe deeply yourself. Using your thumb, apply deep pressure to their solar plexus reflex. You can now spend a few minutes working the solar plexus by:

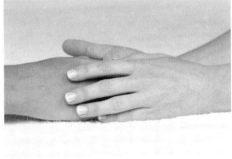

Greeting the hands

- Applying deep pressure with your thumb and maintaining this pressure until you feel your client relax.
- Unwinding it by rotating your thumb in an anticlockwise direction. Do this if the solar plexus feels tight and your client is tense and wound-up.
- Winding it up by rotating your thumb in a clockwise direction. Do this if the solar plexus feels empty and your client is exhausted, run down or depressed.

Effleurage/Stroking

The flowing, warming movements of effleurage relax and warm your client's hands and prepare them for deeper pressure techniques. For more information on the benefits of this technique please turn to page 79.

Effleurage is a natural, instinctive technique. Simply massage your client's hand and forearm with long, flowing strokes. Make sure that the whole of your hand and all your fingers are in contact with your client's skin and establish a rhythm that is in time with both yours and your client's breathing.

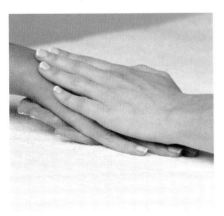

Effleuraging the hands

Opening up the hand/Stretching the metacarpals

Hands hold a great deal of tension, not only because they are constantly being used in a variety of movements ranging from picking up tiny objects to carrying heavy loads, but also because we tend to carry our emotions in our hands (think how common it is for people to clench their fists when angry). It is not surprising, therefore, that the technique used to open up the hand seems to be loved by everyone.

Work on one hand at a time and start by working the palm:

- Hold your client's hand in the fingers of both your hands. Their palm should be facing upwards. Place your thumbs together on their palm, near their wrist.
- Draw your thumbs outward across the palm. The movement should stretch your client's palm open.
- Repeat the movement, but this time start with your thumbs in the centre of the palm, midway between the wrist and fingers.
- Repeat the movement again, but this time start with your thumbs near the fingers.
- Repeat these movements a couple of times and focus on really stretching the palm outwards and opening-up the hand.

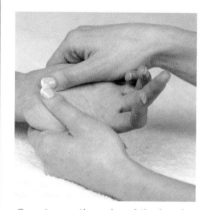 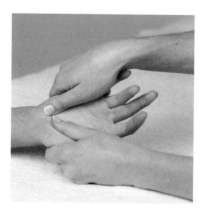 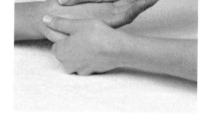

Opening up the palm of the hand

Once you have worked the palm you can turn the hand over and work the top in the same way.

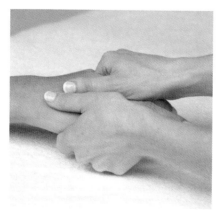 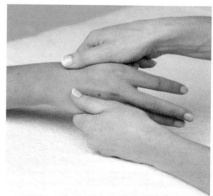

Opening up the top of the hand

Once you have mastered the technique described on the previous page, you can extend it and get more of a stretch into your client's hand by inserting your fingers between theirs. In this way their fingers are stretched outwards while you open up their palm.

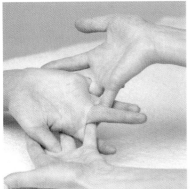 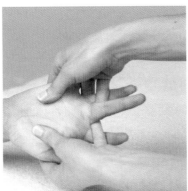 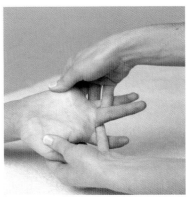

Slip your fingers between your client's fingers to open up the palm

Open up the hand by sliding your thumbs across the palm

Metacarpal manipulation/Longitudinal thumb-stroking and jiggling

Metacarpal manipulation follows on from the technique of opening-up the palm and can also be done with or without your fingers linked into your client's fingers. Hold the hands as you would for opening them up but instead of sliding your thumbs outwards to stretch the hands laterally, slide your thumbs downwards between the metacarpals so that you are stroking them longitudinally.

You can add to this technique by 'jiggling' the metacarpals as you stroke downwards. The idea is to loosen up the hands and get as much movement between the bones as possible.

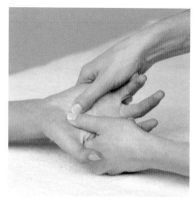
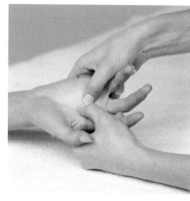
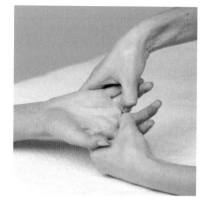

Working the palm of the hand

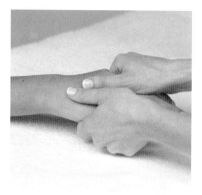
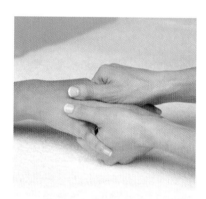
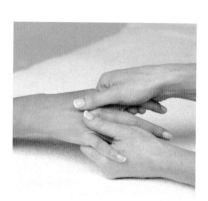

Working the top of the hand

Stretching and rotating the fingers

Stretching and rotating the fingers not only encourages mobility in the joints, it also releases tension and stiffness in the neck and shoulder reflexes. Although this is a beneficial technique, care should be taken with elderly or arthritic clients.

Hold the hand with your support hand and, taking one finger at a time, pull the finger until you have established a good stretch. Then, maintaining that stretch, rotate the finger both clockwise and anticlockwise a few times. Once you have completed the rotations, jiggle the finger to loosen it.

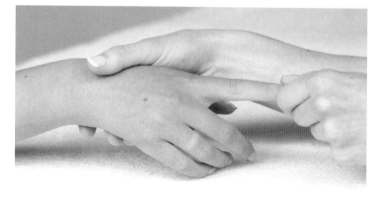

Stretching and rotating the fingers

Finger and thumb wringing/Coin rubbing

Coin rubbing is a technique for encouraging circulation to the fingers and subsequently to the neck and shoulder reflexes. It is also a stress-reliever. Perform this technique on one finger at a time. Begin by holding your client's hand with your support hand and grip one finger between your thumb and index finger, as close to the webbing of your client's hand as possible. Then rub the finger in an outward direction, from the webbing to the tips of your client's finger. When you reach the tip give it a squeeze before releasing the finger and repeating the process on the next finger.

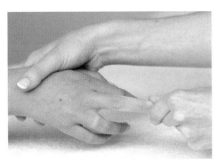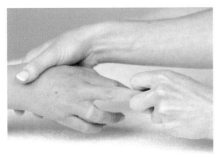

Coin rubbing the fingers

Stretching and rotating the wrist/Wrist circumduction

The wrist is the reflex for the pelvis, so by stretching and rotating the wrist you not only encourage mobility to the joint itself, you are also releasing tension and stiffness in the lower back and hip area. Although this is a beneficial technique, care should be taken with elderly or arthritic clients.

With your support hand lift your client's hand so that their elbow is bent and their hand is off the table:

- Hold your client's wrist with your support hand.
- Link the fingers of your working hand into your client's fingers and, holding their wrist firmly, push their fingers back and forth to bend their wrist backwards and forwards a few times.
- Then gently pull their fingers towards you to stretch their wrist and rotate it both clockwise and anticlockwise a few times.

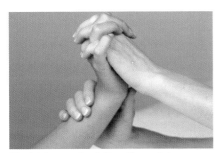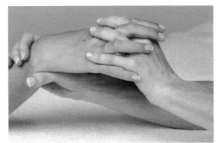

Stretching and rotating the wrist

Pressure techniques

Because pressure techniques are the same whether done on the foot or hand, they are not discussed here. However, photographs demonstrating the techniques on the hands are included on the next page. Please turn to page 87 to learn how to do the techniques demonstrated and how to interpret your findings during the treatment.

Thumb-walking/Caterpillar crawl

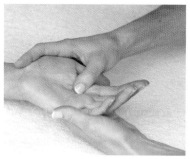 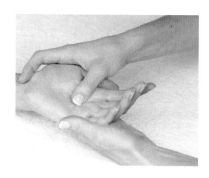 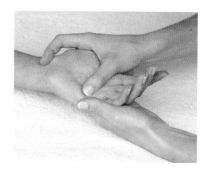

Transverse thumb-walking

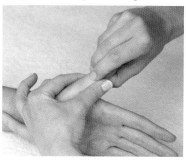 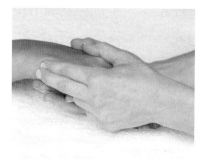 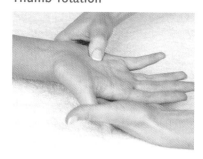

Longitudinal thumb-walking (Zone-walking)

Finger-walking and Finger-rotation

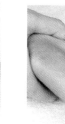 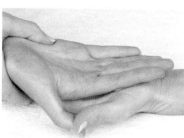

Thumb-rotation

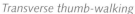

Note how the tip of the thumb joint and not the medial edge is used for thumb-rotations

Thumb-hook/Hook-in, back-up/Bumblebee action

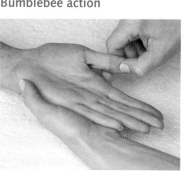

Study Outline

The structure of the forearm and hand

The bones of the forearm are the ulna and radius.
The hand is composed of 8 carpals (trapezium, trapezoid, capitate, hamate, scaphoid, lunate, triquetrum and pisiform), 5 metacarpals and 14 phalanges.
The muscles that move the forearm originate on the humerus, cross over the elbow and insert into the radius and ulna:

- Biceps brachii
- Brachialis
- Brachioradialis
- Triceps brachii
- Pronator teres
- Supinator

The anterior muscles of the forearm flex the wrist and/or fingers:

- Flexor carpi radialis
- Flexor carpi ulnaris
- Flexor digitorum superficialis

The posterior muscles of the forearm extend the wrist and/or fingers:

- Extensor carpi radialis longus
- Extensor carpi radialis brevis
- Extensor digitorum
- Extensor carpi ulnaris

The thenar eminence is the area of firm, raised tissue located on the palm beneath the thumb. It is composed of the muscles that move the thumb which include the:

- Abductor pollicis brevis
- Flexor pollicis brevis

The nerves of the forearm and hand are the:

- Radial nerve
- Median nerve
- Ulnar nerve

The arteries of the forearm and hand are the:

- Radial artery
- Ulnar artery
- Superficial palmar arch
- Deep palmar arch
- Digital arteries

The veins of the forearm and hand are the:

- Cephalic vein
- Median cubital vein (at the elbow)
- Basilic vein

- Median antebrachial vein
- Dorsal metacarpal veins
- Palmar venous arch
- Ulnar vein
- Radial vein

Mapping the body onto the hands

To revise this section please study the diagrams on page 110–111 of this chapter.

Reading and interpreting the hands

- Get a general overview of the hands.
- Look for any local contraindications.
- Look at the colour of the hands.
- Feel the temperature of the hands.
- Feel for excess moisture or dryness.
- Look and feel for changes in skin texture.
- Look and feel for any structural hand disorders.
- Examine the fingernails.

Hand relaxation techniques in a nutshell

Greeting the hands
Hold your client's hand between yours and ask them to take a few deep breaths. Then apply deep pressure to their solar plexus and work it in sync with your client's breath.

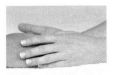

Effleurage
Use long, stroking movements to massage the hand and forearm.

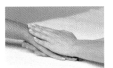

Opening-up the hand
Supporting your client's hand in your fingers or linking your fingers into theirs, place your two thumbs in the middle of their palm and slide your thumbs in opposite directions (laterally) to stretch the palm open. Repeat on the dorsum of the hand.

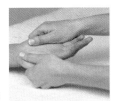
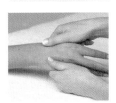

Metacarpal manipulation
Supporting your client's hand in your fingers or linking your fingers into theirs, place your two thumbs in the middle of their palm and slide your thumbs downwards between the metacarpals so that you stroke them longitudinally. You can also jiggle the metacarpals as you stroke. Repeat on the top of the hand.

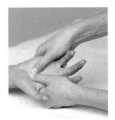
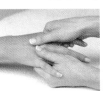

Stretching and rotating the fingers
Stretch, rotate and jiggle each finger individually.

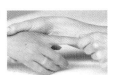

Finger and thumb wringing
Vigorously rub the edges of each finger.

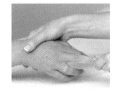

Stretching and rotating the wrist
Bend and flex your client's wrist, then stretch and rotate it.

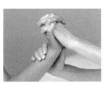

Hand pressure techniques in a nutshell

Thumb-walking
Using the lateral edge of the thumb, bend and straighten it so that it moves along the hand in a tiny crawling movement.

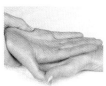

Thumb-rotation
Using the tip of the thumb, apply pressure to a point on your client's hand and then rotate the thumb before releasing the pressure and moving forwards with a tiny movement.

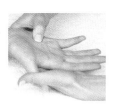

Finger-walking
Using the tip of your index finger to apply pressure, bend and straighten your finger so that it moves along the top of the hand with tiny, crawling movements.

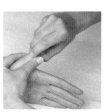

Finger-rotation
Using the tip of the index finger, apply small circular movements to a point on the hand before releasing the pressure and moving it forwards a fraction.

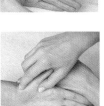

Thumb-hook
Push the tip of your thumb into a reflex and at the same time swing your hand upwards to hook your thumb deeply into the reflex. Use your other fingers for leverage.

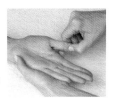

Multiple choice questions

1. **Which of the following veins is not located in the arm?**
   a. Basilic vein
   b. Saphenous vein
   c. Median cubital vein
   d. Ulnar vein.

2. **What is psoriasis?**
   a. A chronic skin disorder characterised by raised, red patches that have silvery scales
   b. An itchy rash that is confined to a specific area and is the result of direct contact with a substance
   c. A thick, scaly, warty growth that develops into an open sore which grows into the underlying tissue
   d. None of the above.

3. **Which of the following are all carpals?**
   a. Lunate, scaphoid, cuboid, trapezium
   b. Pisiform, calcaneus, talus, hamate
   c. Cuneiform, trapezoid, navicular, lunate
   d. Triquetrum, capitate, hamate, pisiform.

4. **Where on the hand would you find the pelvic line?**
   a. It is located where the fingers and thumb join the ball of the hand
   b. It is located on the crease that lies between the ball of the hand and the rest of the palm
   c. It is located on the wrist, where the hand meets the arm
   d. It is located halfway between the ball of the hand and the wrist.

5. **Where on the hand will you find the reflex for the lungs?**
   a. Across the top of the palm where the ball of the hand is
   b. In the webbing between the fingers
   c. In the centre of the thumb
   d. Around the base of the thumb.

6. **Where on the hand will you find the reflexes for the kidneys?**
   a. Left hand only, zone 4, on the diaphragm line
   b. Right hand only, zone 2, on the waistline
   c. Both hands, zone 5, on the diaphragm line
   d. Both hands, zone 3, on the waistline.

7. **If your client presents with deep vertical ridges on their fingers, what could this possibly suggest?**
   a. Headaches
   b. Nausea
   c. Exhaustion
   d. Insomnia.

8. **If your client is elderly and has rheumatoid arthritis in their hands and fingers, which of the following techniques should you not use?**
   a. Stretching and rotating the fingers
   b. Finger walking
   c. Effleurage
   d. Thumb-walking.

9. **What causes carpal tunnel syndrome?**
   a. Compression of the ulnar nerve
   b. Compression of the median nerve
   c. Genetics
   d. A virus.

10. **If your client presents with yellow, chalky fingernails what would you do?**
    a. Diagnose the nail condition your client has
    b. Perform a full reflexology treatment working all areas as normal
    c. Perform a reflexology treatment with additional work directly on the fingernails
    d. Do not perform any reflexology treatment at all and refer to doctor.

4 Applied reflexology

'We are as healthy as the weakest of our glands and organs.'
Laura Norman[1]

Homeostasis is the condition in which the body's internal environment remains relatively constant, within physiological limits. It is when the body is in balance and any imbalances, or a lack of homeostasis, lead to ill health and 'dis-ease'. The fundamental intention of every reflexology treatment is to restore the body to homeostasis and in this chapter we take a look at the systems of the body and how reflexology can help them work together to maintain homeostasis.

Student objectives

By the end of this chapter you will be able to:

- Describe the structure and function of each system of the body.
- Know how, when and why to apply the reflexology techniques you have learned so far in this book.

This chapter briefly introduces the basic concepts of anatomy and physiology and should act as a reminder, not a substitute for proper training in the subject. For more in-depth information on the different systems of the body please refer to *Anatomy & Physiology for Therapists and Healthcare Professionals* by Ruth Hull (ISBN 9780 955 901119).

Overview of the Human Body

The human body consists of delicately balanced systems which depend on one another for their correct functioning. Each system is covered on the following pages:

- Musculo-skeletal system, page 134
- Nervous system, page 150
- Endocrine system, page 160
- Respiratory system, page 172
- Cardiovascular system, page 179
- Lymphatic and immune system, page 185
- Digestive system, page 192
- Urinary system, page 201
- Reproductive system, page 206
- The special senses (including the integumentary system), page 215.

When one system malfunctions it creates an imbalance in all the systems of the body and the result is a physiological disorder or disease. For example, stress does not only affect the nervous system – it can also cause irritable bowel syndrome (affecting the digestive system), breathing difficulties (affecting the respiratory system) and it can put a strain on the heart (affecting the cardiovascular system). Stress also lowers one's immunity (affecting the lymphatic and immune system) and can even affect one's fertility or libido (affecting the reproductive system). From this example you can see how important it is to maintain the delicate balance between all the systems of the body to ensure optimum health.

Cells, tissues and systems

You are going to learn how to apply reflexology to benefit the different systems of the body. However, before that let us briefly return to the very basics of anatomy and physiology.

The body is made up of tiny building blocks called atoms. Atoms such as carbon, hydrogen and oxygen, are essential for maintaining life and combine to form molecules such as fats, proteins and carbohydrates. These molecules then combine to form cells which are the basic structural and functional unit of the body. Cells vary greatly in size, shape and structure according to their function. For example, red blood cells are shaped like saucers to enable them to carry oxygen efficiently while nerve cells have long threadlike extensions for transmitting messages.

Despite their differences, most cells are made up of a nucleus, cytoplasm and a plasma membrane and they are all bathed in interstitial fluid, a dilute saline solution derived from the blood. Interstitial fluid is outside the cell and is also known as extracellular fluid, intercellular fluid or tissue fluid. The fluid inside the cells is called intracellular fluid. Both the interstitial fluid and the intracellular fluid are made up of oxygen, nutrients, waste and other particles dissolved in water.

Cells combine to form tissues. Tissues are groups of cells and the material surrounding the cells. There are four tissue types which perform particular functions. These tissue types are epithelial, connective, muscular and nervous tissue. The table below gives a brief overview of them.

TYPES OF TISSUE IN THE BODY		
Name	Function	Example
Epithelial	• Covers body surfaces and functions in protection, absorption and filtration • Lines hollow organs, cavities and ducts • Forms glands and functions in secretion	Skin
Connective	• Protects and supports the body and its organs • Binds organs together • Stores energy reserves as fat • Provides immunity	Blood, adipose tissue, bone
Muscular	• Provides movement and force	Skeletal muscle
Nervous	• Initiates and transmits nerve impulses	Nerves

Two or more different types of tissue combine to form organs which have very specific functions and recognisable shapes. Examples of organs include the heart, liver, stomach and lungs. Organs that share a common function combine to form systems.

Systems are composed of related organs and they perform a particular function. For example, the digestive system is composed of organs such as the stomach, liver, pancreas and small and large intestines. Its function is to break down and digest food. Finally, systems combine to form an organism, an example of which is a living person.

How to use this chapter
The subject of this chapter is applied reflexology. In other words, it covers how to use the techniques you have learned so far, and apply them to specific systems of the body. Each system is covered as follows:

- There is a basic introduction to the anatomy and physiology of the system. This will help you to get an idea of the role the system plays in the body.
- The main reflexes of the system are then given in detail. You will learn the function of these reflexes, where to locate them on the feet, how to work them with the techniques you have learned, and when and why you should work them.
- Finally, at the end of each system there is an 'In a nutshell' box. This summarises the system, listing its reflexes under the title 'Main reflexes' and giving additional reflexes that are known to help disorders of the system under the title 'Associated reflexes'.

Different books and schools use different terminology so you may know the Main reflexes as 'Direct reflexes' and the Associated reflexes as 'Secondary reflexes' or 'Helper reflexes'.

The Musculo-Skeletal System

The skeletal system

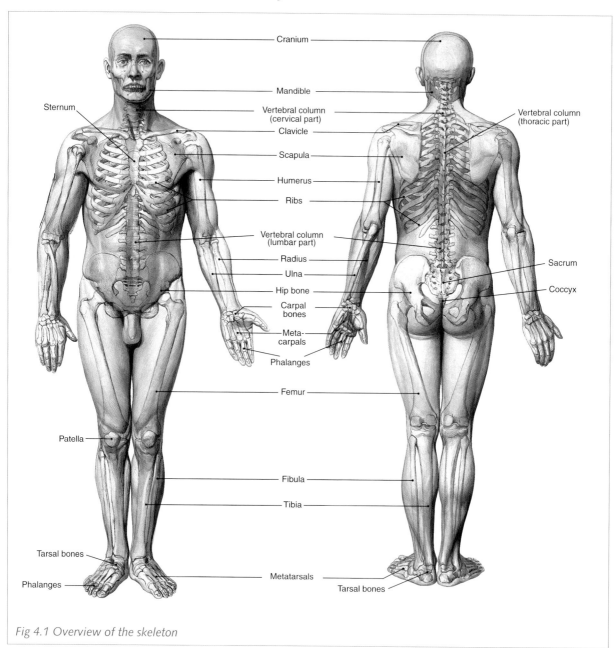

Cranium

Mandible

Vertebral column
(cervical part)

Clavicle

Scapula

Humerus

Ribs

Vertebral column
(lumbar part)

Radius

Ulna

Hip bone

Carpal
bones

Meta-
carpals

Phalanges

Femur

Fibula

Tibia

Metatarsals

Tarsal bones

Sternum

Patella

Tarsal bones

Phalanges

Vertebral column
(thoracic part)

Sacrum

Coccyx

Fig 4.1 Overview of the skeleton

The functions of the skeletal system

The framework of bones and cartilage that supports and protects the body and allows for movement is called the skeleton or skeletal system. It has seven main functions:

- **Support** – Bones are the scaffolding of the body and provide a framework that supports and anchors soft tissues and organs.

- **Shape** – Bones act as a framework to form the basic shape of the body.
- **Protection** – Bones are extremely hard and able to protect the body's vital organs.
- **Movement** – Bones are the sites of attachment for skeletal muscles and so generate movement.
- **Mineral homeostasis** – Bones store most of the calcium present in our bodies and are able to either release it into, or absorb it from, the blood to ensure there is always the correct amount of calcium present in the blood. They also store other minerals such as phosphorous.
- **Site of blood cell production (haemopoiesis)** – Some bones contain red bone marrow which, through the process of haemopoiesis, produces red blood cells, white blood cells and platelets.
- **Storage of energy** – Some bones contain yellow bone marrow which stores lipids (fats) and is an important energy reserve in the body.

Bones

Bone tissue, which is also called osseous tissue, is a connective tissue whose matrix is composed of water, protein, fibres and mineral salts. It can be classified into two types:

- **Compact (dense) bone tissue** – This is a very hard, compact tissue that has few spaces within it and is composed of a basic structural unit called an osteon or Haversian system. The main functions of compact bone tissue are protection and support and it forms the external layer of all bones.
- **Spongy (cancellous) bone tissue** – This is a light tissue with many spaces within it that give it a sponge-like appearance and it does not contain osteons or Haversian systems. Spongy bone tissue contains red bone marrow which is the site of blood cell production and it is found in the hip bones, ribs, sternum, vertebrae, skull and the ends of some long bones.

The body contains many different types of bones which are generally classified according to their shape:

- **Long bones** – Long bones have a greater length than width and usually contain a longer shaft with two ends. Long bones are slightly curved to provide strength and are composed of mainly compact bone tissue with some spongy bone tissue. Examples of long bones include the femur, tibia, fibula, phalanges, humerus, ulna and radius.
- **Short bones** – Short bones are cube-shaped and almost equal in length and width. They are made up of mainly spongy bone with a thin surface of compact bone. Examples of short bones include the carpals and tarsals.
- **Flat bones** – Flat bones are very thin bones consisting of a layer of spongy bone enclosed by layers of compact bone. Thin bones act as areas of attachment for skeletal muscles and also provide protection. Examples of thin bones include the cranial bones, the sternum, ribs and scapulae.
- **Irregular bones** – Bones that cannot be classified as long, short or flat bones fall into the category of irregular bones. They have complex shapes and varying amounts of compact and spongy tissue. An example of an irregular bone is a vertebra.
- **Sesamoid bones** – Sesamoid bones are oval bones that develop in tendons where there is considerable pressure. For example, the patella (knee cap).

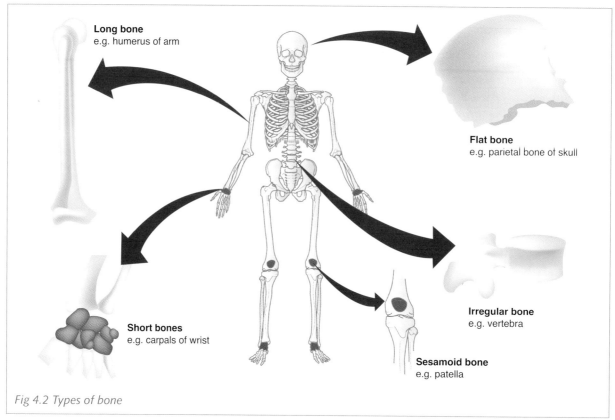

Long bone
e.g. humerus of arm

Flat bone
e.g. parietal bone of skull

Short bones
e.g. carpals of wrist

Irregular bone
e.g. vertebra

Sesamoid bone
e.g. patella

Fig 4.2 Types of bone

The skeleton

There are approximately 206 bones in the human body and the skeleton is made up of:

- **The axial skeleton** – The axial skeleton consists of the 80 bones that are found in the centre of the body, namely the skull, hyoid, ribs, sternum and vertebrae. The auditory ossicles are also usually included in the axial skeleton.
- **The appendicular skeleton** – The appendicular skeleton consists of the 126 bones of the upper and lower limbs and their girdles which connect them to the axial skeleton.

The bones of the skeleton are attached to one another by ligaments. These are tough, fibrous cords of connective tissue that contain both collagen and elastic fibres. They surround joints and bind them together, joining bones to bones.

Joints

Joints are also called articulations and are the points of contact between bones, cartilage and bones or teeth and bones. Without joints, our bodies would be solid structures and we would be unable to move. However, some of the joints of the body, for example the sutures of the skull, do not allow for much movement. Instead, they form firm structures that help protect organs.

Joints can be classified according to their structure. This takes into account the type of connective tissue that binds the joints together and whether or not there is a synovial cavity between the joints.

Structurally, joints can be classified as:

- **Fibrous joints** – Bone ends are held together by fibrous (collagenous) connective tissue and there is no synovial cavity between them. They are strong joints that do not permit movement. For example, the sutures of the skull.
- **Cartilaginous joints** – Bone ends are held together by cartilage and they do not have a synovial cavity between them. They are strong joints that permit only minimal movement. For example, the pubic symphysis.
- **Synovial joints** – Bone ends are separated by a space called a synovial cavity. This space allows for a great deal of movement. For example, the shoulder joint. The articulating surfaces of the bones in a synovial joint are covered by a cartilage that reduces friction between the bones and helps absorb shock. This cartilage is called hyaline cartilage. The entire joint is also enclosed in a dense fibrous capsule containing a lubricating fluid that facilitates movement and is called synovial fluid. There are a number of different types of synovial joint and they are classified according to the shapes of their articulating surfaces. These are discussed in the table on the following page.

Study tip
Cartilage is a strong, resilient connective tissue that is less hard and more flexible than bone.

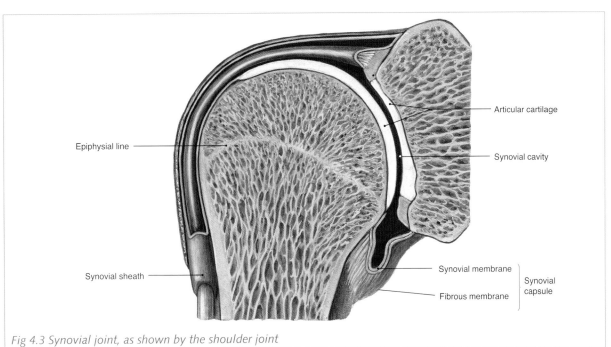

Epiphysial line

Synovial sheath

Articular cartilage

Synovial cavity

Synovial membrane

Fibrous membrane

Synovial capsule

Fig 4.3 Synovial joint, as shown by the shoulder joint

Name of joint	Shapes of articulating surfaces	Movements permitted	Examples	Diagram
Gliding (Plane)	Flat surfaces meet.	Side to side Back and forth Note: no angular or rotary motions are permitted.	Patellofemoral joint at knee. Intercarpal joints. Intertarsal joints. Sacro-iliac joint.	
Hinge	A convex surface fits into a concave one.	Flexion Extension Note: movements are in a single plane only.	Elbow joint. Tibiofemoral joint at knee. Ankle joint. Interphalangeal joints.	
Pivot	A rounded/pointed surface fits into a ring.	Rotation	Atlas and axis. Ulna and radius.	
Condyloid (Ellipsoid)	A condyle is a rounded/oval protuberance at the end of a bone and it fits into an elliptical cavity.	Back and forth Flexion Extension Abduction Adduction Circumduction	Wrist joint. Metacarpophalangeal joints.	
Saddle	A surface shaped like the legs of a rider fits into a saddle-shaped surface.	Side to side, Back and forth, Flexion, Extension, Abduction, Adduction, Circumduction, Opposition of thumbs (where the tip of the thumb crosses the palm and meets the tip of a finger)	Thumb joint.	
Ball and socket (Spheroidal)	A ball fits into a cup-shaped socket.	Flexion Extension Abduction Adduction Rotation Circumduction	Shoulder joint. Hip joint.	

The muscular system

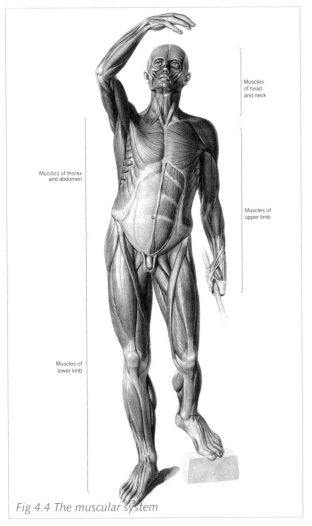

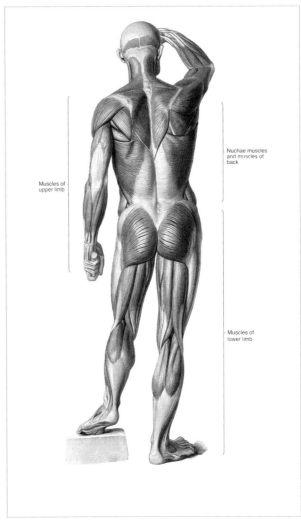

Fig 4.4 The muscular system

In the figures, the following labels appear:

Muscles of head and neck

Muscles of thorax and abdomen

Muscles of upper limb

Muscles of lower limb

Nuchae muscles and muscles of back

Muscles of upper limb

Muscles of lower limb

The functions of the muscular system

Muscles have the unique ability of shortening themselves. This is known as contraction and is the essential function of all muscles. Through contracting, muscles can:

- **Produce movement (locomotion)** – Skeletal muscles are a type of muscle that are mostly attached to bones by strong cords of dense connective tissue called tendons. When these muscles contract, they move the bones at the joints of the body and this produces movement of the skeleton. Some skeletal muscles are not attached to bones. Instead, they are attached to skin. These are the muscles of the face and they enable us to express emotions by smiling, frowning, etc.
- **Maintain posture** – When we are awake, certain skeletal muscles are always partially contracted to keep our bodies in an upright position. For example, the muscles of the neck maintain a sustained partial contraction to keep our heads upright. Muscle tendons also surround, protect and stabilise joints, thus stabilising body positions.

- **Move substances within the body and regulate organ volume** – In addition to skeletal muscle, there are two other types of muscle – smooth and cardiac (more on these in a minute). All three types of muscle function in moving substances within the body and in regulating organ control. For example:
  - *Skeletal muscle* – Skeletal muscle contracts to help return venous blood to the heart and to move lymph through the lymphatic vessels.
  - *Cardiac muscle* – The heart is made up of cardiac muscle tissue which contracts to pump blood around the body. Cardiac muscle also helps regulate blood pressure.
  - *Smooth muscle* – Smooth muscle lining hollow tracts of the body contracts to move food through the gastrointestinal tract, moves urine through the urinary tract and a baby through the birthing canal.
- **Produce heat (thermogenesis)** – Skeletal muscles release a lot of energy as they contract. This energy takes the form of heat which is considered a by-product of muscle contraction. The heat generated by muscular contraction is used to maintain our normal body temperature. If the body needs to increase its temperature, skeletal muscles contract involuntarily (shiver) to increase heat production. The generation of heat in the body is called thermogenesis.

Types of muscle tissue

There are over 600 muscles in the body and they are all under either voluntary or involuntary control. Muscles under voluntary control are under conscious control and can be controlled at will while muscles under involuntary control are not under conscious control and are controlled by neurotransmitters, hormones or autorhythmic cells.

There are three different types of muscle tissue:

- **Skeletal muscle** – This is striated tissue that is voluntarily controlled. It is attached by tendons to bones, skin or other muscles and moves the skeleton, maintains posture and generates heat.
- **Cardiac muscle** – This is striated, involuntarily controlled tissue. It forms most of the heart and pumps blood around the body.
- **Smooth (visceral) muscle** – This is non-striated tissue that is involuntarily controlled. It forms the walls of hollow internal structures such as blood vessels, the gastrointestinal tract and the bladder and it moves substances within the body and regulates organ volume.

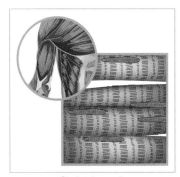

Skeletal muscle

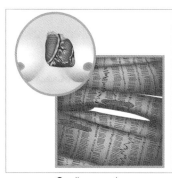

Cardiac muscle

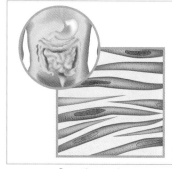

Smooth muscle

Fig 4.5 Types of muscle tissue

Basic anatomy of skeletal muscles

When looking at the musculo-skeletal system, we are mostly concerned with skeletal muscles and how they work together with the skeleton to produce movement. Skeletal muscles generally have the following characteristics:

- **Excitability (irritability)** – they are able to respond to stimuli.
- **Contractility (contractability)** – they can contract and shorten.
- **Extensibility** – they can extend and lengthen.
- **Elasticity** – they can return to their original shape after contracting or extending.

Skeletal muscles are made up of striated fibres. This means that when looked at under a microscope they are made up of light and dark bands, these being the actual contractile elements of the muscles. The striated muscle fibres are generally long and cylindrical-shaped and contain many mitochondria and multiple nuclei which give them their ability to generate so much energy. The muscle fibres are strengthened and reinforced by connective tissue and connected to bones by tendons, other muscles or the skin.

How do skeletal muscles produce movement?

A muscle is usually attached to two bones that form a joint and when the muscle contracts (shortens), it pulls the movable bone towards the stationary bone. All muscles have at least two attachments:

- **Origin** – This is the point where the muscle usually attaches to the stationary bone.
- **Insertion** – This is the point where the muscle usually attaches to the moving bone.

During contraction, the insertion usually moves toward the origin. Most body movements are the result of two or more muscles acting together or against each other so that whatever one muscle does, another muscle can undo. For example, one muscle contracts to bend your forearm (this is called the prime mover or agonist) and another muscle contracts to pull it straight again (this is called the antagonist). This means that muscles at joints are usually arranged in opposing pairs that are also accompanied by other muscles, called synergists, to ensure that movements are smooth and efficient.

Reflexes of the musculo-skeletal system

Note: Although the muscular and skeletal systems are separate anatomical systems, they are discussed together here because they share reflexes on the hands and feet.

The head and neck

The head, or skull, contains twenty-two bones which can be divided into eight cranial and fourteen facial bones. Together these bones protect and support the brain and the special sense organs (vision, taste, smell, hearing and equilibrium) and they form the framework of the face. They also protect the entrances to the digestive and respiratory systems and provide areas of attachment for muscles.

Most of the bones of the head are held together by immovable joints called sutures. However, the jawbone (mandible) is attached to the cranium by a freely movable joint called the temporo-mandibular joint (TMJ). This is a complicated joint and is prone to a number of different disorders which are all classified as temporo-mandibular joint disorder or syndrome.

The muscles of the face generally originate in the fascia or bones of the skull and insert into the skin. They move the skin and enable us to express emotions. There are many muscles in the neck, but the most important one for reflexology is the sternocleidomastoid. This is shaped like a strap, originating in the sternum and clavicle and inserting in the mastoid process behind the ear, and it plays an important role in moving the head. It is often affected in whiplash injury and can also cause headaches and neck pain.

Where are the head and neck reflexes?
The big toes and thumbs are the reflexes for the head:

- The **tips** are the brain reflexes.
- The **pads** are the reflexes for the occipital region (back of the head) as well as for some endocrine glands discussed on page 160.
- The **dorsal aspects** (tops) are the reflexes for the face including the mouth, nose and teeth
- The **sides** are the reflexes for the sides of the head.
- The **necks** are the reflexes for the neck (including the throat, tonsils, thyroid and parathyroid).

Note: the other four toes and fingers also contain reflexes of the head and neck, more specifically the sinuses, eyes and ears. These are discussed in more detail later in this chapter.

How do you work the head and neck reflexes?
Relaxation techniques help to loosen up the head and neck area, especially when there is chronic muscular stiffness and tension. Use techniques such as toe/finger stretching and rotation, or slide your fingers between the toes/fingers to open them up. Relaxation techniques that relax the shoulder area will also benefit the head and neck. Pressure techniques can be performed as follows:

- **The brain** – use your support hand to grip the big toe or thumb and hold it steady while you use either your finger tip or knuckle to work its tip.
- **The occipital region and back of the head** – place the palm of your support hand behind the big toe or thumb and use your thumb to either walk or rotate up its pad. Try to walk up five lines so that you work all five zones of the head. NB if you are working with someone who has very small hands, you may find it easier to work with your finger instead of your thumb.
- **The face** – place the back of your support hand underneath the pad of the big toe or thumb and use your index finger to either walk or rotate down or across its dorsum.
- **The sides of the head** – grip the sides of the big toe or thumb between your thumb and index finger and use small circular movements to move upwards from the base to the top.
- **The neck** – place the palm of your support hand behind the big toe or thumb and use your thumb to either walk or rotate transversely across its neck.

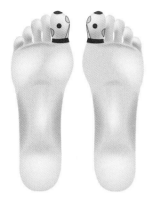
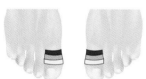

Practical tip
Look at the angle of the big toe – chronic neck and upper back tension often reflects in mis-shapen or angled big toes.

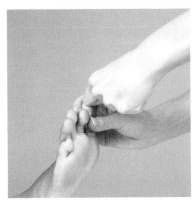

Knuckling the brain reflex

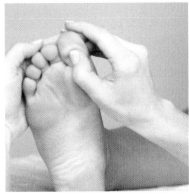

Thumb-walking the back of the head reflex

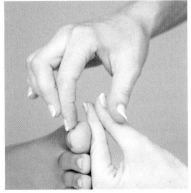

Finger-walking the face reflex

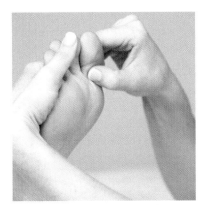

Thumb-walking the neck reflex

Why/When do you work the head and neck reflexes?

Work the head and neck reflexes if there are any problems with the area. For example, eye or ear problems, headaches, neck and shoulder tension or whiplash. In addition, working the neck reflexes benefits any arm or hand problems as the nerves coming off the cervical region feed the arm.

The spine

The spine, or vertebral column, is a strong, flexible structure that is able to bend and rotate in most directions. It supports the head, encloses and protects the spinal cord and is also a site of attachment for the ribs and the muscles of the back.

The spine is composed of thirty-three vertebrae and four curves as follows:

- **Cervical curve** – Seven cervical vertebrae form the neck. The first cervical vertebra (C1) is called the atlas and it supports the head, the second cervical vertebra (C2) is called the axis and it acts as an axis on which the atlas and head can rotate in a side-to-side movement. The third to sixth cervical vertebrae are quite normal, but the seventh (C7) is called the vertebra prominens and is the large prominence that can be seen and felt at the back of the neck.
- **Thoracic curve** – Twelve thoracic vertebrae form the thoracic curve. Ten of these vertebrae articulate with the ribs to form the ribcage.

Practical tip

There is an additional reflex which can be worked for whiplash. It is found on the dorsum of both feet and is the area between zones 1 and 2 that extends from the shoulder line to the diaphragm line – it feels like a groove. Finger-walk or rotate this area a number of times.

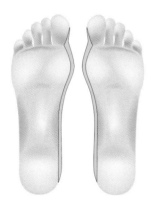

- **Lumbar curve** – Five lumbar vertebrae support the lower back. They are the largest and strongest vertebrae in the spine. They provide attachment for the large muscles of the back and support the weight of the upper body.
- **Sacral/Coccygeal curve** – Five sacral vertebrae fuse to form a triangular bone called the sacrum which is the strong foundation of the pelvic girdle. Four coccygeal vertebrae fuse to form a triangular shape called the coccyx or tailbone.

Altogether, there are 26 separate bones that make up the spine.

Where is the spine reflex?

If you put your two feet together so that the big toes and arches of each foot are touching, you will see the shape of the body reflected in the feet: the toes are the head, the balls of the feet the chest, the waistline is evident and the heels are the pelvis. Now, looking at your feet together, where do you think your spine will be? Quite simply in the middle of the two feet! Just as the spine is the median line of your body, so too is it the median line of your feet when they are placed together.

The reflex for the spine is located on the medial edge of each foot and it runs along the arch of the foot from the base of the big toenail to the heel. On the hand, it runs along the edge of the hand from the base of the thumbnail to the wrist. The right foot or hand represents the right half of the spine while the left foot or hand represents the left half.

The structure of the foot reflects that of the spine: both have 26 bones and 4 curves.

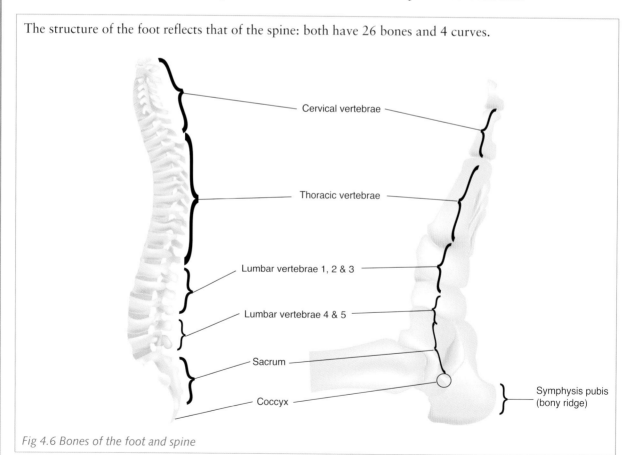

Fig 4.6 Bones of the foot and spine

Just as the spine has four natural curves that give it its flexibility and strength, so too does the spinal reflex on the foot. Each of these curves can be easily located on the foot:

- **Cervical curve** – Run your thumb down the medial edge of the big toe until you feel a bone. This bone is usually in line with the base of the toenail and it is the reflex for cervical 1, the atlas vertebra, which is the start of the spine. The seven cervical vertebrae of the neck are then reflected in the neck of the big toe, from the base of the toenail to the base of the toe (where the toe joins the foot).

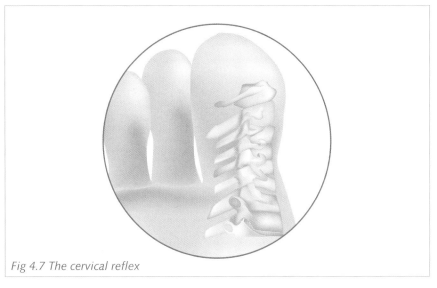

Fig 4.7 The cervical reflex

- **Thoracic curve** – The reflexes for the 12 thoracic vertebrae can be found running from the shoulder line (7th cervical vertebra) to the waistline.
- **Lumbar curve** – The lumbar curve runs from the waistline to the pelvic line. The fifth lumbar vertebra (L5) is located on the medial edge of the foot in line with the pelvic line.
- **Sacral/Coccygeal curve** – The sacral/coccygeal curve is located between the pelvic line and the base of the heel.

How do you work the spine reflex?

There are many different ways to work the spine reflex and a few are suggested below. When working the feet you can use:

- **Relaxation techniques** – Relaxation techniques that focus on the spinal reflex encourage circulation to the spine and also help to release tension in the area. Beneficial techniques include effleurage, foot squeezing, side friction and the spinal twist. Remember to use the spinal twist with care if you have an elderly, frail or arthritic client. Working the ankle will also benefit the spine by relieving tension in the pelvic area. Use techniques such as the ankle boogie and stretching and rotating the ankle. Another technique that benefits the spine is to rub it vigorously with either the heel, palm or knuckles of your hand. Vigorous rubbing of the area produces heat, which improves the circulation. When the area feels warm, place your hand over it and hold it for approximately 15 seconds to allow the heat to disperse slowly.

Practical tip
Take a good look at the shape and muscle tone of the medial longitudinal arches of your client's feet – they reflect the condition of the spine. Turn to page 43 for more information on the importance of the arches.

- **Pressure techniques** – When applying pressure techniques to the spine reflex always work one foot at a time and hold the edge of the foot with your support hand. It sometimes helps to tip the foot outwards so that you have easier access to the spine reflex. You can use either your thumb or finger to either walk or rotate up and down the spine. You can also use the medial edge of your knuckle to massage the length of the spine. If you find any unusually tight or sensitive areas then work these for a while before moving on.

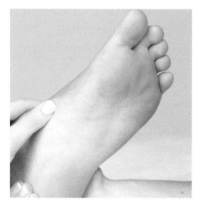

Thumb-walking up the spine

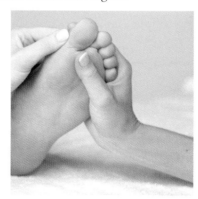

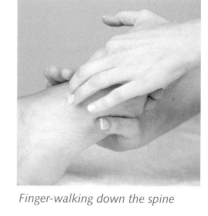

Finger-walking down the spine

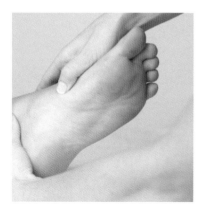

Thumb-walking down the spine

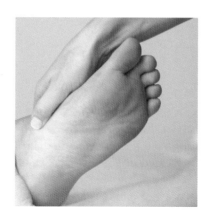

Knuckling down the spine

In hand reflexology, the spine can also be worked with both relaxation and pressure techniques:

- **Relaxation techniques** – Warm up the spinal reflex and improve circulation to the area by rubbing along the edge of the hand from the base of the thumbnail to the wrist. Use either your thumb or knuckle to rub this area and work it vigorously until it is warm. Also use the techniques of effleurage, finger stretching and rotation and finger wringing and focus them specifically on the spinal reflex.
- **Pressure techniques** – Support your client's hand, use either your thumb or finger to either walk or rotate up and down the spine. If you find any unusually tight or sensitive areas then work these for a while before moving on.

Applied reflexology

Why/When do you work the spine reflex?

'Structure governs function.'

Working the spine reflex should be an integral part of every reflexology treatment. The spine houses the spinal cord which is part of the central nervous system and from which 31 pairs of nerves emerge. These nerves influence every organ, structure and, ultimately, every cell in the body. If there is a problem with the structure of the spine then these nerves can become irritated and so negatively affect other parts of the body. For example, tension in the spinal column can lead to knee problems.

Working the spine reflex relaxes the client and releases tension along the length of the spine. Thus, it is beneficial to any disorders of the nervous or musculo-skeletal systems.

Reflexions

The more you work with people, the more you notice how their attitudes and beliefs manifest themselves physically. When working with people with back problems, be aware of the following:

- The neck should be flexible and able to move easily. People who suffer with chronic neck tension and a lack of flexibility in their neck may have more inflexible personalities than most people and be unable to see other points of view.
- People who suffer with shoulder problems often feel as if they are 'carrying the weight of the world on their shoulders'. They may be weighed down by their responsibilities.
- The lower back represents security and chronic lower back ache is common in people who are constantly worrying about their security, especially financial security.

The shoulder

Also called the pectoral girdle and it consists of two bones – the clavicle and scapula. The shoulder joint is a ball-and-socket joint which is bound and strengthened by a group of muscles called the rotator-cuff muscles, composed of the supraspinatus, infraspinatus, teres minor and subscapularis muscles.

Where is the shoulder reflex?

The shoulder reflex is found on both feet and hands lying between the shoulder line and diaphragm line in zone 5. The shoulder line itself is also a reflex for the shoulder.

How do you work the shoulder reflex?

In foot reflexology, the shoulder reflex can be worked with relaxation techniques such as the shoulder sandwich. Foot squeezing, side friction, intercostal sliding, metatarsal manipulation and toe stretching and rotating also benefit the shoulder.

Hand reflexology techniques such as effleurage, metacarpal manipulation and stretching and rotating the fingers (especially the little finger) are all beneficial to the shoulder.

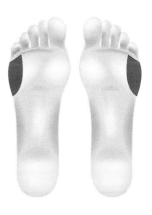

In terms of deeper pressure techniques, the reflex can be thumb-walked or rotated or it can be pinched between the index finger and thumb and rotated deeply.

Why/When do you work the shoulder reflex?

The shoulder reflex should be worked if there are any problems with the shoulder, such as stiffness or tension. It should also be worked for any neck problems or headaches as these problems can often stem from tight shoulders. Working the shoulder reflex will also benefit respiratory disorders and often helps to release tension caused by stress and anxiety. Note that disorders of the shoulders can often be linked to either spinal problems or stress so ensure you work the reflexes for the spine, solar plexus and brain if there are shoulder problems.

> **Reflexions**
> In ayurvedic reflexology great importance is placed on the mobilisation of the joints as it is believed that vital energy gets stuck in these joints and stagnates there.

The elbow/arm

The upper arm is made up of a long bone called the humerus and the forearm is made up of two smaller bones, the ulna and radius. The elbow joint connects the upper arm to the forearm and is a hinge joint.

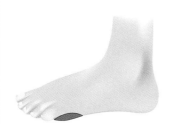

Where is the elbow/arm reflex?

The reflex for the arm is located on the lateral edge of each foot and hand, in zone 5. The arm reflex starts at the shoulder reflex and runs down zone 5 to approximately the 5th metatarsal notch where the elbow joint is located.

How do you work the elbow/arm reflex?

The arm reflex is generally worked by finger-walking or rotating the lateral edge of the foot or hand. Using your fingertips, rotate the elbow reflex.

Why/When do you work the elbow/arm reflex?

Work the arm reflex if there are any problems with the arms or hands. Be sure to also work the neck and cervical reflexes for problems of the arms or hands. Work the elbow reflex if there are any problems with this area, for example, tennis elbow.

The hip/knee/leg

The hip is also called the pelvic girdle and is a strong, stable structure upon which rests the weight of the upper body. It supports both the spine and the visceral organs and is a site of attachment for many muscles. The hip joint is a ball-and-socket joint. The leg is made up of the thigh and lower leg. The thigh is composed of the femur bone which is the longest, strongest and heaviest bone in the body. The lower leg consists of two smaller bones, the tibia and fibula. The knee joint connects the thigh to the lower leg and is actually made up of three smaller joints – one gliding joint and two hinge joints. There is no actual interlocking of bones in the knee joint and it is reinforced by tendons and ligaments only. The kneecap is a bone called the patella.

Where is the hip/knee/leg reflex?

On the feet, the hip, knee and leg are generally treated together and their reflex is located on the lateral edge of both feet, zone 5. It forms a triangle between the heel, fifth metatarsal notch and lateral malleolus. The area around the lateral malleolus can also be worked as a helper to the hip reflex.

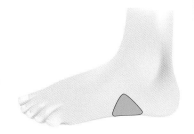

On the hands, the reflex for the hip, knee and leg is located on the lateral edge and dorsum of both hands and is the area between the waistline and pelvic line in zone 5.

How do you work the hip/knee/leg reflex?

Work this reflex on the foot by either finger-walking or rotating the lateral edge of the foot, firstly in a longitudinal direction and then upwards, from the edge of the foot up onto the dorsum. You can also perform deep thumb rotations directly onto the reflex.

On the hands, finger walk or rotate the lateral edge of the hand and then squeeze the reflex between your finger and thumb and rotate it deeply.

Why/When do you work the hip/knee/leg reflex?

The hip/knee/leg reflex should be worked if there are any problems with these areas, including problems with the feet. If a client suffers with hip, knee, leg or foot problems, be sure to also work the lower spine and the sciatic nerve reflexes.

The musculo-skeletal system in a nutshell…

Main reflexes – head, neck, shoulders, elbows/arms, spine, hips/knees/legs

- Disorders of the musculo-skeletal system can often be linked to lifestyle and habits. Exercise, good posture and ergonomics are important to maintaining a healthy musculo-skeletal system, as are nutrition and one's ability to cope with stress. If you have a client suffering with a disorder of these systems, you will need to analyse their habits and recommend changes they can make.
- Disorders of the musculo-skeletal system are usually characterised by symptoms such as pain, inflammation and a loss of bone-density or degeneration. Certain disorders, such as gout or arthritis, also involve a build-up of waste and poor elimination.

Associated reflexes

- Adrenals for pain and inflammation
- Brain for the release of endorphins if there is pain
- Cardiovascular reflexes (heart and recommended relaxation techniques) to improve circulation so that nutrients and oxygen are brought to the affected areas and waste products are removed
- Solar plexus for relaxation
- Lymphatic system to encourage good immunity and help remove waste
- Parathyroids and thyroid glands if the disorder is accompanied by an imbalance in calcium levels
- Kidneys as they help synthesise the hormone calcitriol which is the active form of vitamin D
- Cervical nerves for any problems of the arms, elbows or hands
- Sciatic nerve for any problems of the lower back, legs, knees or feet
- All organs of elimination (lungs, liver, kidneys, large intestine, lymphatic system and skin) to encourage the removal of waste
- Stomach if the client is taking anti-inflammatory medication as this often has a negative effect on the stomach.

Poor posture and tension in the neck, shoulder and thoracic region can cause shallow and difficult breathing which will, in turn, lead to fatigue.

Case study

Joanne was a regular client who came to me on a monthly basis to help her cope with chronic rheumatoid arthritis. One day Joanne came to me for a treatment and I noticed that the toenails of her second toe on both feet were black. I asked her if she had dropped something on them or bruised them in any way. She said no. In traditional Chinese medicine (TCM) the stomach meridian ends on the second toe so I gently pressed the stomach reflex point on the sole of her foot. She found this very painful. After talking to her for a while I learned that she had just started some new anti-inflammatory drugs which were having a very bad effect on her stomach.

The Nervous System

'The first wonder of the world, the human brain, the chief executive of the nervous system and the organ with which the computer is so often compared. … But a computer does not feel emotion; it has no sense of humour; no aesthetic sense; no values; and it cannot re-program itself in the same way as the human computer. In fact it is the reprogramming facility which puts the human brain in a class of its own.'
Dr Christiaan Barnard[2]

Many reflexologists begin their treatments by working the solar plexus, spinal cord and brain reflexes, all of which form the nervous system. This system is made up of millions of nerve cells that communicate with one another to control the body and maintain homeostasis. It is no surprise, therefore, that it is probably the most important system to work in reflexology, not only because of the physical benefits a treatment may bring, but also because of the psychological and spiritual 'reprogramming' it encourages.

Because the nervous system is such a complex system, it is divided into a number of different parts. To begin with, it is divided into the central nervous system (CNS) and the peripheral nervous system (PNS):

- **The central nervous system (CNS)** is made up of the brain and spinal cord. It analyses and stores information, makes decisions and issues orders. It is where memories are made and stored, emotions generated and thoughts conceived.
- **The peripheral nervous system (PNS)** comprises nerve cells that reach every part of the body and consists of:
  - Cranial nerves arising from the brain and carrying impulses to and from the brain.
  - Spinal nerves emerging from the spinal cord to carry impulses to and from the rest of the body. These nerves contain two types of nerve cells (neurones) – sensory, or afferent, neurones which conduct impulses from sensory receptors to the CNS, and motor, or efferent, neurones which conduct impulses from the CNS to muscles and glands.

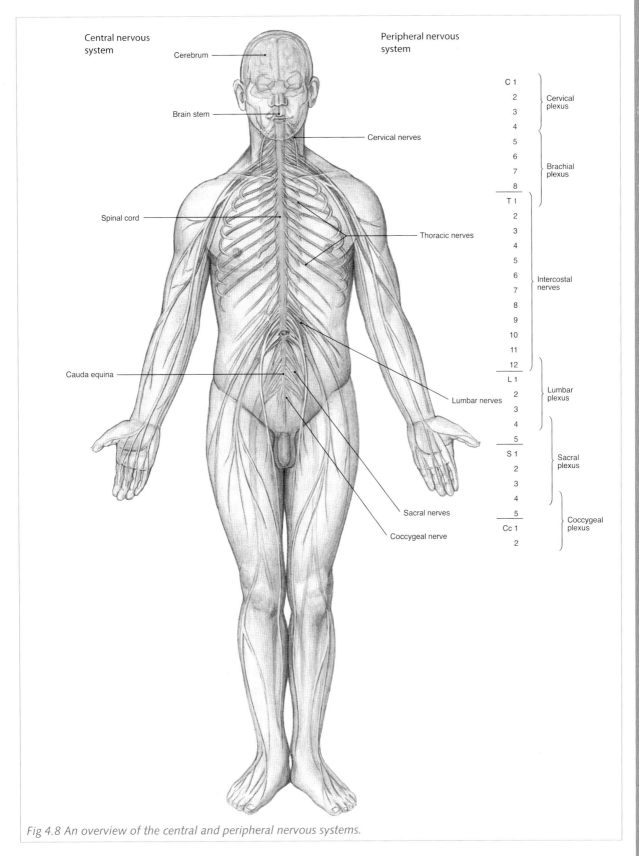

Central nervous system

Cerebrum

Brain stem

Spinal cord

Cauda equina

Peripheral nervous system

Cervical nerves

Thoracic nerves

Lumbar nerves

Sacral nerves

Coccygeal nerve

C 1
2
3
4
} Cervical plexus

5
6
7
8
} Brachial plexus

T 1
2
3
4
5
6
7
8
9
10
11
} Intercostal nerves

12
L 1
2
3
} Lumbar plexus

4
5
S 1
2
3
4
} Sacral plexus

5
Cc 1
2
} Coccygeal plexus

Fig 4.8 An overview of the central and peripheral nervous systems.

Practical tip
Study the big toes and be aware of the angle in which they lie, the condition of their nails and any dryness or corns on them. These can all be indicators of head imbalances such as headaches and migraines.

The PNS is subdivided into the somatic nervous system (SNS) and the autonomic nervous system (ANS):

- **The somatic nervous system** (SNS) allows us to control our skeletal muscles. Thus, it is sometimes called the voluntary nervous system.
- **The autonomic nervous system** (ANS) controls all processes that are automatic or involuntary. Thus, it is sometimes called the involuntary nervous system. It is divided into two branches that help the body adapt to changing circumstances. They work in opposition to one another and so are able to counterbalance each other to maintain homeostasis. They are:
  - The sympathetic nervous system which reacts to changes in the environment by stimulating activity and therefore using energy. For example, the sympathetic nervous system increases the heart beat.
  - The parasympathetic nervous system which opposes the actions of the sympathetic nervous system by inhibiting activity and therefore conserving energy. For example, the parasympathetic nervous system decreases the heart beat.

Reflexology has a profound effect on the nervous system and this is covered in depth on page 25. We will now look at the main reflexes of the nervous system in more depth and discuss the best ways to work them.

The brain

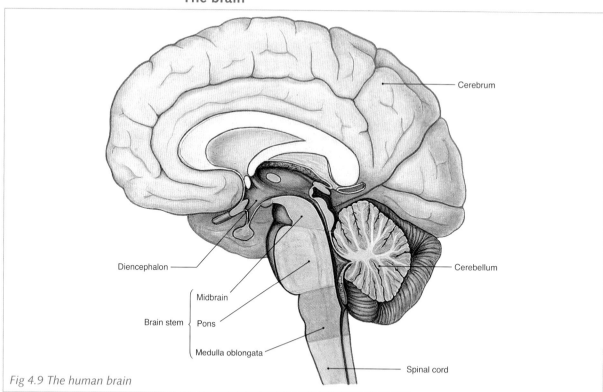

Fig 4.9 The human brain

The brain gives a person the ability to sense changes in both their internal and external environments, to think about these changes, make decisions and act on them. It is divided into the following regions (please note, this is a very simplified version of the brain):

- **Brainstem (medulla oblongata, pons, midbrain)** – this is the link between the brain and spinal cord. It relays motor and sensory impulses between the spinal cord and the other parts of the brain. It also functions in autonomic control such as regulation of the heartbeat, respiration, swallowing, etc.
- **Cerebellum** – this is located at the back of the head and co-ordinates and regulates movement, posture and balance.
- **Diencephalon (epithalamus, thalamus, hypothalamus)** – this lies above the brain stem and is enclosed by the cerebral hemispheres. It relays sensory impulses to the cerebral cortex and regulates homeostasis. It also houses the pituitary and pineal endocrine glands.
- **Cerebrum (cerebral cortex/grey matter, white matter, limbic system, basal ganglia)** – this covers the rest of the brain and is composed of two cerebral hemispheres. It is responsible for emotions and intelligence. It gives us the ability to read, write, speak, remember, create and imagine.

Where is the brain reflex?

The tips/caps of the big toes and thumbs are the main reflexes for the brain: the tip of the right big toe or thumb represents the right side of the brain and the tip of the left big toe or thumb represents the left side of the brain.

However, the tips of toes or fingers 1, 2 and 3 can all be worked to reinforce your treatment as all these digits represent the brain. Although toes and fingers 4 and 5 also represent the head reflex, they are reflexes for the temporal area of the head and not the brain specifically.

Case study

When I first started learning reflexology I was practising on a friend when I noticed what looked like a blood blister on the lateral edge of his big toe. I asked him how he had hurt it and was surprised to learn that he hadn't. Then he asked me if I could tell him exactly where in his body the blood-blister reflected. I said to him that it was the right side of his head, just above his ear. He laughed then, more from shock than anything else, and told me he had recently been hospitalised because a small blood vessel had burst in his brain – on the right side of his head, just above his ear.

How do you work the brain reflex?

Hold the big toe or thumb with the fingers of your support hand and work the brain reflex by applying an on-off pressure with either the tip of your thumb or finger or with the knuckle of your index finger. Be sure to work the tips/caps of the toes and thumbs as close to the nails as possible and do not work the pads as these are different reflexes.

Why/When do you work the brain reflex?

Work the brain reflex in every treatment. In addition, pay particular attention to it if your client has:

- Any stress or stress-related disorders. This is to encourage optimal functioning of the parasympathetic nervous system which helps the body cope with the effects of stress.
- Any pain in their body. This is to encourage the release of endorphins and enkephalins which are the body's natural pain-relievers.

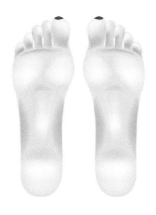

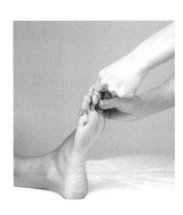

Knuckling the brain reflex

The cranial nerves

There are 12 pairs of cranial nerves, 10 originating from the brain stem and 2 from inside the brain itself. Their names and functions are:

I   Olfactory nerve – nose, smell.
II   Optic nerve – eyes, vision.
III   Oculomotor nerve – eyes, movement.
IV   Trochlear nerve – eyes, movement.
V   Trigeminal nerve (ophthalmic, maxillary and mandibular branches) – eyes, jaw movement, facial skin sensations.
VI   Abducens nerve – eyes, movement.
VII   Facial nerve – (temporal, zygomatic, buccal, mandibular and cervical branches) – facial expression, taste, saliva, tears.
VIII Vestibulocochlear nerve (vestibular and cochlear branches) – ears, hearing, balance.
IX   Glossopharyngeal nerve – tongue, pharynx, saliva.
X   Vagus nerve – thorax, abdomen.
XI   Accessory nerve (cranial and spinal portions) – head, pharynx and larynx.
XII   Hypoglossal nerve – tongue, talking, swallowing.

Where are the cranial nerve reflexes?

The reflexes for the cranial nerves are found along the edges of all the toes and fingers, including the big toe and thumb. In addition, there is a specific reflex for cranial nerve V, the trigeminal nerve. This is a cranial nerve consisting of three branches – the ophthalmic, maxillary and mandibular. It contains fibres which carry sensory information from the face (touch, pain, temperature) and it also controls the action of chewing. Injuries to, or disorders of, this nerve will affect these functions. The reflex for the trigeminal nerve is found on the dorsal aspect of the big toe. It begins at the base of the toe nail, on the lateral side, and runs down to the base of the distal phalange.

How do you work the cranial nerve reflexes?

In foot reflexology, the easiest way to work the cranial nerves is to hold the medial edge of the ball of the foot with your support hand (your thumb will be on the ball of the foot under the big toe, your fingers will be on the top of the foot and the medial edge of the foot where the spinal reflex is will be

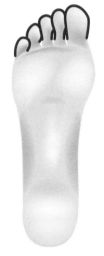

The cranial nerve reflexes

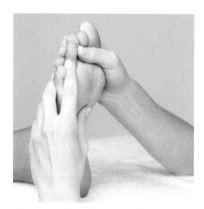
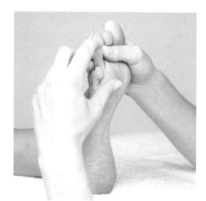
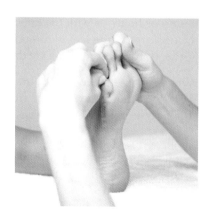

Finger-walking the cranial nerves

at the webbing between your thumb and fingers) and, starting with the little toe, finger walk up the lateral edge of the toe, across the top of it and down the medial edge. You can always use the fingers of your support hand to open up the toes if necessary. Then finger walk toe 4 the same way, then toe 3, toe 2 and finally toe 1. Now repeat this entire process but this time finger walk from toe 1 first and end with toe 5. This walk is called the cranial nerve walk.

The cranial nerve walk can be carried out in exactly the same way on the hands. In addition, the technique of finger wringing also works the cranial nerves.

Why/When do you work the cranial nerve reflexes?

The cranial nerve walk is very good for any stress or stress-related conditions as well as for depression. In addition, it should be used for any disorders related to the cranial nerves, such as Bell's Palsy or problems with the eyes, ears or nose.

The spinal cord and spinal nerves

The spinal cord, which is housed inside the spinal column, is continuous with the brain stem and has two main functions that help maintain homeostasis. It transports nerve impulses from the periphery of the body to the brain and from the brain to the periphery and it receives and integrates information and produces reflex actions.

Thirty-one pairs of spinal nerves originate in, and emerge from, the spinal cord. These nerves form part of the peripheral nervous system and connect the central nervous system to receptors in muscles and glands. These nerves are:

- 8 pairs of cervical nerves.
- 12 pairs of thoracic nerves.
- 5 pairs of lumbar nerves.
- 5 pairs of sacral nerves.
- 1 pair of coccygeal nerves.

Branches of spinal nerves form networks called plexuses. All nerves emerging from a specific plexus will innervate specific structures. In the table on the following page you will find details of the spinal plexuses and the areas they innervate. Take note where in the spinal column the nerves emerge from as these will be the reflex areas you will need to work.

THE SPINAL PLEXUSES			
Plexus	**Origin**	**Distribution**	**Reflexology notes**
Cervical plexus	C1–C4/5	Serves the head, neck and the top of the shoulders	Work the origins of this plexus for disorders of the head, including eye, ear, mouth, nose and throat problems.
Brachial plexus	C5–C8, T1	Serves the shoulder and arm	Work the origins of this plexus for disorders of the shoulder and arm, including weakness, numbness or tingling in the hands and fingers, wrist drop, weak thumb movements, inability to pronate the forearm or flex the wrist or carpal tunnel syndrome).
Lumbar plexus	L1–L4	Serves the abdominal wall, external genitals and part of the legs	Work the origins of this plexus for disorders of the legs and external genitals, including loss of sensation, inability to extend the leg or nerve-related disorders of the genitals.
Sacral plexus	L4–L5, S1–S4	Serves the buttocks, perineum and legs	Work the origins of this plexus for disorders of the sciatic nerve as well as foot drop; the inability to dorsiflex the foot; and a loss of sensation over the leg and foot.

Note, there is no thoracic plexus. Instead, the thoracic nerves T2–T12 directly innervate the chest, armpit and part of the arm. Their origins should be worked in any disorders of these areas.

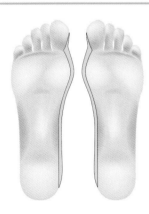

Where is the spinal cord reflex and why/when do you work it?
The reflex for the spinal cord and nerves is the same as the reflex for the spine/vertebral column. Please refer to page 144 to find out how to locate and work the spine reflex on both the hands and feet. In addition, the following reflex can be used during your treatment:

- **Occiput/Occipital reflex** – The occipital region is the back of the head and people often suffer with tension headaches in this area, especially if they have stiffness and tension in their neck and shoulders. The occipital reflex is located on the plantar aspect of the foot, at the base of the pad of the big toe, just above the reflex for the neck. You may find a thickening or hardening of the skin over this area, especially if your client suffers with tension headaches at the back of their head. Work this area with deep pressure techniques and also work the reflexes for the neck and shoulders.

The solar plexus (coeliac ganglion)

'the solar plexus – your own internal sun'
Dr Rudolph Ballentine[3]

The solar plexus is the most important reflex to work for calming and relaxing a person. The solar plexus (also called the coeliac ganglion or plexus) is a network of autonomic nerves that is located in the abdomen that innervates the digestive organs. It plays a role in the functioning of the autonomic nervous system which controls all the automatic processes of our body such as digestion. Because of its integral role, the solar plexus is often referred to as the abdominal brain or the nerve switchboard.

Reflexions

The solar plexus reflex on the foot is located in the same place as the first point on the kidney meridian which is called 'Bubbling Spring' (Well point). This is a vital point in traditional Chinese medicine because the 'kidneys store the jing and rule birth, development, and maturation.'[4] The solar plexus reflex on the hand lies in the same place as acupoint pericardium 8 (PE-8). Working this point has a very calming effect on the mind and it is used with disorders such as hysteria.

Where is the solar plexus reflex?

The reflex for the solar plexus lies just below the diaphragm line between zones 2 and 3. To find the reflex on the foot, use one hand to squeeze the toes/metatarsals together until you see a deep crease in the middle of the foot. Place your thumb below the ball of the foot and in the centre of this crease. When you release your squeeze on the toes/metatarsals you will see that your thumb fits comfortably into a natural hollow that lies just below the ball of the foot (the diaphragm line) in line with the gap between toes 2 and 3. To find it on the hand, locate the diaphragm line (the natural crease where the ball of your hand ends) and the solar plexus lies just below the diaphragm line between the second and third finger. It often feels tight and can be sensitive on someone suffering from stress and tension.

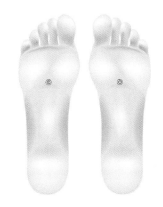

How do you work the solar plexus reflex?

The solar plexus is most commonly worked with the thumb and either one or both feet/hands can be worked at a time. If working one foot/hand at a time, be sure to support its dorsum with your support hand and pull the foot/hand into your thumb to gain a deeper pressure. If working both feet/hands at the same time, use the fingers of your working hand in opposition to your thumbs to bring greater pressure to your techniques.

When you first place your thumbs on the solar plexus, take a few seconds to relax and 'feel' the state/energy of the reflex. You can then decide how to work it. Please turn to page 78 to review the technique of first contact. Here you will learn a variety of techniques that can be used on the solar plexus. In addition, pages 91–92, which cover interpreting reflex points, give more options on how to work this vital point.

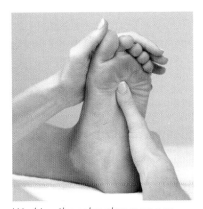

Working the solar plexus on one foot at a time

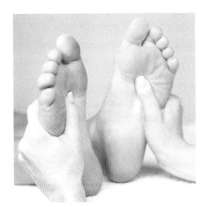

Working the solar plexus on both feet at the same time

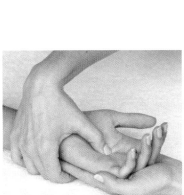

Working the solar plexus on the hand

Why/When do you work the solar plexus reflex?

As with the brain and spine, the solar plexus should be worked in every reflexology treatment. It is usually the first point worked because it has such a calming and balancing effect on the nervous system. It can then be worked during the treatment, especially if a client suffers with any disorders of the nervous or digestive systems, and again it is often used as part of the relaxation techniques that are used at the end of a treatment. In addition, the solar plexus can be worked or held gently if your client has any negative reactions, such as crying, during the treatment.

Case study

I was once with a friend who had an anxiety attack and was struggling to breathe. I took her hand and firmly pressed the solar plexus reflex for approximately two minutes. She calmed down and her breathing returned to normal. I now teach this point to all my clients who suffer with anxiety or who are going through very stressful times. They find that when they begin to feel stressed they simply hold the point and focus on their own breathing. The point will often feel sensitive and I recommend to them that they hold it until the sensitivity eases. It is also a great point to help you calm yourself before an exam!

The sciatic nerve

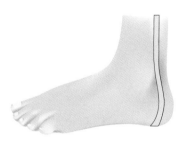

'For reflexologists this nerve is of particular interest because this is the very nerve conducting all touch and pain sensations from the feet. Each foot contains 75,000 free nerve endings registering everything we do as reflexologists. That incredible amount of information is relayed to the central nervous system via the sciatic nerve. Therefore, it makes sense assuming that a proper functioning of the sciatic nerve is necessary for a good effect of reflexology.'
Dorthe Krogsgaard and Peter Lund Frandsen[5]

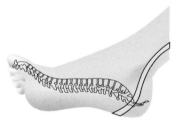

The sciatic nerve arises from the sacral plexus of the spinal cord and descends down the back of the thigh before splitting into the tibial and common peroneal nerves. The sciatic nerve is the largest nerve in the body and is responsible in some way for innervating most of the leg and foot. It is therefore a very important reflex to work during a reflexology treatment as problems with the nerve can affect most of the area from the buttock down the back of the leg and into the foot itself.

Where is the sciatic nerve reflex?

On the foot, the reflex for the sciatic nerve begins behind the medial malleolus (ankle bone) and runs down the side of the foot, then directly across the heel and up the other side of the foot where it ends behind the lateral malleolus. It is shaped like a stirrup.

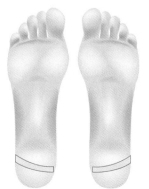

On the hand, the reflex for the sciatic nerve begins above the wrist, on the edge of the forearm. It runs down the forearm to the pelvic line on the palmar aspect of the hand, directly across the pelvic line and then up the other side of the forearm. Again, it is shaped like a stirrup or a 'U'.

How do you work the sciatic nerve reflex?

In foot reflexology, there are two ways to work the sciatic nerve reflex – you can either knuckle the entire pelvic reflex (the heel of the foot) in which the sciatic nerve reflex is found or you can do the sciatic nerve walk. This walk is done as follows:

- Support the right foot in your right hand by placing the palm of your hand underneath the heel, with your fingers up the lateral side of the foot and your thumb up the medial side.
- Using the thumb of your left hand, lift your elbow and move your body slightly so that you can comfortably place the pad of your thumb beneath your client's lateral malleolus. Ensure the tip of your thumb is pointing towards you and not toward your client's head.
- Now thumb-walk in a straight line downwards from the anklebone to the heel. At the heel you will thumb-walk horizontally across the centre of the heel.
- At the medial edge of the heel change hands so that your left hand becomes the support hand and your right thumb becomes the working thumb.
- Now, using your right thumb, thumb-walk in a straight line up the edge of the foot until you are beneath the medial malleolus.
- Repeat the entire walk backwards and forwards a few times before repeating it on the left foot.

The sciatic nerve walk described above also applies to hand reflexology.

Practical tip
Sciatica has many causes, especially tension in the lumbar and sacral regions and hip problems. It is important, therefore, to always work the lumbar and sacral reflexes as well as the hip reflexes if a client suffers from sciatica.

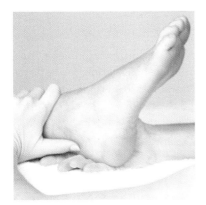
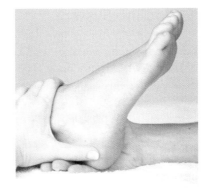
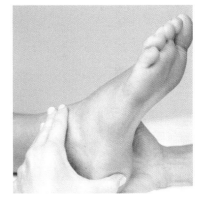

Thumb-walking the sciatic nerve

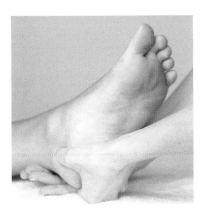

Why/When do you work the sciatic nerve reflex?

If your client suffers from sciatica or any problems with the legs and feet, spend some time focusing on the sciatic nerve reflex. Sciatica is inflammation of the sciatic nerve and is characterised by pain, numbness or pins-and-needles along the nerve path running down the back of the leg. Complications of sciatica can include foot drop, the inability to dorsiflex the foot or loss of sensation in either the leg or foot.

Balancing the parasympathetic nervous system

To balance the parasympathetic nervous system apply pressure to both the brain and sacral reflexes at the same time and maintain this pressure for approximately 30 seconds.

The nervous system in a nutshell

Main reflexes – brain, cranial nerves, spinal cord, solar plexus, sciatic nerve. The system that most obviously benefits from reflexology is the nervous system. Reflexology relaxes a person and enhances the functioning of the parasympathetic nervous system and so helps us cope with stress. It also helps with many stress-related conditions such as irritable bowel syndrome and eczema. Therefore, the reflexes of the nervous system are often important associated reflexes for many other systems.

Associated reflexes

- Reflexes of the musculo-skeletal system to ensure there is no entrapment or impingement of nerves
- Reflexes of the cardiovascular system to bring oxygen and nutrients to nerves and remove their waste
- Adrenal glands if we are under stress.

The Endocrine System

The endocrine system, together with the nervous system, is responsible for most of the activities in the body. The endocrine system is composed of a number of ductless glands which secrete chemical messengers, called hormones, into the extracellular space around their cells. These secretions then diffuse into blood capillaries and are transported by the blood to target cells located throughout the body. Hormones regulate cellular activity.

Functions of the endocrine system

The endocrine system has many functions as it affects a variety of cells and tissues in the body. A simplistic view of its functions is that it co-ordinates body functions such as:

- Growth
- Development
- Reproduction
- Metabolism
- Homeostasis.

It also helps regulate activities of the immune system and the process of apoptosis. This is the normal, ordered death and removal of cells as part of their development, maintenance and renewal.

Control of hormone release

The secretions of hormones into the bloodstream need to be controlled otherwise there will be an underproduction or overproduction of a

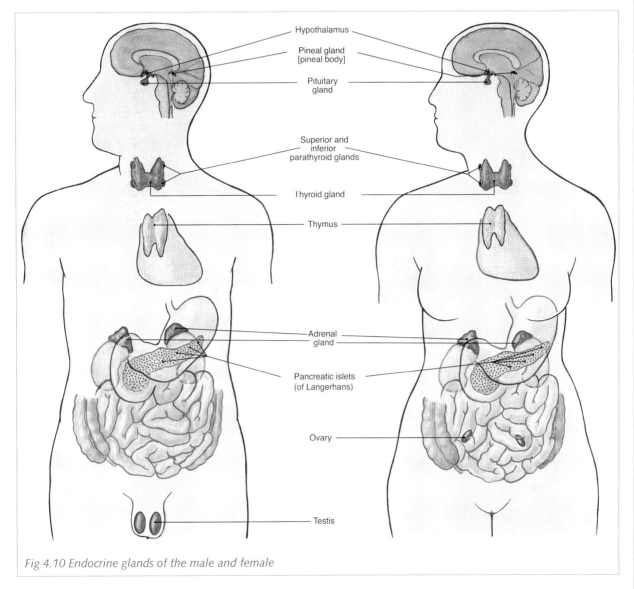

Fig 4.10 Endocrine glands of the male and female

hormone that can result in disease. Hormone secretion is controlled by signals from the nervous system, chemical changes in the blood and other hormones.

Neural stimulation – Signals from the nervous system can stimulate the release of hormones into the bloodstream. For example, sympathetic nervous stimulation causes the release of adrenaline.

Chemical changes in the blood – Changes in the levels of certain ions, for example calcium, or nutrients can stimulate the release of hormones. For example, blood calcium levels regulate the secretions of the parathyroid glands.

Hormonal stimulation – The presence of a hormone can stimulate the release of another hormone. For example, hormones secreted by the anterior pituitary gland stimulate the release of other hormones into the bloodstream.

Once hormones have been released into the body, their levels are controlled by a negative feedback mechanism. This is a system in which rising levels of a hormone will inhibit the further release of that hormone.

The hypothalamus

The hypothalamus is not always considered an endocrine gland as it is actually part of the nervous system and is an area of the brain near the pituitary gland. However, it is included here because of its vital connection to the pituitary gland. It releases a number of hormones that control the secretions of the pituitary gland. It also synthesises two hormones that are then transported to, and stored in, the posterior pituitary gland. These hormones are oxytocin and antidiuretic hormone.

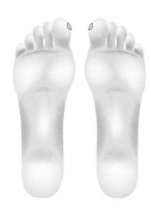

Where is the hypothalamus reflex?
The reflex for the hypothalamus is in the same place as the reflex for the pineal gland which we will discuss shortly. It is located at the top of the spine reflex. To find it, run your thumb down the medial edge of the big toe until you feel a bone. This bone is usually in line with the base of the toenail and the top of this bone is the reflex for the hypothalamus. On the hand, the hypothalamus/pineal reflex is located at the top of the spine reflex on the edge of the thumb.

Note that some foot maps show the hypothalamus/pineal gland reflex as being in the middle of the pad of the big toe or thumb, just above the pituitary gland. This is an energetic reflex which can be worked with great success.

How do you work the hypothalamus reflex?
To work the hypothalamus reflex simply place your thumb on the reflex (it should be resting on the top of the bone) and push gently downwards.

Why/When do you work the hypothalamus reflex?
Because of its vital connection to the pituitary gland, the hypothalamus should be worked in any circumstances where it is necessary to work the pituitary gland. Please turn to page 164 for more details on when to work the pituitary gland. Both the hypothalamus and pituitary glands should always be worked for the hormonal balance of the whole body.

The pituitary gland

The pituitary gland is the size and shape of a large pea, yet it is the master gland of the body. Despite its small size, its hormones control most of the other glands of the body.

The pituitary gland is also called the hypophysis and is located in the brain behind the nose and between the eyes. It is attached to the hypothalamus and is composed of an anterior and posterior lobe.

The tables on the next two pages detail the hormones secreted by the pituitary gland.

HORMONES OF THE PITUITARY GLAND

HORMONE	TARGET TISSUE	ACTIONS	DISORDERS AND DISEASES
Anterior pituitary gland All the hormones released by the anterior pituitary gland, except for human growth hormone, regulate other endocrine glands.			
Human growth hormone (hGH) or Somatotropin	Bone, muscle, cartilage and other tissue.	Stimulates growth and regulates metabolism.	**Hyposecretion**: Pituitary dwarfism **Hypersecretion**: Gigantism, Acromegaly
Thyroid-stimulating hormone (TSH) or Thyrotropin	Thyroid gland	Controls the thyroid gland.	**Hyposecretion**: Myxoedema **Hypersecretion**: Graves' disease (NB: These diseases are more commonly caused by a problem with the thyroid gland itself).
Follicle-stimulating hormone (FSH)	Ovaries and testes	**In females**: stimulates the development of oocytes (egg cells or immature ovums). **In males**: stimulates the production of sperm.	**Hyposecretion**: Sterility
Luteinizing hormone (LH)	Ovaries and testes	**In females**: stimulates ovulation, the formation of the corpus luteum and secretion of oestrogens and progesterone **In males**: stimulates the production of testosterone.	**Hyposecretion**: Sterility **Hypersecretion**: Stein-Leventhal syndrome (Polycystic ovary syndrome)
Prolactin (PRL) or Lactogenic hormone	Mammary glands	**In females**: stimulates the secretion of milk from the breasts. **In males**: action is unknown.	**Hypersecretion** in females: Galactorrhoea (abnormal lactation) Amenorrhoea (absence of menstrual cycles)
Adrenocorticotropic hormone (ACTH) or Corticotropin	Adrenal cortex	Stimulates and controls the adrenal cortex.	**Hyposecretion**: Addison's disease **Hypersecretion**: Cushing's syndrome
Melanocyte-stimulating hormone (MSH)	Skin	Exact actions are unknown, but can cause darkening of the skin.	

HORMONES OF THE PITUITARY GLAND			
HORMONE	**TARGET TISSUE**	**ACTIONS**	**DISORDERS AND DISEASES**

Posterior pituitary gland
The posterior pituitary gland does not synthesise hormones. Instead, it stores and releases hormones synthesised by the hypothalamus.

HORMONE	TARGET TISSUE	ACTIONS	DISORDERS AND DISEASES
Oxytocin (OT)	Uterus, mammary glands	Stimulates contraction of uterus during labour and stimulates the 'milk let-down' reflex during lactation.	
Antidiuretic hormone (ADH) or Vasopressin	Kidneys, sudoriferous glands, blood vessels	Antidiuretic effect (i.e. conserves water by decreasing urine volume and perspiration), raises blood pressure.	**Hyposecretion**: Diabetes insipidus

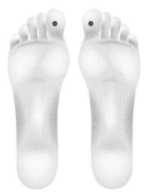

Where is the pituitary reflex?

Although foot maps often show the pituitary gland as being in the centre of the pad of the big toe or thumb, it is not always there as people's toes differ. To find the exact location of the gland, look closely at the pad of the big toe or thumb and you will see the whorls of the print. The pituitary gland is in the centre of the whorl and this centre point can often appear as a slightly raised area.

How do you work the pituitary reflex?

The pituitary gland can be worked in two ways:

* Use the thumb-hook technique described on page 89.
* Or, support the back of the big toe or thumb with the palm of your support hand, and locate the pituitary reflex. Once you have found it, apply a deep pressure to it with the knuckle of your index finger if you are working the toe or the tip of your index finger if you are working the thumb.

Why/When do you work the pituitary reflex?

Once you have an understanding of all the different hormones the pituitary gland secretes, you will realise why it is such a vital gland and why it should be worked in most situations. It should be worked in any conditions concerning growth, development, metabolism or reproduction and it is especially beneficial for people with low energy levels and women with menstrual or reproductive disorders.

A famous reflexologist, Dwight Byers, wrote: 'I have found the pituitary gland reflex is excellent for reducing fevers and also useful in fainting spells. This gland is also responsible for cellular growth and it should be worked in

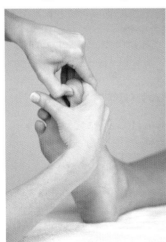

Thumb-hook on the pituitary

all cases of extracellular growth whether the growth be benign or malignant. It should also be worked as a normal procedure in children.'[6]

The pineal gland

The pineal gland is located in the centre of the brain and although its physiological role in the body is still unclear, it is known to produce the hormone melatonin. Melatonin is thought to affect the timing of the body's biological clock and its release is stimulated by darkness and inhibited by sunlight.

Where is the pineal reflex and how do you work it?

The pineal reflex is in the same place as the hypothalamus reflex and is worked in the same way. Please turn to page 162 for more information on how to locate and work this reflex.

Why/When do you work the pineal reflex?

Working the pineal reflex helps to set the body's biological clock and is beneficial for sleep disorders such as insomnia as well as for conditions such as jet-lag. In addition, working the pineal reflex has been found to help with mood disorders, depression and seasonal affective disorder (SAD).

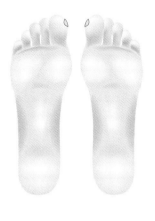

The thyroid gland

The thyroid is a butterfly-shaped gland that is wrapped around the trachea, just below the larynx. It secretes two hormones that play a vital role in the body's metabolism. These are tri-iodothyronine (T3) and thyroxine (T4). Together they are often referred to as 'thyroid hormone'. Thyroid hormone affects all the cells and tissues of the body and controls cellular metabolism, growth and development. It also controls oxygen use and the basal metabolic rate which is the minimum amount of energy used by the body to maintain vital processes. The thyroid gland also secretes the hormone calcitonin which lowers blood calcium levels.

Where is the thyroid reflex?

Because the thyroid gland is located in the neck, its reflex is found in the neck of the big toe or thumb. In addition, a helper reflex for the thyroid gland is found on the ball of the foot. It starts in the space between the big toe and the second toe and curves down the ball of the foot, in a C shape, to where the diaphragm line intersects the spine reflex.

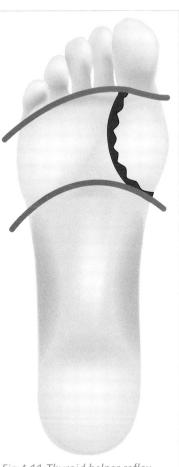

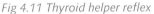

Fig 4.11 Thyroid helper reflex

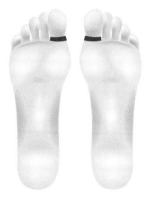

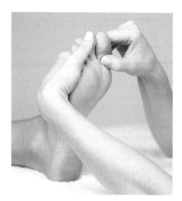

Thumb-walking the neck area works the reflexes for both the thyroid and parathyroid glands

Study tip

If a person has an underactive thyroid you will find the neck of the big toe will be quite soft and saggy. You may also find calluses on the thyroid helper reflex.

How do you work the thyroid reflex?

Both the thyroid reflex and the thyroid helper reflex are usually walked by either thumb-walking or thumb-rotating the reflex.

Why/When do you work the thyroid reflex?

The thyroid gland is a vital reflex to work as it plays such a significant role in metabolism, growth and development. It is quite common for this gland to go out of balance and when it does the person can be affected both physically and mentally. For example, if the thyroid is underactive (hypothyroidism/myxoedema) symptoms can include oedema, slow heart rate, low body temperature, weight gain and a feeling of constant tiredness and mental sluggishness. If, on the other hand, the thyroid is overactive (hyperthyroidism/thyrotoxicosis), the body's vital functions can speed up resulting in a rapid heartbeat, constant sweating, weight loss and anxiety. Therefore, it is important to maintain the balance of the gland.

The thyroid is sometimes referred to as the third ovary and it is an important reflex to work in cases of menstrual disorders or sub-fertility. Susanne Enzer, a leading maternity reflexologist and practising midwife, wrote: 'In many of the cases of sub-fertility with which I have worked I have often discovered imbalances in the thyroid reflexes – leading in particular to a suspicion of low thyroid function. Some common symptoms of low thyroid function include no ovulation, a short luteal phase … and sometimes an increase in the hormone prolactin – an excess of which has a negative impact on pregnancy.'[7] In addition, in *Better Health with Foot Reflexology*, Dwight Byers says that the thyroid gland 'has also been called the third ovary because of its important effect on those glands in the female'.[8]

The parathyroid glands

The parathyroids are four small, round masses of tissue found on the posterior surfaces of the thyroid gland. They release only one hormone, parathormone (parathyroid hormone/PTH), which works together with calcitonin from the thyroid gland and calcitriol from the kidneys to control blood calcium levels. Parathormone increases blood calcium and magnesium levels, decreases blood phosphate levels and promotes the formation of calcitriol by the kidneys.

Where are the parathyroid reflexes?

The parathyroid reflexes are found with the thyroid reflexes in the necks of the big toes and thumbs.

How do you work the parathyroid reflexes?

The parathyroid reflexes are worked together with the thyroid and neck reflexes through either thumb-walking or thumb-rotating the reflexes.

Why/When do you work the parathyroid reflexes?

The reflexes for the parathyroid glands should be worked to maintain the correct amounts of minerals in the blood and bones and for any problems of bone density, such as osteoporosis. Take note that these minerals are not only essential for the strength and density of bones, but also for all nervous

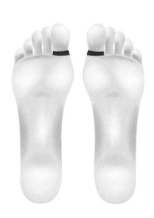

and muscular functions. Thus, the parathyroids should also be worked for disorders of the nerves and muscles such as spasms and tetany. Finally, they are also important reflexes to be worked if a person has kidney stones.

The thymus gland

The thymus gland is located in the thorax, behind the sternum and between the lungs. It is large in infants and reaches its maximum size around puberty. It then begins to decrease with age. The thymus gland plays an important role in the immune system and secretes a number of hormones involved in immunity. One such hormone is thymosin which promotes the growth and maturation of T-Cells. These are a type of lymphocyte (white blood cell) that directly attack antigens and which are vital to immunity. The thymus gland also functions as part of the lymphatic system.

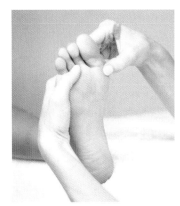

Working the thymus reflex

Where is the thymus reflex?
The reflex for the thymus gland is actually quite difficult to locate. It is on the thoracic spine reflex and is best found by very slowly running your thumb down this reflex. Start at the neck reflex and run your thumb down the thoracic spine until you feel a slight hollowing/concave dip (this is where the proximal phalange joins the first metatarsal or metacarpal). This is the thymus reflex.

How do you work the thymus reflex?
Use your thumb to apply a deep pressure to the thymus reflex.

Why/When do you work the thymus reflex?
The thymus reflex is generally worked in cases of poor immunity and recurrent infections.

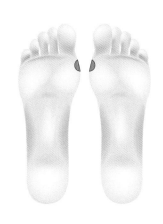

The pancreas (Pancreatic islets/Islets of Langerhans)

The pancreas is an organ found behind and slightly below the stomach and it is described as having a head and body that taper into a tail. It is part of both the endocrine and digestive systems. Only its endocrine functions are discussed here. Scattered in the pancreas are small groups of endocrine tissue called pancreatic islets or islets of Langerhans. They secrete four different hormones which generally help regulate blood glucose levels. Three of these hormones that are important to you are glucagon, insulin and somatostatin. Glucagon raises blood glucose levels by accelerating the breakdown of glycogen into glucose and stimulating the release of glucose into the blood. Insulin lowers blood glucose levels by accelerating the transport of glucose into the cells and converting glucose into glycogen. Somatostatin inhibits the release of both glucagon and insulin and also slows the absorption of nutrients from the gastrointestinal tract.

Where is the pancreas reflex?
In foot reflexology, the pancreas reflex is located on both feet, but mainly the left. The head of the pancreas lies on the right foot, just above the waistline in zone 1. The pancreas then extends across into the left foot where it is also located just above the waistline from zones 1–4. It overlaps with the stomach and kidney reflexes.

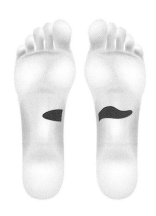

Study tip
Remember that if you wish to work on someone who has diabetes mellitus you must get their doctor's permission first. Turn to page 31 for more information on diabetes mellitus.

In hand reflexology, the pancreas reflex is also located on both hands, but mainly the left. Its head lies on the right hand, just above the waistline in zone 1 and it extends across into the left hand where it is located above the waistline from zones 1–4.

How do you work the pancreas reflex?

The pancreas reflex is best worked with either thumb-walking or thumb-rotations. Use these techniques to work transversely across the reflex in one direction a couple of times before repeating the transverse work in the other direction. The area can also be knuckled.

Why/When do you work the pancreas reflex?

The pancreas reflex should be worked if there are blood sugar imbalances such as diabetes mellitus, hypoglycaemia or hyperglycaemia. In addition, it is an important reflex of the digestive system (this will be discussed shortly).

The adrenal glands

The adrenal glands (also called the suprarenal glands) are found above the kidneys. Although an adrenal gland looks like a single organ, it contains two regions that are structurally and functionally different. The outer adrenal cortex surrounds the inner adrenal medulla. The table on the next page details the hormones secreted by the adrenal gland.

Where are the adrenal reflexes?

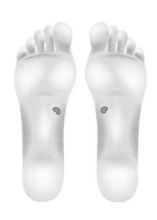

Although anatomically the adrenal glands rest above the kidneys and many foot maps show them seated directly on top of the kidneys, you actually need to feel around for them. The adrenal glands are found in the same way on both feet. Find the kidney reflex on the foot (see page 203) and then move your thumb upwards and medially towards the spine. Located approximately half way between the diaphragm line and waistline in zone one, medial to the flexor hallucis longus tendon, you will find the adrenal reflex. In many people these are sensitive and in stressed people they tend to feel like small, tight balls.

The easiest way to find the adrenal glands on the hands is to draw a line downwards from the webbing between the thumb and index finger towards the waistline. You will find the glands on this line, slightly above the waistline. They are in the centre of the thenar eminence, the area of firm, raised tissue below the thumb and are usually sensitive to pressure.

How do you work the adrenal reflexes?

You can work these reflexes in a number of different ways. For example, you can apply direct pressure to the reflex, hold the reflex, rotate or unwind the reflex or use the pin-pointing technique. Be aware that the adrenal glands are often very sensitive, especially when a person is under stress, so take care not to hurt your client.

Why/When do you work the adrenal reflexes?

You will see from the table on the next page what an important role the adrenal glands have. Their reflexes should be worked for any metabolic disorders, the regulation of fluid balance and blood pressure, sub-fertility and in all stress-related conditions. See page 26 for information on the

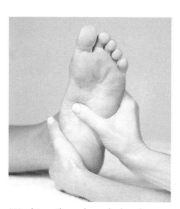

Working the adrenal glands

HORMONES OF THE ADRENAL GLANDS

Adrenal cortex
The adrenal cortex produces steroid hormones that are essential to life and loss of them can lead to potentially fatal dehydration or electrolyte imbalances. These hormones are grouped into mineralcorticoids, glucocorticoids and sex hormones.

HORMONE	TARGET TISSUE	ACTIONS	DISORDERS AND DISEASES
Mineralcorticoids (mainly aldosterone)	Kidneys 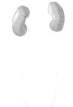	Regulate mineral content of the blood by: Increasing blood levels of sodium and water. Decreasing blood levels of potassium.	**Hyposecretion** of glucocorticoids and aldosterone: Addison's disease **Hypersecretion** of aldosterone: Aldosteronism
Glucocorticoids (mainly cortisol)	All body cells 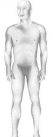	Regulate metabolism. Help body resist long-term stressors. Control effects of inflammation. Depress immune responses.	**Hyposecretion** of glucocorticoids and aldosterone: Addison's disease **Hypersecretion**: Cushing's syndrome
Sex hormones (androgens and oestrogens)	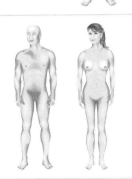	Very small contribution to sex drive and libido.	Presence of feminising hormones in males: Gynaecomastia (enlargement of breasts) **Hypersecretion**: Hirsutism

Adrenal medulla
The adrenal medulla is innervated by neurones of the sympathetic division of the autonomic nervous system and can very quickly release hormones that are collectively referred to as *catecholamines*. These hormones are, to a large extent, responsible for the fight-or-flight response of the body and they help the body cope with stress.

HORMONE	TARGET TISSUE	ACTIONS	DISORDERS AND DISEASES
Adrenaline (epinephrine) and **Noradrenaline** (norepinephrine)	All body cells 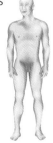	Fight-or-flight response: • Increase blood pressure • Dilate airways to the lungs • Decrease rate of digestion • Increase blood glucose level • Stimulate cellular metabolism.	**Hypersecretion**: Prolonged fight-or-flight response

Study tip
Always work the adrenal glands for any inflammation in the body. This can range from swollen joints to allergies. Note that the suffix -*itis* denotes inflammation. Therefore, work the adrenals for any conditions ending in the letters -*itis*. For example, arthritis, diverticulitis, urethritis, sinusitis and tendonitis.

function of the adrenal glands in the stress response. Also work the adrenal glands for any pain or inflammatory responses, including allergies.

The ovaries and testes

Please turn to the reproductive system discussed on page 206.

> **Reflexions – the chakra system**
> The chakra system is a way of explaining the concept of energy work – it makes sense of phrases such as a lump in the throat or butterflies in the stomach. Chakras are energy centres found along the central axis of a person and their characteristics include emotional, physical and spiritual qualities. These qualities are all one and the same energy which cannot be separated and when this energy is in balance, we have healthy minds, bodies and emotions. As you will see from the chart below, the chakra system is closely aligned to the endocrine system.

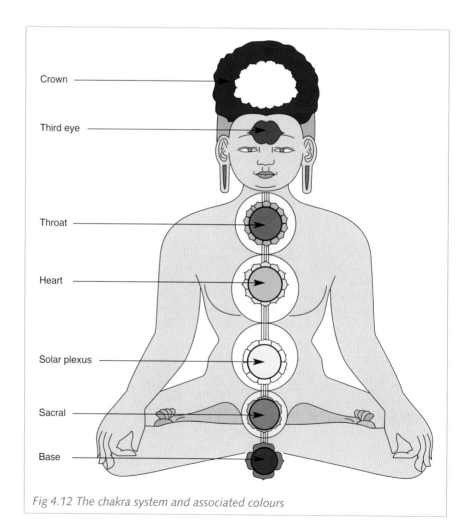

Crown

Third eye

Throat

Heart

Solar plexus

Sacral

Base

Fig 4.12 The chakra system and associated colours

THE CHAKRAS		
CHAKRA	**GLAND**	**ENERGY CONNECTIONS**
Crown	Pineal	Spiritual awareness – perfection, integration, wisdom and purpose, universal consciousness, enlightenment
Third Eye	Pituitary	Connections between emotions and the physical body – inner vision, intuition, insight, perception, imagination, concentration, peace of mind, projection of will
Throat	Thyroid	Communication – creative self expression, inspiration, wisdom, confidence, integrity, truth, freedom, independence
Heart	Thymus	Relationships – unconditional love, harmony, forgiveness, healing, compassion, understanding, personal transformation, warmth, sharing, devotion, selflessness
Solar Plexus/ Stomach	Pancreas	Confidence – personal power, social identity, influence, authority, self-control, energy, will, peace, radiance, joy, inner harmony, vitality, inner strength
Sacral/Splenic	Gonads	Courage – primal feelings, awe, enthusiasm, openness to others, personal creativity
Base	Adrenals	Vitality – survival, power to achieve goals, grounding, material security, stability, stillness, courage

The endocrine system in a nutshell

Main reflexes – Hypothalamus, pituitary, pineal, thyroid, parathyroids, thymus, pancreas, adrenals, gonads (ovaries/testes). The endocrine system works closely with the nervous system to control all the functions of our bodies, including metabolism, growth, development and reproduction. It is, however, quite easily unbalanced through poor habits and lifestyle, especially poor nutrition, stress and lack of sleep so all these areas need to be assessed when working with a client with a hormonal imbalance.

Associated reflexes
- Cardiovascular reflexes, as all hormones are transported by the blood
- Nervous system, as it works so closely with the endocrine system

The Respiratory System

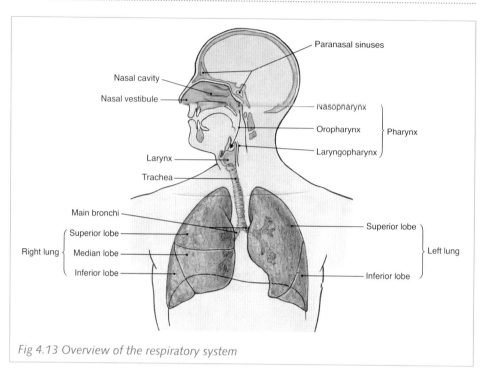

Fig 4.13 Overview of the respiratory system

The main function of the respiratory system is to take in oxygen and eliminate carbon dioxide. This exchange of gases is called respiration and it takes place between the atmosphere, the blood and cells in different phases:

- **Pulmonary ventilation** – the word *pulmo* refers to the lungs and pulmonary ventilation is another term for breathing. Air is inspired or breathed in to the lungs and expired or breathed out of the lungs.
- **External respiration** (pulmonary respiration) – gaseous exchange between the lungs and the blood. In external respiration, the blood gains oxygen and loses carbon dioxide.
- **Internal respiration** (tissue respiration) – gaseous exchange between the blood and tissue cells. In internal respiration the blood loses oxygen and gains carbon dioxide.

Note: Cellular respiration (oxidation) is a metabolic reaction that takes place within a cell. It uses oxygen and glucose and produces energy in the form of adenosine triphosphate. A by-product of cellular respiration is carbon dioxide.

The respiratory system also functions in olfaction, which is the sense of smell. One of its structures, the nose, houses the olfactory receptors and the sense of smell is discussed in more detail on page 219. Finally, the respiratory system functions in sound production. Vibrating air particles produce sound. As we breathe out, air passes through the larynx (voice box) where there are specialised membranes called vocal cords. The air causes these to vibrate and produce sounds which are converted into words by the muscles of the pharynx, face, tongue and lips. The pharynx, mouth, nasal cavity and paranasal sinuses also act as resonating chambers for sound.

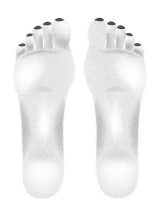

The sinuses

The sinuses, or paranasal sinuses, are air-filled spaces located within the cranial and facial bones. They are found near the nasal cavity and serve as resonating chambers for sound and are lined with a mucous membrane. They have tiny openings into the nasal cavity called ostia.

There are three pairs of paranasal sinuses named after the bones in which they are located – the frontal, maxillary and sphenoid sinuses. There are also the ethmoid sinuses which consist of many spaces inside the ethmoid bone.

Where are the sinus reflexes?
The reflexes for the sinuses are the very tips of all the toes and fingers.

How do you work the sinus reflexes?
The sinus reflexes can either be knuckled or you can apply deep pressure to them with either a thumb or finger tip. Remember to support the toes or fingers while working these reflexes.

Why/When do you work the sinus reflexes?
Work the sinus reflexes if your client suffers with sinusitis, headaches, hay-fever or colds and flu.

The nose

The nose is a framework of bone and hyaline cartilage that is covered by skin and lined internally with a mucous membrane. Air enters the respiratory system through the nose, whose functions include inhaling, filtering, warming and moistening air, receiving olfactory stimuli and acting as a resonating chamber for sound.

Where is the nose reflex?
The reflex for the nose is found with the reflex for the mouth. They are located on the dorsal aspect of the big toe or thumb, below the nail.

How do you work the nose reflex?
It is easiest to finger-walk or finger-rotate across the nose/mouth reflex in a transverse direction. Otherwise simply apply deep, maintained pressure with a fingertip. Remember to support the plantar aspect of the big toe or thumb when you work the nose/mouth reflex.

Why/When do you work the nose reflex?
Work the nose/mouth reflexes for any problems related to these areas.

The throat (pharynx)

The throat/pharynx is a funnel-shaped tube whose walls are made up of skeletal muscles lined by mucous membranes and cilia. The mucous traps dust particles and the cilia move the mucous downwards. The throat acts as a passageway for air, food and drink as well as a resonating chamber for sound and houses the tonsils which function in immunity.

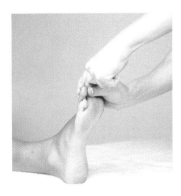

Knuckling the sinuses

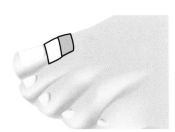

The nose/mouth reflex

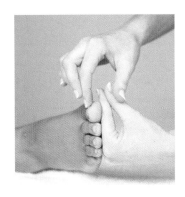

Finger-walking the nose/mouth reflex

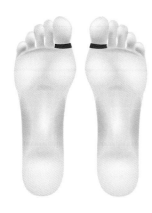

Where is the throat reflex?

The reflex for the throat is located in the neck of the big toe and thumb.

How do you work the throat reflex?

The throat reflex can be worked by either thumb-walking or thumb-rotating the reflex in a transverse direction.

Why/When do you work the throat reflex?

The throat reflex should be worked for any throat problems such as sore throats, laryngitis, tonsillitis and Eustachian tube problems.

The larynx (voicebox)

The larynx is a short passageway between the pharynx and the trachea and it plays two important roles in the respiratory system. It routes air and food into their correct channels and it produces sound.

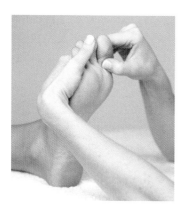

Thumb-walking the throat

Where is the larynx reflex?

The reflex for the larynx is also in the neck of the big toe or thumb. In addition, a helper reflex for the larynx can be found on the foot in the webbing between the big toe and the second toe.

How do you work the larynx reflex?

The larynx reflex is worked when the neck reflex is either thumb-walked or thumb-rotated. The helper reflex can be worked by pinching the webbing between toes 1 and 2 between your thumb and index finger.

Why/When do you work the larynx reflex?

The larynx reflex should be worked if there are any disorders of the voicebox. For example, hoarseness, loss of voice or laryngitis.

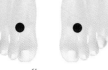

The larynx reflex

> *'(An) incident was reported in a newspaper on April 29, 1934, under the headline 'Mystery of Zone Therapy Explained.' The article tells of a dinner party at which one of the guests was Fitzgerald, and another a well-known concert singer who had announced that the upper register tones of her voice had gone flat. Throat specialists had been unable to discover the cause of this affliction. Dr Fitzgerald asked to examine the fingers and toes of the singer. He told her that the cause of the loss of her upper tones was a callus on her right big toe. After applying pressure to the corresponding part in the same zone for a few minutes, the patient remarked that the pain in her toe had disappeared. Then, to quote from the article: 'the doctor asked her to try the tone of the upper register. Miraculously, it would seem to us, the singer reached two tones higher than she had ever done before.'[9] (Dougans)*

The trachea (windpipe) and the bronchi

The trachea is a long tubular passageway which transports air from the throat into the bronchi. The trachea lies in front of the oesophagus and is composed of incomplete C-shaped rings of hyaline cartilage. The open parts of the C-shape are held together with transverse smooth muscle fibres and elastic connective tissue and lie against the oesophagus, allowing for expansion of the oesophagus during swallowing. The closed cartilage parts of the C-shape are solid so that they can support the trachea and keep it open despite changes in breathing. The trachea is lined with mucous membranes and cilia that move any dust particles still in the respiratory system upwards away from the lungs to the throat where they can be swallowed or spat out.

Having travelled down the trachea, air flows into branch-like passageways called bronchi (singular = bronchus). These bronchi repeatedly divide inside the lungs into smaller and smaller branches that finally carry the air into the alveoli. Their division is similar to the branching of a tree from a large central trunk (trachea) into branches (bronchi), twigs (bronchioles) and finally leaves (alveoli). This continual dividing of the passageways means that air can be transported to literally millions of alveoli where gaseous exchange can take place.

Where is the trachea/bronchi reflex?

The reflex for the trachea is the same as the reflex for the bronchi. It is found on the medial edge of the balls of the feet, or the edge of the hand, running between the throat and lung reflexes. It is often not shown on foot or hand maps because it is such a small reflex. Instead, a helper reflex is commonly found on foot maps. This is located running vertically from the shoulder line to the waistline between the big toe and the second toe (zones 1 and 2). This reflex is often callused or hardened in people who have respiratory problems and also those who suffer with recurrent sore throats.

How do you work the trachea/bronchi reflex?

The helper reflex is usually worked by either thumb-walking or thumb-rotating the reflex in a longitudinal/vertical direction.

Why/When do you work the trachea/bronchi reflex?

Work the trachea/bronchi reflex for any problems with this area, including asthma and bronchitis.

> **Study tip**
>
> A quick reminder of the ways the respiratory system defends itself from foreign particles:
>
> - Coarse hairs inside the nostrils filter out large dust particles.
> - A mucous membrane lines the respiratory passages and traps foreign particles.
> - Cilia line the respiratory passages and move dust-laden mucous towards the pharynx where it can be swallowed or spat out.
> - Particles that have not been removed by the mucous and cilia are engulfed by scavenger cells, or macrophages, in the alveoli.

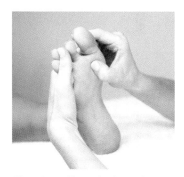

Thumb-walking the bronchi helper

The lungs

The lungs are cone-shaped organs that occupy most of the thoracic cavity. They extend from the diaphragm to slightly above the clavicles and are surrounded and protected by the ribs. The right lung is shorter, thicker and broader than the left. This is because the diaphragm is higher on the right

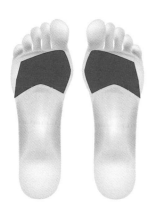

side to accommodate the liver beneath it. The lungs are separated from one another by the heart and the mediastinum, which is a mass of tissue extending from the sternum to the vertebral column, and they are covered with and protected by the pleural membrane.

Once air has travelled through the conducting passageways of the respiratory system, it arrives at the air sacs, or alveoli, inside the lungs. These are cup-shaped pouches where the exchange of gases occurs. There are approximately 300 million alveoli in the lungs, which provide a huge surface area for gaseous exchange. The walls of the alveoli are extremely thin and together with the walls of the pulmonary capillaries they form the respiratory membrane. This is the site of gaseous exchange between the lungs and the blood. It is an extremely thin membrane so that the gases can diffuse rapidly across it.

Where are the lung reflexes?

In foot reflexology, the reflexes for the lungs lie in the ball of the foot, between the shoulder line and diaphragm line, zones 1–4. They can be worked on both the dorsal and plantar surfaces of the foot.

In hand reflexology the lung reflexes are more difficult to locate as the reflex for the thoracic region is often quite small. However, they are found between the shoulder line and diaphragm line, zones 1–4, on both hands.

How do you work the lung reflexes?

Because the lung reflexes are so large and easy to access on the feet, they can be worked in a number of different ways:

- **Relaxation techniques** – There are many relaxation techniques that help relieve muscular tension in the thoracic area, encourage deeper breathing, increase circulation and help relieve stress. Focus on opening up the thoracic area by encouraging movement in the ball of the foot and between the metatarsals. Try techniques such as the shoulder sandwich, metatarsal manipulation and intercostals sliding. Working the solar plexus and the diaphragm is also extremely beneficial to the lungs.
- **Breathing techniques** – A technique that encourages deep breathing is a reversal of the metatarsal manipulation/chest relaxation technique you learned on page 83. Ask your client to take a deep breath then, as they breathe out, apply pressure to the lung reflexes with a closed fist. Be aware that this technique is different to the usual relaxation techniques in which you apply pressure with the in-breath. Here you are applying pressure with the out-breath and you are encouraging your client to empty their lungs fully and release their internalised tension.
- **Pressure techniques** – The lung reflexes can be worked deeply through knuckling, using thumb-walking or thumb-rotations on the plantar aspect of the foot or finger-walking or finger-rotations on the dorsal aspect. The reflexes can be worked in either transverse or longitudinal directions.

In hand reflexology, the lungs are best worked through relaxation techniques such as opening up the hand and metacarpal manipulation. These reflexes can also be worked with pressure techniques such as thumb or finger walking or rotations.

Practical tip

A deep vertical line on the lung reflex often indicates lung disorders such as asthma.

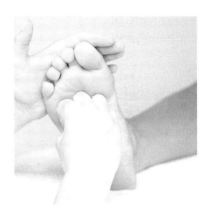

Knuckling the lungs

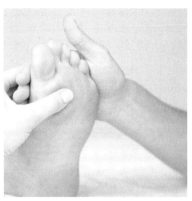

Transverse thumb-walking on the lungs

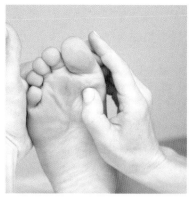

Longitudinal thumb-walking on the lungs

Why/When do you work the lung reflexes?

Work the lung reflexes if there are any problems associated with the area, such as chest infections or emphysema. In addition, the lungs should always be worked if a person is suffering from depression or any stress-related condition. Deep breathing encourages relaxation on all levels and enables a person to let go of tension and anxiety. It also provides more oxygen which is vital to the body and without which healing cannot take place.

Working the lung reflexes will also help with fatigue and exhaustion as these conditions are often accompanied by shallow breathing. If your client does suffer with lung conditions, stress or fatigue be sure to also work the shoulder, neck and thoracic spine reflexes as tension in these areas and poor posture can make deep breathing difficult.

Practical tip

Remember that one of the main aims of working on the lung reflexes is to encourage deep breathing and improve the quality of your client's breath. To do this, ensure you work with their breathing when working on the lung reflexes. Ask your client to breathe deeply and focus on their own breathing.

> **Reflexions**
> Metaphysically the lungs are associated with sadness, grief and the inability to let go and I have found veruccas and calluses to be common on the chest reflexes of people who have suffered a great sadness in their lives.

The diaphragm

The diaphragm is a large muscle that forms the floor of the thoracic cavity. It functions in inhalation and produces approximately 60% of one's breathing capacity. In its relaxed state, the diaphragm is dome shaped. However, when it contracts it flattens and this increases the vertical dimension of the thoracic cavity. The dimensions of the thoracic cavity are further increased by the contraction of the external intercostal muscles which elevate the ribs. As the dimensions of the thoracic cavity increase, the pressure inside the lungs actually decreases. When this pressure becomes less than the atmospheric pressure, a partial vacuum is created inside the lungs and this vacuum pulls air into the lungs. This is the process of inhalation/inspiration.

Normal exhalation (expiration) is a passive process that does not involve any muscular contraction. After being stretched during inspiration, the muscles of the lungs and chest contract to their natural state and the volume

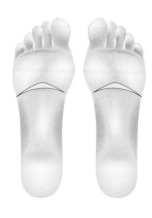

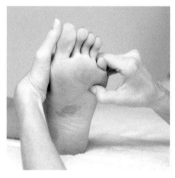

Working the diaphragm. Note the birthmark on this client's digestive reflexes. She is a young person who has no digestive problems herself, but both her mother and grandmother do.

Practical tip

The diaphragm is a key reflex to work in the last trimester of pregnancy if a woman is suffering from fatigue, constipation or fluid retention.

of the lungs decreases. This increases the pressure within the lungs and once this pressure is greater than the atmospheric pressure, the air will move out of the lungs to the area of lowest pressure.

Where is the diaphragm reflex?

The reflex for the diaphragm is the diaphragm line itself.

How do you work the diaphragm reflex?

The diaphragm reflex can be thumb-walked or thumb-rotated in a transverse direction.

Why/When do you work the diaphragm reflex?

The diaphragm reflex should be worked for all respiratory conditions. In addition, it is a vital reflex to work for stress or stress-related conditions as it encourages deep breathing and helps to slow a person down.

The diaphragm also plays a fundamental role in both the digestive and lymphatic systems. The movement of the diaphragm helps encourage peristalsis, a wave-like motion that pushes the contents of the gastrointestinal tract forward. When the diaphragm does not move effectively, constipation often results. Similarly, the movement of the diaphragm increases and decreases the dimensions of the thoracic cavity. This causes pressure changes in the thoracic cavity which help move lymph through the lymphatic vessels. Without the movement of the diaphragm lymph tends to collect and stagnate, usually in the peripheries of the body (hands and feet). It is important, therefore, to work the diaphragm reflex in cases of constipation or poor lymphatic drainage and deep breathing should also be encouraged.

The Respiratory System in a Nutshell

Main reflexes – sinuses, nose/mouth, throat/pharynx, larynx, trachea/bronchi, lungs, diaphragm. The respiratory system is intricately linked to the cardiovascular system and together they bring oxygen and nutrients to every cell in the body and remove waste. In addition, the respiratory system functions in sound production and the sense of smell.

This system is easily unbalanced by environmental pollution, smoking, mucous-producing foods such as dairy and wheat, a lack of exercise, stress and emotional turmoil. Inge Dougans said about the lungs, 'The lungs are called the 'tender' organ because they are the most easily influenced by environmental factors'.[10]

Associated reflexes
- Cervical nerve plexus – the phrenic nerve which emerges from this plexus innervates the diaphragm
- Lymphatics of the upper body, especially if there is an infection, to stimulate the immune system and help the body eliminate waste
- Adrenals for any inflammation of the airways (e.g. in bronchitis)
- Ileocaecal valve if there is excess mucous. **Note:** if your client has a respiratory condition that involves excess mucous, such as sinusitis, coughs, runny noses, etc it is best that they limit their intake of mucous-producing foods such as dairy and wheat products

- Liver and spleen, especially if there is an infection, to stimulate the immune system and help the body eliminate waste
- Organs of elimination (liver, kidneys, large intestine, lymphatic system and skin) to support the eliminatory function of the lungs
- Large intestine – in TCM the lungs and large intestine are partnered (you will learn more about this on page 240) and they directly affect one another so if your client suffers from a lung condition be sure to work the large intestine and vice versa
- Solar plexus to help relax your client and encourage them to deal with any emotional issues and breathe deeply
- Neck, shoulders and thoracic spine to relax any muscular tension in this area that may be limiting your client's ability to breathe deeply.

The Cardiovascular System

The cardiovascular system is composed of the heart, blood and blood vessels and it is responsible for transporting blood to every cell in the body. In reflexology there is only one reflex you need to learn for the cardiovascular system – the heart. However, certain relaxation techniques are also beneficial to the cardiovascular system as a whole.

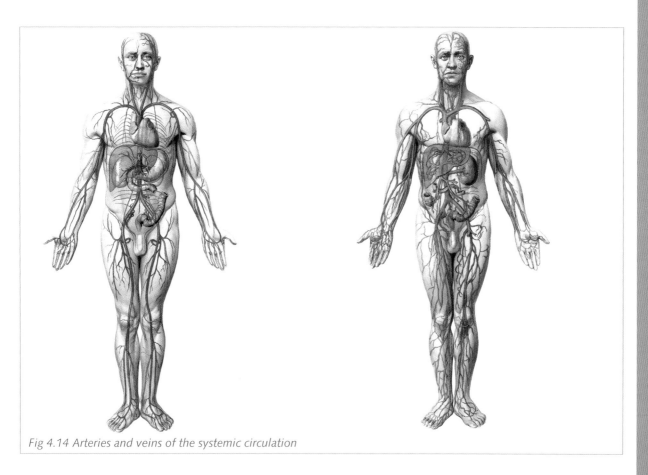

Fig 4.14 Arteries and veins of the systemic circulation

Blood

Blood is a liquid connective tissue that is slightly sticky, heavier, thicker and more viscous than water. It is a vital substance that transports oxygen from the lungs to cells, carbon dioxide from cells to the lungs, nutrients from the gastrointestinal tract to cells, heat and waste products away from cells, and hormones from glands to cells. Blood also regulates the pH of the body, its temperature, and the water content of cells. It also protects cells against foreign microbes and toxins. Finally, blood has the ability to clot and so protect the body against excessive blood loss.

Blood plasma is a watery, straw-coloured liquid that comprises 55% of blood. This liquid contains water and dissolved substances such as proteins, electrolytes, nutrients, enzymes, hormones, gases and wastes. The other 45% of blood is composed of cells and cell fragments. Together these are referred to as formed elements. Red blood cells make up 99% of formed elements and only 1% are white blood cells and platelets.

Red blood cells, or erythrocytes, are produced in the red bone marrow of long bones and are biconcave in shape, have no nucleus and few organelles. This ensures there is maximum space within the cells for oxygen transportation. Oxygen is carried by red pigment protein molecules called haemoglobin and each red blood cell contains approximately 280 million haemoglobin molecules. Red blood cells do not have a long life span and are broken down in the spleen and liver where their breakdown products are then recycled.

White blood cells, or leucocytes, function primarily in protecting the body against foreign microbes and in immune responses. There are many different types of white blood cells, including lymphocytes, phagocytes, macrophages, thrombocytes and T-cells.

Study tip

As a reflexologist it is important that you are aware of the connection of the cardiovascular system to the liver and spleen.

The liver:
- Maintains normal blood glucose levels
- Synthesises all the major plasma proteins
- Detoxifies the blood
- Destroys worn-out red blood cells, white blood cells and some bacteria through a process known as phagocytosis
- Stores iron from broken down cells
- Stores extra blood that is not usually in circulation.

The spleen:
- Acts as a reservoir of blood
- Filters and cleans blood
- Destroys worn-out red blood cells
- Stores platelets
- Produces lymphocytes – white blood cells that function in immunity.

Blood vessels

Blood is pumped by the heart into vessels that then transport it throughout the body. These vessels form a closed system of tubes that is made up of:

- **Arteries and arterioles** – Arteries are thick, strong vessels that carry blood away from the heart towards the tissues. They consist of a lumen, which is a hollow centre through which the blood flows, surrounded by a triple-layered wall. Blood from arteries flows into smaller vessels called arterioles and then finally into capillaries.
- **Capillaries** – Capillaries are tiny vessels that form branching networks throughout tissues and they are supplied by arterioles and drained by venules. The walls of capillaries are only one cell thick and this allows for the exchange of gases, nutrients and wastes between the blood and tissues.
- **Veins and venules** – Blood from several capillaries drains into small vessels called venules. These then feed veins which carry blood away from the tissues towards the heart. Veins have thinner walls than arteries and are found closer to the surface of the body. They also contain valves which prevent the backflow of blood.

Blood vessels are organised into routes that transport blood throughout the body. The word systemic refers to the body as a whole and systemic circulation is the route blood follows from the heart to the tissues and organs of the body and back to the heart.

Blood pressure

The force exerted by blood on the walls of a blood vessel is referred to as blood pressure. It is the force that keeps blood circulating and it is generated by the contractions of the left ventricle. Blood pressure is measured in millimeters of mercury (mm Hg) and is measured near the large systemic arteries. In a normal, young adult blood pressure is 120/80 mm Hg while at rest. When measuring blood pressure it is important to remember that it can vary slightly according to:

- **Time of day** – blood pressure drops during night-time sleep.
- **Posture** – blood pressure is lower when lying down.
- **Gender** – men usually have a slightly lower blood pressure than women.
- **Age** – blood pressure tends to increase with age.

The heart

Structure of the heart

The heart is a hollow, muscular organ located in the mediastinum (the partition between the lungs) in the thoracic cavity. It is approximately the same size as a person's fist and two-thirds of it lies to the left of the median line. The heart is divided into two halves:

- The right side of the heart receives deoxygenated blood from the body and pumps it to the lungs for oxygenation.
- The left side of the heart receives oxygenated blood from the lungs and pumps it to the rest of the body.

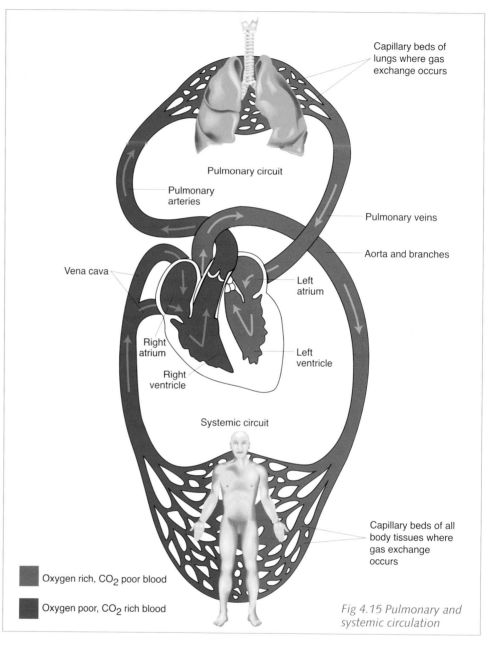

Capillary beds of lungs where gas exchange occurs

Pulmonary circuit

Pulmonary arteries

Pulmonary veins

Aorta and branches

Vena cava

Left atrium

Right atrium

Left ventricle

Right ventricle

Systemic circuit

Capillary beds of all body tissues where gas exchange occurs

Oxygen rich, CO_2 poor blood

Oxygen poor, CO_2 rich blood

Fig 4.15 Pulmonary and systemic circulation

Each of these halves both receives and delivers blood and so each has a receiving chamber called an atrium and a delivering chamber called a ventricle. Separating these chambers are valves. These valves are specially designed to prevent blood from flowing backwards.

The heart has an extremely strong wall which is composed of three layers – the outer epicardium which is a thin membrane that surrounds the heart, the middle myocardium which is composed of cardiac muscle tissue and is the layer that actually contracts to pump blood, and the inner endocardium which is the thin, smooth lining of the inside of the heart. In addition, the heart is surrounded and protected by a triple-layered sac called the pericardium.

Pulmonary, systemic and coronary circulation

The heart is basically a double-pump which pumps blood into two different circulations:

- **Pulmonary circulation** – The right side of the heart receives deoxygenated blood from the body and pumps it to the lungs where it is oxygenated. This is referred to as pulmonary circulation.
- **Systemic circulation** – The left side of the heart receives oxygenated blood from the lungs and pumps it to the rest of the body. This is referred to as systemic circulation.

The heart is composed mainly of muscle and, like all muscles, it needs a constant supply of oxygen and nutrients and the removal of its waste products in order to function. Thus, it also needs its own blood supply and this supply is called the coronary circulation (cardiac circulation).

Regulation of the heart rate

Cardiac muscle cells are unique in that they contract independently of nervous stimulation and thus have what is called a myogenic rhythm. However, although the cells contract regularly and continuously, the rhythm of their contraction needs to be controlled to ensure the heart functions as a co-ordinated whole. This rhythm is controlled by a 'pacemaker' which consists of specialised cells called autorhythmic cells. The autonomic nervous system and certain hormones also help control the rate at which the heart beats.

The number of times the heart beats in one minute is called the heart rate and in the average resting male it is approximately 70 beats per minute while in the average resting female it is slightly higher, approximately 75 beats per minute. Although the heart's pacemaker establishes the fundamental rhythm of the heart beat, it can be modified by the nervous and endocrine systems:

- **Autonomic regulation of the heart rate** – In the medulla oblongata of the brain is the cardiovascular centre which receives information from sensory receptors such as proprioceptors which monitor the positions of limbs and muscles, chemoreceptors which monitor chemical changes in the blood, and baroreceptors which monitor blood pressure changes in the arteries and veins. Information from higher brain centres such as the cerebral cortex and limbic system also send signals to the cardiovascular system. Once all this information has been interpreted the autonomic nervous system responds either sympathetically or parasympathetically to adjust the heart beat:
  - **Sympathetic stimulation** – Cardiac accelerator nerves stimulate the release of noradrenaline which, acting as a neurotransmitter, increases the heart rate.
  - **Parasympathetic stimulation** – Cranial nerve X, the vagus nerve, stimulates the release of the neurotransmitter acetylcholine which decreases the heart rate.
- **Chemical regulation of the heart rate** – Different chemicals can also affect the heart rate:
  - Hormones such as adrenaline and noradrenaline, released by the adrenal medulla, increase the heart rate. Their release is stimulated by

Study tip
Some cardiovascular conditions are contraindications to reflexology. Please double-check these contraindications on page 28.

exercise, stress and excitement. Thyroid hormones also increase the heart rate.

- Ions are electrically charged molecules that play an integral role in the production of impulses in both nerve and muscle fibres. If there is an imbalance in their concentrations the heart rate will be affected.
- Certain drugs and dissolved gases can also alter the heart rate.

Reflexions
Statistics show that your lifestyle influences your risk of suffering from heart disease and simple changes to your lifestyle can often reduce your chances of developing heart disease. Factors that increase your chance of suffering from a disease are called risk factors and the following are major risk factors in heart disease:

- Obesity
- Lack of regular exercise
- High blood cholesterol level
- High blood pressure
- Cigarette smoking
- Diabetes mellitus
- Family history of heart disease at an early age
- Gender – men are more at risk of heart disease than women. However, after the age of 70 years the risk is equal in both genders.

Where is the heart reflex?

In foot reflexology, the heart reflex is found on the balls of both feet, between the shoulder line and the diaphragm line. On the right foot the heart reflex is in zone 1 only and on the left foot it extends across to zone 3.

In hand reflexology, the heart reflex is located in the same way as it is on the feet. It is found between the shoulder and diaphragm lines in zone 1 on the right hand and zones 1–3 on the left hand.

How do you work the heart reflex?

The heart reflex is usually worked when you work the lung reflexes and you use the same techniques – thumb-walking or rotating the plantar aspect of the foot or hand and finger-walking or rotating the dorsal aspect. In addition, the following foot relaxation techniques help improve circulation – effleurage, side-to-side, foot-squeezing, lower leg massage, hacking and pummelling. Fast, vigorous rubbing of the entire foot also improves circulation and is beneficial to the heart. Once you have rubbed the foot and warmed it up, hold it in both of your hands for approximately 15 seconds to allow the heat to disperse slowly.

Why/When do you work the heart reflex?

The heart reflex is worked for cardiovascular conditions such as hypertension. Working it is also beneficial to circulatory disorders such as oedema and it is an important associated reflex for many other systems of the body including the endocrine, respiratory, digestive and musculo-skeletal systems.

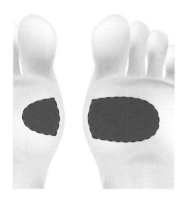

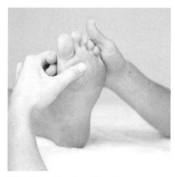

Working the heart reflex

The cardiovascular system in a nutshell

Main reflexes – heart. Every cell depends on the efficient functioning of the cardiovascular system to bring it nutrients and oxygen and remove its waste. The regulation of body temperature and the transportation of all hormones are also dependent on this system so it is vital that it functions well. The cardiovascular system is easily affected by stress, poor diet and a lack of exercise and these factors will need to be assessed if your client suffers from a cardiovascular condition. You will often need to get a doctor's permission when dealing with disorders of this system.

Associated reflexes
- Cranial nerves – cranial nerve X, the vagus nerve, innervates the heart
- Cervical and thoracic vertebrae to relieve musculo-skeletal tension in the thoracic area
- Shoulder reflexes – especially the left shoulder as heart conditions often cause discomfort in this area
- Solar plexus for relaxation
- Adrenals for stress relief
- Diaphragm to encourage the return of venous blood
- Kidneys and adrenals to help control blood pressure
- Respiratory, nervous, lymphatic and musculo-skeletal systems.

The Lymphatic and Immune System

The lymphatic system is a type of circulatory system. Every cell in the body is bathed in a dilute saline solution called interstitial fluid. Blood plasma and its components, such as protein particles, fat molecules and debris, leak out of blood vessels and into the interstitial fluid. Not all of this fluid is reabsorbed back into the bloodstream, instead it is drained by the lymphatic system. The functions of the lymphatic system are to:

- Drain excess interstitial fluid and return it to the bloodstream.
- Transport dietary fats and fat-soluble vitamins (A, D, E and K) from the small intestine into the bloodstream.
- Protect the body against invasion through the immune response.

The lymphatic system consists of:

- **Lymph** – This is a clear, straw-coloured fluid derived from interstitial fluid. It is similar in composition to blood plasma and contains protein molecules, lipid molecules, foreign particles, cell debris and lymphocytes. Lymph is only found in lymphatic vessels.
- **Lymphatic capillaries** – These are tiny, closed-ended vessels similar to blood capillaries that transport lymph into lymphatic vessels. They have a larger diameter than blood capillaries and a unique structure that permits fluid to flow into them but not out of them. Lymphatic capillaries are found throughout the body except in avascular tissue, the central nervous system, splenic pulp and bone marrow.
- **Lymphatic vessels and trunks** – Lymphatic vessels carry lymph from the capillaries through a number of lymphatic nodes into large vessels called

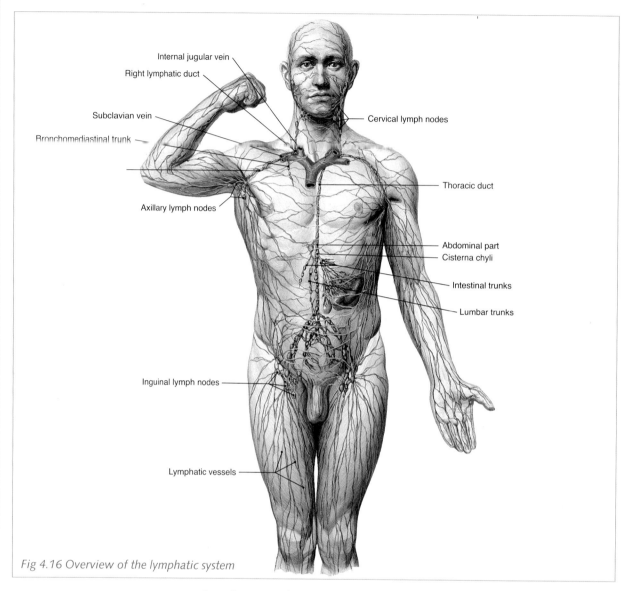

Fig 4.16 Overview of the lymphatic system

lymphatic trunks. These trunks are named after the areas they serve, such as the intestinal trunk.

- **Lymphatic ducts** – Lymphatic trunks carry lymph into two main channels: the thoracic duct (left lymphatic duct) and the right lymphatic duct. These eventually empty their contents into the left and right subclavian veins respectively.
- **Lymphatic nodes, lymphatic organs and lymphatic nodules (the tonsils, ileocaecal valve and appendix)** – all of these are discussed on the following pages.

Reflexions

Unlike blood, which is pumped around the body by the heart, lymph has no pump to move it through its vessels and it can become stagnant, resulting in fluid retention. However, certain mechanisms combine to help lymph move through its vessels. These are:

- The contraction of the smooth muscles in the walls of the vessels
- The contraction of skeletal muscles
- Pressure changes in the thoracic cavity caused by breathing
- One-way valves which prevent the backflow of lymph in the vessels.

If you have a client suffering with a disorder of the lymphatic system try to encourage them to exercise and breathe deeply. This will help move lymph.

Immunity

Our bodies are constantly at war, fighting off pathogens trying to invade them. Bacterial attack, fungal attack, viral attack, chemical attack... and so on. The body has two ways of defending itself against these invaders:

- **Non-specific resistance to disease** – The body has a number of defence mechanisms that are in place to firstly ward off invading microbes and secondly help the body deal with any microbes that manage to enter the system. These mechanisms include mechanical and chemical barriers, natural killer cells and phagocytes, inflammation and fever.
- **Immune response or immunity** – The body employs specialised lymphocytes that recognise and combat specific pathogens. Immunity involves a very specific and focused recognition and response to foreign molecules and it involves what is known as immunological memory or acquired immunity. This is the body's ability to remember and recognise antigens that have triggered an immune response.

Reflexions

The role of the immune system is to attack foreign substances that have entered the body. Occasionally, however, the body attacks its own tissues. When this occurs a person is said to have an autoimmune disorder. Autoimmune disorders include rheumatoid arthritis, pernicious anaemia, Addison's disease, Graves' disease, insulin-dependent (Type I) diabetes mellitus, myasthenia gravis, multiple sclerosis and systemic lupus erythematosus. For more information on these diseases, please look them up in Chapter 6, Diseases and Disorders.

Study tip

Here is a reminder of some important vocabulary:

- **Antibody** – a specialised protein that is synthesised to destroy a specific antigen.
- **Antigen** – any substance that the body recognises as foreign.
- **Lymphocyte** – a type of white blood cell involved in immunity. B cells and T cells are types of lymphocytes.
- **Macrophage** – a scavenger cell that engulfs and destroys microbes.
- **Microbe** (micro-organism) – an organism that is too small to be seen by the naked eye. Microbes include bacteria, viruses, protozoa and some fungi.
- **Pathogen** – a disease-causing micro-organism.
- **Phagocyte** – a cell that is able to engulf and digest microbes. Phagocytes include macrophages and some types of white blood cell.

Study tip

A fever is an abnormally high temperature and it is the body's way of dealing with infection as an elevated body temperature increases the body's defence mechanisms. Normal body temperature is between 36–37°C (96.8–98.6°F) and a temperature over 37.8°C (100°F) is generally regarded as a fever. Fevers are a symptom of an illness, most often an infection, and are contra-indicated to reflexology.

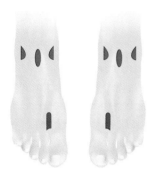

Lymphatic nodes (Glands)

As lymph travels through its vessels towards the lymphatic ducts, it passes through a number of nodes, or glands, before it is returned to the bloodstream. The function of these nodes is to filter the lymph and remove or destroy any potentially harmful substances before it is returned to the blood. The nodes also produce lymphocytes that function in the immune response.

Where are the lymphatic node reflexes?

Although there are many lymphatic nodes in the body, we only work two of them in reflexology – the lymphatics of the upper body and the lymphatics of the lower body and groin (often called the inguinals):

- **Lymphatics of the upper body** – The lymphatic reflexes for the upper body (including the chest, breast, head and neck regions) are found in the webbing between all the toes and fingers in zones 1–5. The webbing between toes 1 and 2 represent where the lymphatic ducts empty their contents into the bloodstream at the subclavian veins.
- **Lymphatics of the lower body and groin (inguinals)** – The lymphatic reflexes for the lower body (including the legs and groin) are found on the dorsal aspects of both feet and hands and are in the same place as the Fallopian tube/vas deferens reflexes. On the feet they are a band running from the ovaries/testes reflex, which is a depression midway between the lateral malleolus and the heel area, across the top of the ankle to the uterus/prostate reflex, a depression midway between the medial malleolus and the heel area.

On this band are two points which are important lymphatic reflexes. They are located on the band in front of each malleolus and can be felt as small depressions into which your fingers slip easily. They can be quite tender on some clients. On the hands they are a narrow band running from the ovaries/testes reflex beneath the the wrist to the uterus/prostate reflex.

How do you work the lymphatic node reflexes?

Lymphatics of the upper body – To work the lymphatics of the upper body, squeeze the webbing of the toes or fingers between your thumb and index finger. Use small, repetitive, squeezing movements that slowly move up and down 'milking' the webbing between the toes or fingers.

Lymphatics of the lower body and groin – Work this reflex by finger-walking or rotating the band from the lateral side to the medial side. Repeat this action a number of times. These reflexes can also be worked with the following techniques on the feet:

- **Relaxation techniques** – If you are working your client's right foot, place the thumb of your left hand on your client's ovary/testes reflex and your index finger on their uterus/prostate reflex. With your hand in this position, the webbing between your thumb and index finger should be pressed firmly along the lymphatic reflex band. Now, use your right hand to grip the ball of the foot and rotate the entire foot in both directions. You can also stretch the ankle back and forth. What is important here is that you maintain pressure over the lymphatic reflexes whilst mobilising the foot.

- **Pressure techniques** – Using the middle finger of each of your hands, apply pressure to the points located on the lymphatic band that lie under the malleoli and apply an on-off pressure so that you are 'pumping' these reflexes. Once you have pumped them a number of times, finger-walk the band from the lateral side to the medial side a few times.

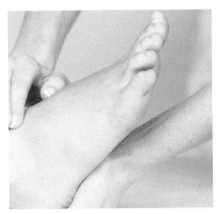

Finger-walking the lymphatic band of the lower body and groin

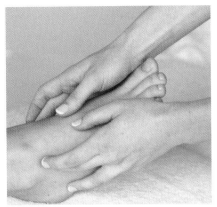

Pumping the lymphatics of the lower body and groin

Why/When do you work the lymphatic node reflexes?

Lymphatic nodes are areas in the body that filter and destroy harmful substances and they can become congested or inflamed, especially when a person is not well. It is therefore important to work these reflexes in any conditions associated with poor lymphatic drainage such as water retention or oedema, poor immunity such as repeated infections, lethargy and exhaustion.

The thymus gland

The thymus gland also forms part of the endocrine system and is discussed in detail on page 167.

The spleen

The spleen is the largest single mass of lymphatic tissue in the body. It is located in the abdomen, behind and to the left of the stomach. Although it is an organ of the lymphatic system, it is important to remember that the spleen does not filter lymph. Instead, it filters and stores blood. Functions of the spleen include filtering and cleaning blood, destroying worn-out red blood cells, storing platelets and blood and producing lymphocytes.

Where is the spleen reflex?

The reflex for the spleen is found on the left foot and hand only. It lies below the diaphragm line in zones 4–5 of the left foot and hand and it is overlapped by the lateral edge of the stomach and the tail of the pancreas.

How do you work the spleen reflex?

The spleen reflex can be worked by thumb-walking, thumb-rotations or by knuckling.

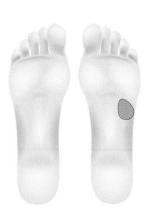

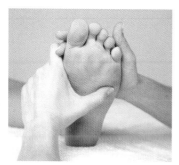

Working the spleen

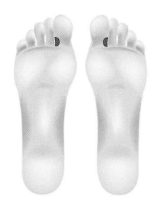

Why/When do you work the spleen reflex?

The spleen should always be worked in cases of poor immunity or infection. In addition, it is an important reflex to work if a person is anaemic because of the role it plays in filtering, cleaning and storing blood.

The tonsils

Lymphatic nodules, or mucosa-associated lymphoid tissue (MALT), are concentrations of lymphatic tissue that are strategically positioned to help protect the body from pathogens that have been inhaled, digested or have entered the body via external openings. They are scattered throughout the mucous membranes that line systems exposed to the external environment.

The tonsils are lymphatic nodules in the back of the mouth. They help protect the body against pathogens that may have been inhaled or digested.

Where are the tonsil reflexes?

The reflexes for the tonsils are found on the lateral edge of the neck of the big toe or thumb, close to the second digit.

How do you work the tonsil reflexes?

Simply apply pressure to the reflexes with the tip of either a thumb or finger. You can also rotate this reflex.

Why/When do you work the tonsil reflexes?

The tonsil reflexes are generally worked if a person is suffering from tonsillitis or a sore throat.

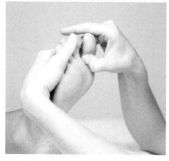

Working the tonsils

The ileocaecal valve

Peyer's patches are lymphatic nodules located in the ileum of the small intestine and they help protect the body against pathogens that have been digested. In reflexology, Peyer's patches are accessed via the reflex of the ileocaecal valve which is located where the ileum of the small intestine meets the caecum of the large intestine.

Where is the ileocaecal valve reflex?

The reflex for the ileocaecal valve is in the same place as the reflex for the appendix, which is at the start of the large intestine. The ileocaecal valve/appendix reflex is found on the right foot and hand only. It lies just above the pelvic line in zone 5.

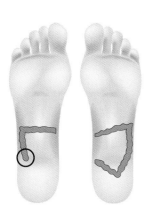

How do you work the ileocaecal valve reflex?

Place your thumb on the reflex and either apply deep on-off pressure, hold the reflex or rotate it.

Why/When do you work the ileocaecal valve reflex?

The ileocaecal valve reflex should be worked in any instances of excess mucous as it helps to control its production and elimination. Conditions include respiratory infections such as runny noses, coughs, colds and sinusitis as well as food allergies or intolerances. In addition, the ileocaecal valve is an important reflex to work if a person suffers with sluggish bowel movements or constipation.

The appendix

The appendix is located at the end of the caecum. Its physiological function is not yet known. Please see the information on the previous page on the ileocaecal valve to learn how to locate and work the appendix.

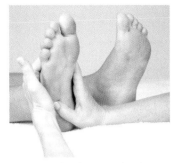

Working the ileocaecal valve

The lymphatic and immune system in a nutshell

Main reflexes – lymphatics of the upper body, lymphatics of the lower body and groin, thymus gland, spleen, tonsils, ileocaecal valve, appendix. The lymphatic system plays a vital role in the transportation of fats and fat-soluble vitamins (A, D, E and K), in the repair of injuries and in immunity and it is closely linked to the cardiovascular system. It is also considered an organ/system of elimination and supports the lungs, liver, kidneys, large intestine and skin in removing wastes from the body.

Clients suffering from frequent infections, fluid retention, fatigue/exhaustion, depression, mood swings and allergies all need to have the reflexes of their lymphatic and immune system worked. To help support the lymphatic and immune system, you should discuss the following:

- **Bed rest** – if a client has an infection it is often best that they rest as much as possible to give their bodies a chance to heal.
- **Exercise** – clients who suffer with poor lymphatic drainage, fluid retention or frequent infections need to exercise. Because the lymphatic system does not have a heart to pump lymph around the body, exercise is vital in helping lymph move.
- **Dry brushing** – lymphatic vessels lie very close to the surface of the skin and lymph can be encouraged to move through the vessels by dry brushing. This is a simple technique which takes only a few minutes and can be done on a daily basis. Take a soft-bristled body brush and, starting at the feet, use long, sweeping, upward movements and brush towards the heart. Work from the feet upwards to the heart and then from the hands upwards to the heart. Try to work the entire body, always in the direction of the heart. The brushing should be gentle and not affect the skin. This is a very stimulating technique and it should be done in the morning rather than the evening. Clients will find that after a few weeks of dry brushing their lymphatic drainage will improve, their energy will increase and they will be less prone to common infections such as coughs and colds. Although dry brushing is beneficial to the lymphatic system, if a person has had a lymph node surgically removed or has medical oedema they must check with their doctor first to ascertain whether or not it is safe for them to use this technique.

Associated reflexes
- Heart reflex and relaxation techniques to benefit the cardiovascular system
- Organs of elimination (lungs, liver, kidneys, large intestine and skin) to help the body remove its waste
- Diaphragm to encourage the movement of lymph
- Spleen and liver to help the body fight infections
- Adrenals if there is any inflammation in the body
- Kidneys if there is fluid retention as they regulate the volume and composition of the blood.

The Digestive System

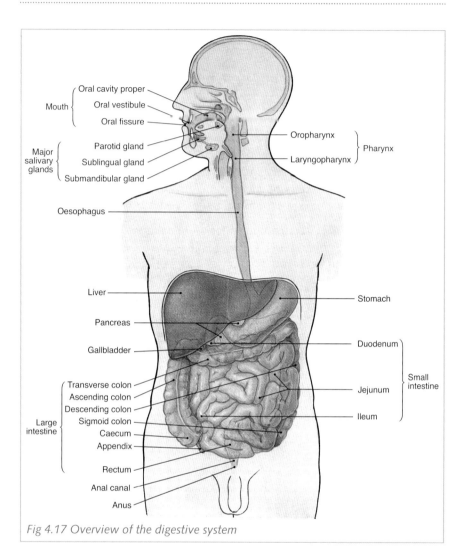

Fig 4.17 Overview of the digestive system

The digestive system is composed of a long tube that passes from the mouth to the anus. This is the gastrointestinal tract (also called the alimentary canal). This continuous tube forms the following organs and structures:

- Mouth
- Pharynx
- Oesophagus
- Stomach
- Small intestine – composed of the duodenum, jejunum and ileum
- Large intestine
- Anus.

In addition to the gastrointestinal tract, the digestive system includes accessory structures which help with the digestion of food. Most of them produce and/or store secretions that help with the chemical breakdown of food. These accessory structures are the:

- Teeth, tongue and salivary glands – all located in the mouth
- Liver
- Gallbladder
- Pancreas.

Digestion is the process by which large molecules of food are broken down into smaller molecules that can enter cells. Food is digested both mechanically and chemically. In mechanical digestion, food is physically broken down and ground into smaller substances by the teeth, tongue and physical movements such as peristalsis. It is then mixed with fluids until it finally becomes a liquid. Once in a liquid state, it is easier for chemical digestion to take place. In chemical digestion, food molecules are broken down into smaller molecules by enzymes. Enzymes speed up reactions but do not actually become involved in the reactions themselves. The chart below outlines the breakdown of carbohydrates, fats and proteins.

CHEMICAL DIGESTION OF CARBOHYDRATES, FATS AND PROTEINS			
NUTRIENT	ENZYMES	FROM	TO
Carbohydrates	Amylases	Starches and polysaccharides into disaccharides	Monosaccharides
Fats	Lipases	Triglycerides	Fatty acids and glycerol
Proteins	Proteases	Peptones and polypeptides	Amino acids

The functions of the digestive system can be broken down into six basic processes: ingestion, secretion, mixing and propulsion, digestion, absorption and defecation.

The mouth

The mouth is a mucous-membrane lined cavity formed by the cheeks, hard and soft palates and the tongue. Its opening is protected by the lips and the mouth houses the teeth and salivary glands. The mechanical digestion of food begins in the mouth. The tongue moves food, the teeth grind it and saliva mixes with the food and begins to dissolve it. Finally, it is reduced to a soft, flexible mass called a bolus. Chemical digestion of carbohydrates by the enzyme salivary amylase also begins in the mouth. However, because the food is in the mouth for such a short time, the digestion of these continues in the stomach.

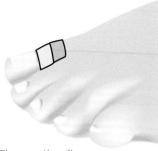

The mouth reflex

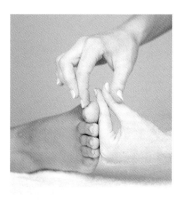

Working the mouth reflex

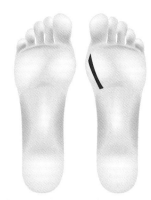

The oesophagus reflex

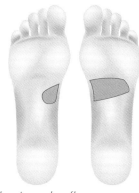

The stomach reflex

Where is the mouth reflex?
The reflex for the mouth is the same reflex as that of the nose. It is located on the dorsal aspect of the big toe and thumb, below the nail. This area can be divided into reflexes of the upper and lower jaw with the teeth of the upper jaw being located closest to the nail and the teeth of the lower jaw being beneath those of the upper jaw.

How do you work the mouth reflex?
It is easiest to finger-walk or finger-rotate across the mouth/nose reflex in a transverse direction. Otherwise simply apply deep, maintained pressure with a fingertip. Remember to support the plantar aspect of the big toe or thumb when you work this reflex.

Why/When do you work the mouth reflex?
Work the mouth reflex for any problems of the mouth, jaws and teeth.

The oesophagus

The oesophagus is a muscular tube approximately 25 cm long connecting the mouth to the stomach.

Where is the oesophagus reflex?
The oesophagus reflex is located on the left foot and hand only, running from the throat reflex to the stomach reflex in zone 1.

How do you work the oesophagus reflex?
The oesophagus reflex can be worked with either the thumb-walking or thumb-rotating techniques.

Why/When do you work the oesophagus reflex?
Work the oesophagus reflex if your client suffers with acid reflux or indigestion, a hiatus hernia or any problems of the oesophagus.

The stomach

The stomach is a J-shaped organ lying below the diaphragm and in the left-hand side of the abdominal cavity. In the stomach food is mixed, pummelled and churned into a thin liquid called chyme. In the presence of food, endocrine cells in the walls of the stomach secrete the hormone gastrin which stimulates the production of gastric juice. Gastric juice is secreted by gastric glands and contains water which liquefies food, hydrochloric acid which kills microbes, intrinsic factor which is necessary for the absorption of vitamin B12, pepsinogen which is converted into pepsin, an enzyme that begins the breakdown of proteins and gastric lipase which is an enzyme that breaks down lipids. The main chemical digestion that takes place in the stomach is the breakdown of proteins by the enzyme pepsin.

Where is the stomach reflex?
The stomach reflex is located between the diaphragm line and waistline on both feet and hands. However, it is only found in zone 1 on the right foot and hand while it extends across to zone 4 on the left foot and hand.

How do you work the stomach reflex?

The stomach reflex can be worked with either the thumb-walking or thumb-rotating technique. In addition, the reflexes on the feet can be knuckled.

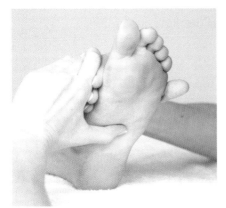

Thumb-walking the digestive reflexes

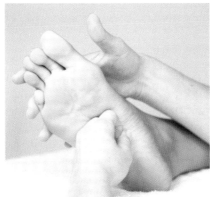

Knuckling the digestive reflexes

Why/When do you work the stomach reflex?

The stomach reflex should be worked if there are any problems with the stomach, for example, gastric ulcers. In addition, this is an important reflex to work when a person is suffering with stress or anxiety – think of that 'butterflies in the stomach' feeling.

Practical tip

The reflexes of the digestive system tend to overlap one another and some of them, such as the stomach and liver, are large and extend across many zones. For these reasons, it is important to work the abdominal area very well. In order to do this, try to use a few different techniques and work in all directions. For example:

- Work the entire abdominal area with the thumb-walking technique going in a transverse direction from right to left.
- Swop hands and rework the area with the same thumb-walking technique in a transverse direction from left to right.
- Using the thumb-rotation technique this time, work the area longitudinally or in a diagonal direction up and down a few times.
- Finish off with some knuckling of the entire area.

Practical tip

On some clients you may find what feels like a hard knot on the stomach reflex on the left foot. Chat to your client about their stress levels as this knot can often be linked to chronic stress or stress-related disorders such as ulcers or indigestion.

The pancreas

The pancreas is a long, thin gland lying behind the stomach and connected to the duodenum by two ducts. The pancreas has a head, body and tail and is 12–15 cm long. Some 99% of pancreatic cells are exocrine cells that secrete pancreatic juice. This is a clear, colourless liquid composed mainly of water, some salts, sodium bicarbonate and enzymes. Pancreatic juice is slightly alkaline and so buffers the acidic chyme coming from the stomach, stops the action of pepsin and creates the correct pH in the small intestine in which the enzymes can work. There are many different enzymes in pancreatic juice, including pancreatic amylase which continues the breakdown of carbohydrates, trypsin which continues the breakdown of proteins, pancreatic lipase which continues the breakdown of lipids, and enzymes that digest nucleic acids. The remaining 1% of pancreatic cells are endocrine cells found in clusters called pancreatic islets (islets of Langerhans). These are discussed in more detail on page 167.

The liver

The liver is a large organ located in the top right portion of the abdominal cavity, below the diaphragm. It is a vital organ with many important functions in the body. These include the metabolism of carbohydrates to maintain normal blood glucose levels, the metabolism of both lipids and proteins, the detoxification of alcohol and certain drugs, the storage of nutrients (glycogen, vitamins A, B12, D, E and K, and the minerals iron and copper), phagocytosis of worn-out red blood cells, white blood cells and some bacteria, the activation of vitamin D and the production of bile. Bile contains water, bile acids, bile salts, cholesterol, phospholipids, bile pigments and some ions. The liver secretes bile into the gallbladder where it is stored. The gallbladder then intermittently releases it into the duodenum where it functions in the emulsification and absorption of fats.

Practical tip
The feet of a person with a liver imbalance tend to be yellowish in colour.

Study tip
The liver has a unique double blood supply:

- It receives oxygenated blood via the hepatic artery.
- It also receives deoxygenated blood from the gastrointestinal tract via the hepatic portal vein. This blood contains newly absorbed nutrients as well as drugs, toxins or microbes that may have been absorbed from the gastrointestinal tract. This blood needs to be cleaned before it can be circulated to the rest of the body.

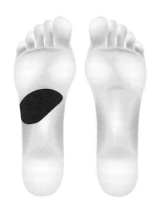

Where is the liver reflex?
The liver reflex is found on the right foot and hand only. It is a large reflex, extending across the entire area (zones 1–5) between the diaphragm line and the waistline.

How do you work the liver reflex?
The liver reflex can be worked with either the thumb-walking or thumb-rotating technique. In addition, the area on the feet can be knuckled. Be sure to keep reworking this area in as many different directions as possible (transverse, longitudinal and diagonal) and try to use a variety of techniques.

Why/When do you work the liver reflex?
Because it has such a variety of functions, the liver reflex is a crucial reflex to work for many disorders. In addition to working this reflex for any disorders directly associated with it, such as hepatitis, work the liver reflex to detoxify the body, for blood sugar disorders such as hypo/hyperglycaemia and diabetes mellitus, for blood disorders such as anaemia, for headaches and migraines, for problems with the spleen and if the body is struggling to eliminate its waste, e.g. constipation.

The organs of elimination

The body has different ways in which it gets rid of its wastes and there are six primary organs/systems of elimination. These are the lungs, liver, kidneys, large intestine, lymphatic system and skin. If one of these organs is not functioning properly and is struggling to excrete waste, it is important to pay extra attention to the other organs to help the body eliminate its waste. For example, if your client suffers from a skin disorder such as acne, ensure you work the reflexes for the lungs, liver, kidneys, large intestine and lymphatics. Likewise, if your client suffers with constipation, ensure you work the lungs, liver, kidneys and lymphatics in addition to the large intestine. How do we work the skin reflex? The best way to help the skin eliminate waste is by encouraging sweating – either by cardiovascular exercise or in a sauna.

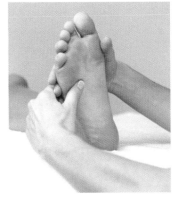

Working the liver reflex

Reflexions

Metaphysically, the liver and gallbladder are thought to store emotions such as anger, frustration and resentment and it is interesting how a link between these organs and emotions is common in different cultures. The word gall refers to bitterness and impudence while a liverish person is irritable. In Oriental diagnosis the liver controls anger and a person who harms their liver (usually through unhealthy eating and drinking) is thought to be prone to outbursts of anger and irritability. Liverish people are quite easy to recognise as they tend to have deep vertical lines between their eyebrows (see Oriental Facial Diagnosis page 313).

The gallbladder

The gallbladder is a pear-shaped, green sac that is located behind the liver and attached to it by connective tissue. The gallbladder receives bile from the liver and concentrates and stores it. It then releases bile into the duodenum via the common bile duct.

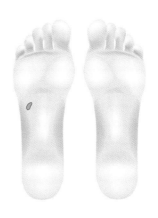

Where is the gallbladder reflex?

The reflex for the gallbladder is located on the right foot and hand only. It is a small reflex in the top right corner of the liver reflex, underneath the diaphragm line and between zones 4 and 5. In foot reflexology you can locate the reflex on the plantar aspect of the foot. Draw a line straight through the foot to the dorsum and then work the gallbladder reflex on the plantar aspect and dorsum of the foot at the same time.

How do you work the gallbladder reflex?

There are a few ways to work this reflex. You can apply deep pressure to the reflex with the tip of your thumb, then maintain this pressure, use an on-off pumping action or rotate the reflex. Another way to work the gallbladder reflex is to 'pinch' it. Place your thumb on the plantar reflex and your index finger on the dorsal reflex and squeeze.

Why/When do you work the gallbladder reflex?

Work the gallbladder reflex if there are any problems with the gallbladder, such as gallstones. In addition, work this reflex if a client feels nauseous after eating rich or fatty foods.

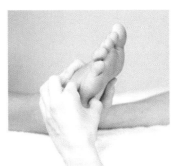

Pinching the gallbladder

The small intestine

The small intestine is made up of three segments:

- **The duodenum** is the first segment of the small intestine and is also the shortest. It is approximately 25 cm long and receives food from the stomach, bile from the gallbladder and pancreatic juice from the pancreas.
- **The jejunum** is approximately 1m long and lies between the duodenum and the ileum.
- **The ileum** is the longest segment of the small intestine and is about 2m long. It receives food from the jejunum and passes it into the large intestine via the ileocaecal valve.

In the small intestine, the thin liquid chyme is mixed with digestive juices and brought into contact with finger-like projections on the wall of the intestine called villi and microvilli. Here it is further digested by a combination of pancreatic juice, bile, intestinal juice and brush border enzymes. Digestion and absorption of most nutrients is usually completed in the small intestine. Most substances are absorbed into the blood capillaries of the villi and are then carried in the bloodstream to the liver via the hepatic portal vein. Fatty acids, glycerol and the fat-soluble vitamins (A, D, E and K), however are absorbed into lacteals (lymphatic vessels) in the villi, before being transported in the lymph to the bloodstream. The small intestine absorbs nutrients as well as water, electrolytes and vitamins. Any remaining undigested or unabsorbed matter passes into the large intestine.

Where is the small intestine reflex and the duodenum reflex?
The reflex for the small intestine is found on both feet and hands between the waistline and the pelvic line. It is outlined/edged by the large intestine reflex. Note that the first part of the small intestine, the duodenum, has its own reflex area. This is a C-shaped reflex located on the right foot and hand only, just above the waistline and below the pancreas reflex. It extends across zone 1 and slightly into zone 2.

How do you work the small intestine reflex?
The small intestine reflex can be worked with either the thumb-walking or thumb-rotating technique. In addition, the area on the feet can be knuckled.

Why/When do you work the small intestine reflex?
The small intestine reflex should be worked if there are any disorders of the small intestine or any general digestive problems. The bile and pancreatic ducts open into the duodenum so this is a very important digestive reflex.

The large intestine

The large intestine is a wide tube running from the ileum to the anus. It is divided into four regions:

- **Caecum** – The caecum is a 6 cm long pouch that receives food from the small intestine via the ileocaecal valve (ileocaecal sphincter). Attached to the caecum is the vermiform appendix.
- **Colon** – forms most of the large intestine. It is a long tube made up of the:
  - *Ascending colon* – ascends from the caecum up the right side of the

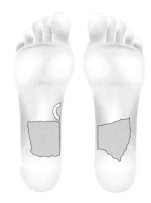

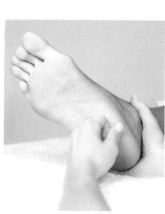

Knuckling the small intestine

abdomen to just beneath the liver. Here it turns to the left, forming the right colic (hepatic) flexure.
- *Transverse colon* – continues across the abdomen to beneath the spleen where it curves downwards at the left colic (splenic) flexure.
- *Descending colon* – descends to the level of the iliac crest where it turns inwards to form the last part of the colon.
- *Sigmoid colon* – joins the rectum at the level of the third sacral vertebra.
- **Rectum** – approx. 20 cm long, it lies in front of the sacrum and coccyx.
- **Anal canal** – The last 2–3 cm of the rectum is called the anal canal. Its external opening is called the anus and it is guarded by both internal and external sphincter muscles. These are closed except during defecation.

Small amounts of undigested nutrients can pass into the large intestine and these are digested by bacteria living in the lumen. These bacteria also produce some B vitamins as well as vitamin K. These nutrients, together with water and electrolytes are absorbed in the ascending and transverse colon. Having spent 3–10 hours in the large intestine and having had most of its water content absorbed by the walls of the colon, the liquid chyme has now become a solid or semi-solid mass called faeces. Faeces contain water, inorganic salts, dead epithelial cells from the mucosa of the gastro-intestinal tract, bacteria, products of bacterial decomposition and undigested foods. Faeces are eliminated from the body by a process called defecation.

Where is the large intestine reflex?

The reflex for the large intestine is quite complicated. It is found on the plantar aspects of both feet, and the palmar aspects of both hands, between the waistline and pelvic line. It runs from the right foot/hand to the left foot/hand. The large intestine reflex begins with the reflexes for the appendix/ileocaecal valve/caecum. These are located on the right foot/hand, in zone 5, just above the pelvic line.

The ascending colon reflex then runs up zone 5 from the pelvic line to the waistline. Here the reflex turns medially at the colic/hepatic flexure. The transverse colon runs along the waistline straight across zones 5 to 1 on the right foot/hand and into the left foot/hand. On this foot/hand it also runs straight across the waistline from zones 1 to 5. At zone 5 it turns downwards at the colic/splenic flexure.

Note that when working the transverse colon you will be working with your left thumb which should be held transversely so that the tip of it points towards your right. The top edge of your thumb should be in line with the waistline, not on top of it. This means that the reflex for the transverse colon lies just beneath the waistline and not directly on top of it.

The descending colon runs downwards in zone 5 until it reaches the pelvic line. At the pelvic line it angles inwards and descends, diagonally, to the centre of the heel of the foot/hand where it then turns upwards towards the bladder reflex. Where the colon turns in the heel is a v-shaped reflex. This is the sigmoid flexure and the portion that runs between this flexure and the end of the colon is called the sigmoid colon. The large intestine reflex ends with the reflexes for the rectum and then anus which are on the medial edge of the foot/hand next to the bladder.

Practical tip
If the feet have an offensive odour your client's body may not be eliminating waste effectively. This is often a sign of constipation.

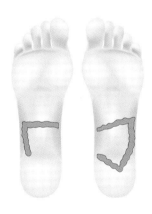

Practical tip

Although dry and cracked heels are often linked to lower back problems or reproductive disorders, they can also be signs of haemorrhoids.

How do you work the large intestine reflex?

The reflex for the large intestine can be either thumb-walked or rotated and must be worked sequentially, always from the right foot or hand to the left. The description below focuses on working the feet but can be followed for hand reflexology as well:

- Start by supporting your client's right foot with your support hand and use your other hand as the working hand.
- Place your working thumb on the appendix/ileocaecal valve/caecum reflex and work up along the ascending colon and then transversely across the transverse colon.
- When you get to the end of the transverse colon on the right foot, hold the client's left foot with your right hand and, using your left thumb, continue to walk/rotate the transverse colon until you reach zone 5.
- Now change hands so that your left hand supports the foot and your right thumb becomes the working thumb.
- Walk/Rotate down the descending colon and follow its angle until you get to the sigmoid flexure.
- At this flexure spend a bit of time using deep pressure techniques such as an on-off pumping action or deep rotations on this flexure.
- Then continue walking/rotating up to the rectum and anus.
- Repeat this entire process at least three times.

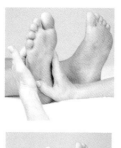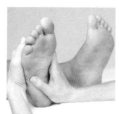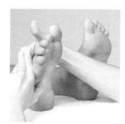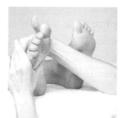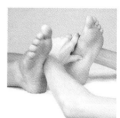
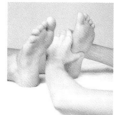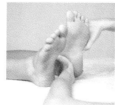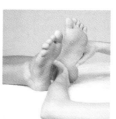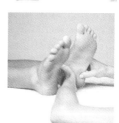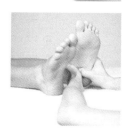

Walking the large intestine

Why/When do you work the large intestine reflex?

The large intestine is one of the main excretory organs of the body and should be worked in all conditions in which the body is struggling to eliminate waste. This includes digestive disorders such as constipation, as well as skin disorders such as acne, headaches, bad breath (halitosis) and fluid retention. In addition, it is an important reflex to work if a person suffers with fatigue or depression. Note that the sigmoid flexure is an important reflex to work if a person suffers with bloating or flatulence.

Reflexions

On a metaphysical level people who suffer with disorders of the large intestine, such as constipation, often struggle to let go of issues or feel trapped under a great deal of pressure.

The digestive system in a nutshell

Main reflexes – mouth, oesophagus, stomach, pancreas, liver, gallbladder, small intestine, large intestine. There is a saying that when life is palatable, digestion is easy and many disorders of the digestive system can be linked to stress and emotions, such as eating disorders, irritable bowel syndrome (IBS) and ulcers. In addition, what a person eats and the exercise they do have a huge impact on their digestive system and when working with a client who has a problem with this system, they need to take responsibility for their lifestyle and make any necessary changes to it.

Obvious symptoms of digestive disorders are constipation and diarrhoea but fatigue, headaches, depression and mood swings can also result from an imbalanced digestive system. If a client presents with any of these it is important to work their digestive reflexes and assess their eating and exercise habits.

Associated reflexes
- Solar plexus to relax the client
- Nervous system to relax the client
- Adrenals for stress and also if there is any inflammation (e.g. in colitis)
- Cranial nerves – cranial nerve X, the vagus nerve, innervates the digestive organs
- Thyroid gland as its hormones control metabolism
- Lungs – in TCM the lungs and large intestine are partnered (you will learn more about this on page 240) and they directly affect one another so if your client suffers from a digestive condition be sure to work the lungs and vice versa
- Organs of elimination (lungs, liver, kidneys, lymphatics and skin) to help the body remove its waste when the large intestine is not functioning properly
- Diaphragm to encourage peristalsis if there is constipation
- Cardiovascular system to encourage the distribution of nutrients by the blood
- Lymphatics, spleen and kidneys if there is any infection

The Urinary (Renal) System

The urinary system has the vital function of filtering waste products from the blood and processing them into urine. Urine is a clear to pale yellow fluid that is produced in the kidneys and excreted from the body via the urethra. Although the kidneys filter approximately 180 litres of fluid every day, only 1–2 litres is excreted as urine and the rest is reabsorbed into the blood. The chart on the following page identifies the characteristics and content of normal urine in a healthy person.

The analysis of urine gives many clues to the internal state of the body and substances that should not normally be present in urine include glucose, proteins, pus, red blood cells, haemoglobin and bile pigments. The presence of any of these substances needs to be investigated further.

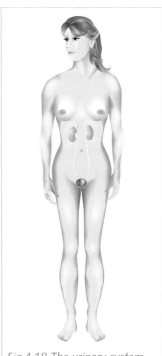

Fig 4.18 The urinary system

ANALYSIS OF NORMAL URINE	
CHARACTERISTIC	**DESCRIPTION**
Volume	1–2 litres every 24 hours
Colour	Clear to pale yellow. The colour of urine is due to the presence of pigments and can vary depending on the concentration of the urine and on diet and health.
Odour	Initially slightly aromatic but it quickly becomes ammonia-like upon standing. As with colour, the odour of urine can vary depending on the concentration of the urine and diet and health.
pH	Varies considerably according to diet and ranges between 4.6–8.0. Diets high in protein produce more acidic urine while vegetarian-based diets produce more alkaline urine.
SOLUTE	**DESCRIPTION**
Urea	The main product of protein metabolism.
Creatinine	Product of muscle activity.
Uric acid	Product of nucleic acid metabolism.
Urobilinogen	Bile pigment derived from the breakdown of haemoglobin.
Inorganic ions	These vary according to diet.

Practical tip

A sweet odour to the feet can indicate a kidney imbalance, or most commonly, diabetes.

The kidneys

The kidneys are a pair of reddish, kidney-bean shaped organs located just above the waistline. They are approximately 10–12 cm long, 5–7 cm wide and 2.5 cm thick and are uniquely structured to filter blood and produce urine. The right kidney is slightly lower than the left because the liver occupies a large area on the right side of the abdominopelvic cavity.

If you cut a kidney lengthwise, you will see that it has three distinct regions: an outer renal cortex, a middle renal medulla composed of cone-shaped structures called renal (medullary) pyramids and an inner renal pelvis which is connected to the ureter. Together the renal cortex and renal pyramids form the functional part of the kidney. They are composed of approximately one million microscopic structures called nephrons. These are the functional units of the kidney and are where urine is formed.

The kidneys filter blood and remove from it any substances that the body no longer needs, e.g. waste products, toxic substances and excess essential materials such as water. During this filtering process, they also restore certain amounts of water and solutes to the blood if and when it needs it. In this way the composition and volume of blood is constantly regulated.

In addition to regulating the composition and volume of blood, the kidneys also filter out and excrete differing quantities of hydrogen (H+) ions from the blood. This helps to regulate its pH. They also secrete an enzyme called renin which causes an increase in blood pressure and blood volume. Thus they help to regulate blood pressure.

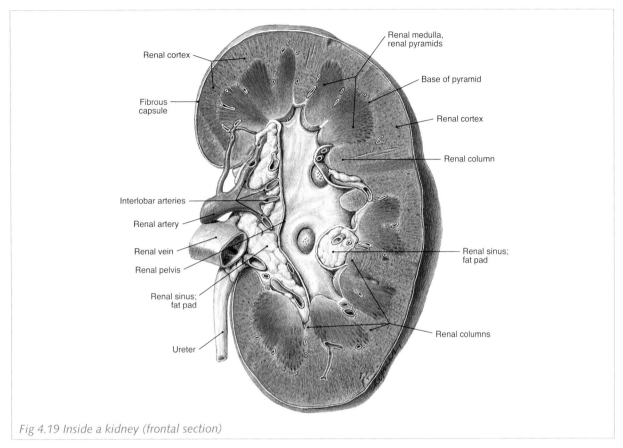

Fig 4.19 Inside a kidney (frontal section)

The kidneys have other functions in the body. They help to synthesise the hormone calcitriol which is the active form of vitamin D, they secrete the hormone erythropoietin which stimulates the production of red blood cells and during periods of starvation they can synthesise new glucose molecules in a process called gluconeogenesis.

Where are the kidney reflexes?
The reflexes for the kidneys are located on the plantar aspect of both feet and the palmar aspect of both hands. They are found on the waistline and in zones 2 and 3. On the foot they are lateral to the flexor hallucis longus tendon. The kidney reflexes are best worked together with the other organs of the urinary system. This will be discussed shortly.

The ureters

The ureters are two 25–30 cm long tubes that carry urine from the kidneys to the bladder. Each ureter drains the renal pelvis of a kidney and inserts into the posterior aspect of the bladder.

Where are the ureter reflexes?
The ureter reflexes are located on both feet and hands, running down from the kidney reflexes to the bladder reflexes.

Practical tip
The kidney reflexes are often quite sensitive.

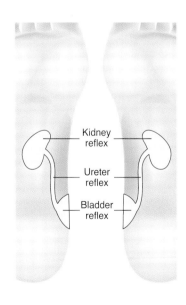

Practical tip

Broken capillaries over the bladder reflex often suggest an imbalance in this region such as incontinence or frequent urinary tract infections.

The bladder

The urinary bladder is a freely movable, hollow muscular organ that acts as a reservoir, storing urine until it is excreted from the body. The bladder changes its shape depending on how much urine it is holding. When empty it is pear-shaped and when full it is more oval. The location of the bladder also varies according to gender. In females the bladder lies in front of the vagina and below the uterus while in males it lies in front of the rectum. Furthermore, the size of the bladder varies depending on one's gender – females have smaller bladders than males because of the uterus above it.

Where is the bladder reflex?

In foot reflexology, the reflex for the bladder is located on the medial edge of both feet, on the pelvic line. It often appears as a slightly raised or puffy area. In hand reflexology, the reflex for the bladder is located on the edge of the hand, on the pelvic line.

The urethra

At the end of the urinary system is a passageway that discharges urine from the body. This passageway is the urethra and it is a small tube leading from the internal urethral orifice in the bladder to the external environment.

Just as the size and location of the bladder differs according to gender, so does the size and location of the urethra. In females the urethra is a 4 cm tube lying behind the pubic symphysis and opening to the outside between the clitoris and vaginal opening. In males the urethra is a 15–20 cm tube that runs through the prostate gland, then through the urogenital diaphragm and finally through the penis. The urethra also differs between genders in what it transports. In females the urethra only transports urine while in males it transports urine and reproductive secretions.

Where is the urethra reflex?

There is no direct reflex for the urethra on the feet or hands. Instead, it is worked as part of the bladder reflex.

How do you work the reflexes for the urinary system?

The reflexes for the urinary system on the feet can be worked as follows and this description can be adapted for working the reflexes on the hands:

- Start by working your client's right foot. Hold the heel of their right foot in your right hand and use your left hand as the working hand.
- Place your left thumb on the kidney reflex and spend some time working this reflex deeply. You can apply an on-off pressure to the point, rotate it or simply apply a deep pressure and maintain that pressure for a while. Some reflexologists also like to thumb-walk the kidney reflex area a number of times.
- Having worked the kidney reflex, angle your thumb so that the tip of it is pointing downwards and thumb-walk or rotate down the ureters to the bladder reflex.
- At the bladder reflex change hands so that your left hand is now supporting the lateral edge of the foot and your right thumb is now the working thumb.

- Thumb-walk or rotate the bladder reflex a number of times.
- Repeat the entire process on your client's left foot. Remember that your left hand will now be the support hand and your right thumb the working thumb until you get to the bladder reflex when you will swop hands.

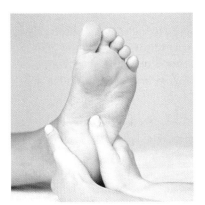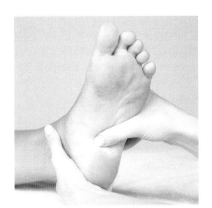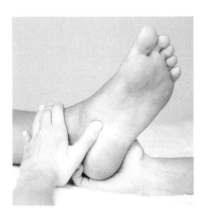

Working the urinary system on the left foot: start at the kidneys, thumb-walk down the ureters and then work the bladder

Why/When do you work the reflexes for the urinary system?

Because the urinary system helps the body eliminate waste, its reflexes should be worked if a client suffers with excretory problem or if any of the other organs of elimination (such as the lungs, liver, large intestine and skin) are not functioning properly. This system also plays an essential role in maintaining the correct volume, composition and pressure of the blood and so its reflexes should be worked if there are any disorders of the blood such as high or low blood pressure or a build-up of uric acid in the blood (in the case of gout). Finally, the reflexes for this system should be worked if there are problems with the system itself, for example urinary tract infections, cystitis, incontinence or kidney stones.

The urinary system in a nutshell

Main reflexes – kidneys, ureters, bladder, urethra. The urinary system plays a far greater role than simply eliminating waste from the body. It controls the composition and volume of the blood and so helps regulate blood pressure. It synthesises the active form of vitamin D and so plays an indirect but essential role in the growth and maintenance of bones and it secretes hormones responsible for the production of red blood cells. Common disorders of this system include infections, incontinence and kidney stones but remember that disorders such as high or low blood pressure and oedema are also linked to the functioning of the kidneys.

Associated reflexes
- Work the entire pelvic region by knuckling the heel
- Lumbar and sacral regions of the spine for their innervations to this area
- Adrenals for inflammation
- Organs of elimination (lungs, liver, large intestine, lymphatics and skin) to help the body remove its waste when the kidneys are not functioning properly
- Lymphatics, spleen and liver if there is any infection.

The Reproductive System

Reproduction occurs in all living organisms and is the process by which a new member of a species is produced. Reproductive cells are called gametes and are produced in the gonads (ovaries or testes) of men and women.

In men sperm are produced in the testes. These are highly specialised cells that are able to travel the long journey from the testes, through the male reproductive ducts, into the female reproductive system and finally into an ovum. In women, ova (sing = ovum) are produced in the ovaries. Ova are commonly called eggs.

A sperm, formed in the male reproductive system, enters the female reproductive system through sexual intercourse. The sperm and ovum unite and fuse in a process called fertilisation. This produces a zygote which is a new cell that now contains two sets of chromosomes (46 chromosomes) – one set from the mother and one from the father. The zygote then begins to divide by a process called mitosis and develops into a new organism.

The Male Reproductive System

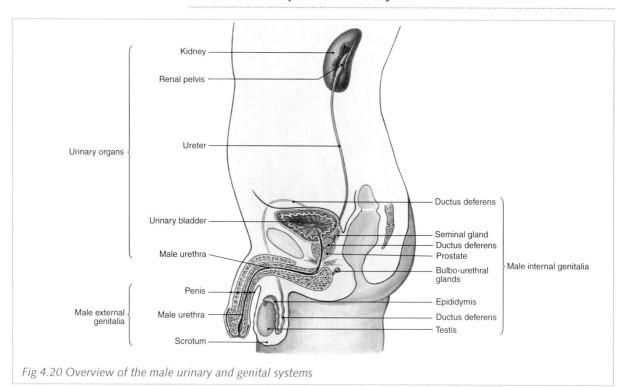

Fig 4.20 Overview of the male urinary and genital systems

The male reproductive system consists of the testes, which are the gonads where sperm are formed, a system of ducts for transporting and storing sperm and accessory organs that produce supporting substances.

Ageing and the male reproductive system

Before puberty, a boy has low levels of the reproductive hormones luteinising hormone (LH), follicle stimulating hormone (FSH) and testosterone. At puberty the levels of these hormones begin to increase and specialised cells in the testes mature to secrete testosterone. The production of sperm now begins and the increased levels of testosterone bring about the development of secondary sexual characteristics, the enlargement of the reproductive glands and both muscular and bone growth.

From around the age of 55, testosterone levels begin to decline and men lose their muscular strength. Their sperm also becomes less viable and their libido decreases. However, healthy men are still able to reproduce into their eighties and sometimes even their nineties.

The testes

The testes (singular = testis), or testicles, are a pair of oval glands located in the scrotum. This is a sac of loose skin and superficial fascia hanging from the root of the penis and divided internally into two sacs. Each sac contains one testis. The testes are the gonads of the male reproductive system and they produce sperm in a series of tightly coiled tubules called the seminiferous tubules.

From the seminiferous tubules in each testis, sperm travel down a series of tubules and ducts into a comma-shaped organ lying along the posterior border of each testis. This is the epididymis and is composed of a series of coiled ducts that empty into a single tube called the ductus epididymis. The epididymis is the site of sperm maturation. It stores sperm until they are fully mature and then helps propel them via peristaltic contractions.

The testes produce male sex hormones called androgens. The principal androgen is testosterone which:

- Stimulates the development of masculine secondary sex characteristics such as the development of pubic, axillary, facial and chest hair, a general thickening of the skin, the skeletal and muscular widening of the shoulders and narrowing of the hips, an increase in sebaceous oil gland secretion and the enlargement of the larynx and subsequent deepening of the voice.
- Promotes growth and maturation of the male reproductive system and sperm production.
- Promotes male sexual behaviour and stimulates libido (sex drive).
- Stimulates anabolism which is protein synthesis. This results in heavier muscle and bone mass.

Where are the testes reflexes?

In foot reflexology, the reflexes for the testes are located on the lateral aspect of both feet, in the depression midway between the lateral malleolus (ankle bone) and the heel area. In hand reflexology, the reflexes for the testes are located on the lateral edges of both hands in the depression where the wrist meets the forearm, zone 5. Note that these reflexes are located in the same place as the reflexes for the ovaries in a woman.

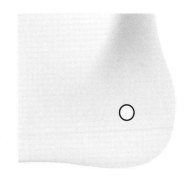

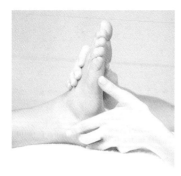

Working the testes/ovaries reflex

How do you work the testes reflexes?

Work the testes reflexes with the tip of either a thumb or finger and try to use a variety of techniques such as on-off pressure, circular rotations or a deep, direct pressure. Be aware that these reflexes can be sensitive.

Why/When do you work the testes reflexes?

The testes reflexes should be worked if there are any problems with the testes. This can include sub-fertility or impotence.

The Vas Deferens/Spermatic cords

The end of the ductus epididymis straightens and widens and continues as the vas deferens. This is a very long duct which runs from the epididymis into the pelvic cavity where it loops over the ureter and then over the side and down the posterior surface of the bladder. It finally ends in the urethra. The vas deferens transports sperm via peristaltic contractions from the epididymis to the urethra. Running alongside the vas deferens is a supporting structure consisting of blood vessels, lymphatic vessels, nerves and muscles. This structure is called the spermatic cord.

Where is the vas deferens reflex?

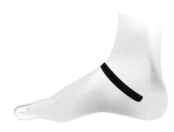

The vas deferens reflex is located in the same place as the reflex for the lymphatics of the lower body and groin. They are found on each foot as a band running from the ovaries/testes reflex, which is a depression midway between the lateral malleolus and the heel area, across the top of the ankle to the uterus/prostate reflex, a depression midway between the medial malleolus and the heel area. In hand reflexology, they are a narrow band running beneath the wrist on the dorsal aspect of the hand.

How do you work the vas deferens reflex?

Please turn to page 188 to see how to work the reflex for the lymphatics of the lower body and groin. The vas deferens reflex is worked in the same way.

Why/When do you work the vas deferens reflex?

Work this reflex if there are any problems with male fertility.

The prostate gland

The prostate gland is a doughnut shaped gland that surrounds the prostatic urethra. It secretes a milky, slightly acidic fluid that contributes to sperm mobility and viability.

Where are the prostate gland reflexes?

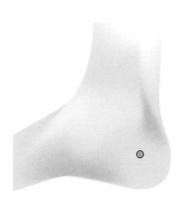

In foot reflexology, the reflexes for the prostate gland are found on the medial side of both feet, in the depression midway between the medial malleolus and the heel area. In hand reflexology, the reflexes for the prostate glands are located on the medial edges of both hands in the depression where the wrist meets the forearm, zone 1.

How do you work the prostate gland reflexes?

The prostate gland reflexes can be worked in the same way as the testes reflexes. You can use the tip of your thumb or finger to apply deep pressure on the reflex. Use an on-off pressure or rotate on the point.

Why/When do you work the prostate gland reflexes?

The prostate gland reflex should be worked if there are any problems directly associated with the prostate gland. In addition, they should be worked for any disorders of the male reproductive system.

The penis

The penis is a cylindrical organ composed of erectile tissue permeated by blood sinuses. When sexually stimulated, arteries supplying the penis dilate and large quantities of blood enter the sinuses which then expand. In doing so, these sinuses compress any veins that normally drain the penis and so the blood in the penis becomes trapped. This is an erection of the penis.

The function of the penis is to excrete urine and ejaculate semen. During ejaculation, the sphincter muscle at the base of the urinary bladder closes to prevent any urine passing into the urethra.

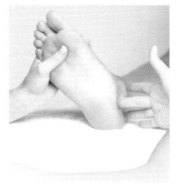

Working the prostate/uterus reflex

Where is the penis reflex?

The reflex for the penis is located on the medial aspect of both feet, running from the prostate gland reflex to the bladder reflex. This reflex is often too small to be located on the hands and so is usually worked through the prostate and bladder reflexes.

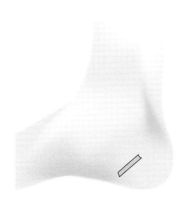

How do you work the penis reflex?

The reflex for the penis can be thumb-walked or rotated in the direction it runs – downwards from the prostate gland reflex to the bladder reflex.

Why/When do you work the penis reflex?

The penis reflex should be worked if there are any problems with the penis or if the client suffers from impotence.

The Female Reproductive System

The female reproductive system is specially structured not only to produce ova, but also to house, nourish and nurture a growing foetus.

The reproductive/menstrual cycle

Before puberty, a girl has low levels of reproductive hormones (LH and FSH) and oestrogens. However, at the onset of puberty, LH and FSH stimulate the ovaries to produce oestrogens and girls then develop secondary sexual characteristics and begin menstruating. This event is marked by menarche which is a girl's first menses around the age of 12 years. Once a female has begun to menstruate, she is capable of becoming pregnant.

Every month after the onset of puberty a woman's body prepares itself for a possible pregnancy through a series of events called the reproductive cycle. A woman's reproductive cycle lasts anywhere from 24–35 days. The details given below are based on an average 28-day reproductive cycle:

- The word *menses* means 'month' and menstruation marks the beginning of a woman's monthly cycle. Menstruation normally lasts approximately 5 days and the first day of menstruation is termed Day 1 of a woman's cycle. Before menstruation begins, a woman's uterus is prepared to

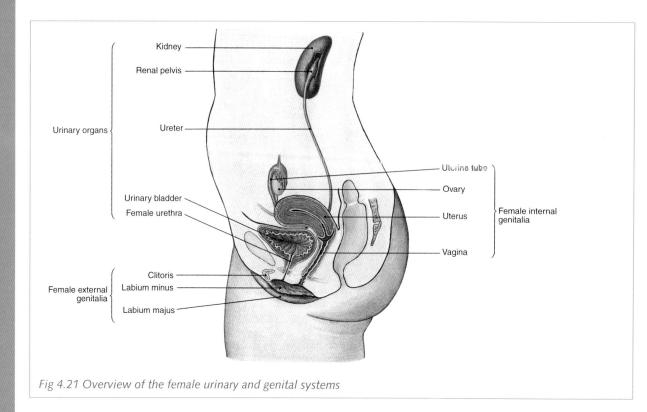

Fig 4.21 Overview of the female urinary and genital systems

Practical tip

Problems of the menstrual cycle are quite common and important reflexes to work are the hypothalamus, pituitary, thyroid and adrenal glands as well as the ovaries and uterus. It is also helpful to be aware that metaphysically the menstrual cycle represents the essence of womanhood and women who have problems embracing or accepting their womanhood, or who are not recognised/accepted by those around them, can have problems with their menstrual cycle.

receive a fertilised ovum. If it does not receive a fertilised ovum, levels of oestrogens and progesterone decline and a layer of the lining of the uterus (called the stratum functionalis of the endometrium) dies and is discharged from the body via menstrual flow.

- The time between menstruation and ovulation is called the preovulatory phase. In a 28-day cycle it can vary between 6 and 13 days in length. In this phase a large ovarian follicle containing an ovum forms (this is called a Graafian follicle) and the endometrium proliferates.
- Ovulation usually occurs around day 14 of a 28-day cycle and involves the rupture of the mature Graafian follicle and the release of an ovum into the pelvic cavity. It is during this phase that a woman can become pregnant.
- The postovulatory phase lasts for approximately 14 days after ovulation. During this time the endometrium awaits the arrival of a fertilised ovum. It is thickened, highly vascularised and secreting tissue fluid and glycogen.
- If fertilisation has occurred, the ovum takes approximately a week to arrive at the endometrium where it becomes embedded and develops into a foetus. At this stage a woman is now pregnant. If fertilisation has not occurred, menstruation and the reproductive cycle begin again.

Pregnancy

Pregnancy is the sequence of fertilisation, implantation, embryonic growth and foetal growth. An average pregnancy lasts 40 weeks from the first day of the woman's last menstrual period (approximately 38 weeks from conception) and is divided into three trimesters, each trimester comprising approximately three months:

- Trimester 1, months 0–3

During the first trimester the embryo implants and secures itself in the uterus. It grows from a single cell into a fully formed foetus in only 12 weeks and by the end of the first trimester it has all its organs, muscles, limbs and bones.

- Trimester 2, months 4–6

The foetus is now fully formed and just growing and maturing. During the second trimester it develops its individual fingerprints, toe and finger nails, eyebrows and lashes and a firm hand grip. It is in this trimester that it even starts grimacing and frowning.

- Trimester 3, months 7–birth

During the third trimester the foetus develops its sense of hearing, practises its breathing motions and learns to focus and blink its eyes. It is fully formed and puts on a great deal of weight in the last few weeks.

Menopause

Although men are capable of reproducing into old age, women are only capable of reproducing into their forties or fifties. At this age they go through menopause which is the cessation of the menses. Menopause is often called the 'change of life' and can be accompanied by a number of symptoms, including hot flushes, headaches, hair loss, sweating, vaginal dryness, insomnia, weight gain and mood swings. After menopause, a woman's reproductive organs begin to atrophy.

The ovaries

The female gonads, or ovaries, are paired almond-shaped organs located in the superior portion of the pelvic cavity on either side of the uterus. The ovaries have two functions – oogenesis and ovulation.

Oogenesis is the process through which the ovaries produce ova, or eggs. This occurs in two stages. Firstly, during foetal development germ cells differentiate into millions of immature eggs called primary oocytes and at birth a girl has all the oocytes she will ever have. Secondly, the release of gonadotropic hormones at puberty stimulates meiosis of a primary oocyte. This occurs in one oocyte in one follicle each month after puberty. The primary oocyte develops into a secondary oocyte, or ovum, and the follicle in which this development occurs is the mature Graafian follicle.

Ovulation is the process in which a mature Graafian follicle releases an ovum. The released ovum then travels down the Fallopian tube towards the uterus. The ovaries also function in the production of hormones. Oestrogens and progesterone are the principal female sex hormones and are produced mainly by the ovaries although small amounts are also produced by the adrenal cortex, testes and placenta. Oestrogens:

- Stimulate the development and maintenance of feminine secondary sex characteristics such as enlarged breasts, the pattern of hair growth on the hair and body, a broadened pelvis and the distribution of adipose tissue over the abdomen and hips.
- Help regulate fluid and electrolyte balance and lower cholesterol levels.
- Increase protein anabolism.

Practical tip

Reflexology is wonderful in pregnancy and can help with many of the discomforts associated with this special time. However, if you want to work with pregnant women it is best to first complete a reflexology course that specialises in pregnancy care.

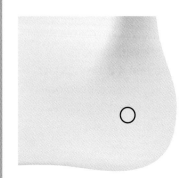

Progesterone works together with oestrogens to prepare the uterus for pregnancy and the mammary glands for lactation. Inhibin is a hormone that inhibits the secretion of follicle stimulating hormone (FSH) and relaxin is a hormone that is produced by both the ovaries and placenta during pregnancy. It helps dilate the cervix and increase the flexibility of the pubic symphysis during childbirth.

Where are the ovaries reflexes?

The reflexes for the ovaries are in the same place as the reflexes for the testes on a man. In foot reflexology they are located on the lateral aspect of both feet, in the depression half-way between the lateral malleolus and the heel. There is also a helper reflex for the ovaries. This is found on the plantar aspect of both feet in the middle of the heel area. In hand reflexology, the reflexes for the ovaries are located on the lateral edges of both hands in the depression where the wrist meets the forearm, zone 5.

> **Practical tip**
> Running up either side of the Achilles tendon on both feet is the chronic reproductive area. This houses many vital acupoints including spleen 6 (the meeting point of the three yin leg meridians). The chronic reproductive area should be massaged with deep effleurage and kneading techniques if there are any problems with your client's reproductive system or if they are struggling to become pregnant. However, this area is contraindicated if your client is pregnant as some of the acupoints it houses are used to encourage uterine contractions.

Practical tip
Remember that the thyroid gland is also called the 'Third Ovary' and should be worked if there are any problems with the ovaries or fertility issues. For details on how to work this gland please turn to page 166.

How do you work the ovaries reflexes?

Work the ovaries reflexes with the tip of either a thumb or finger and try to use a variety of techniques. For example, on-off pressure, circular rotations or a deep, direct pressure. Be aware that these reflexes can be sensitive.

> **Practical tip**
> If your client is menstruating, do not apply deep pressure to the ovaries or uterus reflexes as this can cause a slightly heavier period than usual. You can still work these reflexes, but only gently.

Why/When do you work the ovaries reflexes?

The ovary reflexes should be worked if there are any problems directly associated with them, if your client has problems with her menstrual cycle, or if she is trying or struggling to become pregnant (sub-fertile).

The Fallopian (Uterine) tubes

The Fallopian tubes are two thin tubes running from the ovaries to the uterus. They are the site of fertilisation and it is here that sperm and ovum unite and fuse to form a zygote. They also transport the zygote to the uterus. It takes approximately seven days for the zygote to travel down the tubes and into the uterus.

Where are the Fallopian tube reflexes?

The reflexes for the Fallopian tubes are the same as the reflexes for the vas deferens and the lymphatics of the lower body and are worked in the same way. Please turn to page 188 to see how to work these reflexes.

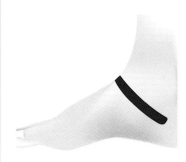

Why/When do you work the Fallopian tube reflexes?
The Fallopian tube reflexes should be worked if there are problems with the Fallopian tubes and if your client is trying to become pregnant.

The uterus

The uterus, or womb, is a muscular sac located between the bladder and rectum. Before fertilisation, the uterus acts as a pathway through which sperm travel into the Fallopian tubes where they attempt to fertilise an ovum. If fertilisation is successful, then the uterus becomes the site of implantation of a zygote and houses the developing foetus throughout pregnancy. It then contracts forcefully during labour to expel the foetus. If, however, fertilisation is not successful, the uterus becomes the site of menstruation.

Where is the uterus reflex?
The reflex for the uterus is in the same location as the reflex for the prostate gland on a man. In foot reflexology it is found on the medial aspects of both feet, in the depression between the medial malleolus and the heel.

In hand reflexology, the reflexes for the uterus are located on the medial edges of both hands in the depression where the wrist meets the forearm, zone 1.

How do you work the reflex?
The uterus reflex can be worked in the same way as the ovary, testes and prostate reflexes are worked. The ovaries/testes and uterus/prostate reflexes can also be worked together as follows:

- Cross your arms over so that your right hand will work your client's right foot and your left hand will work your client's left foot.
- Place the heel of your client's right foot in the palm of your right hand and wrap your fingers around the heel so that your middle finger touches the ovary/testis reflex and your thumb touches the uterus/prostate reflex. Place the heel of your client's left foot in the palm of your left hand so that your middle finger touches their ovary/testis reflex and your thumb touches their uterus/prostate reflex.
- Using both hands at the same time apply pressure and squeeze the reflexes between your middle finger and thumb. Maintain this pressure or use an on-off pumping action.

Why/When do you work the reflex?
Work the uterus reflex if your client has any problems with their uterus, any menstrual disorders or if they are trying to become pregnant. This is also an important reflex to work when a woman is in labour.

The vagina

The vagina is a muscular tube between the bladder and rectum and attached to the uterus. The vagina acts as a passageway for blood during menstruation, semen during sexual intercourse and the foetus during childbirth.

Where is the vagina reflex?
The reflex for the vagina is in the same place as the reflex for the penis in a man. It is on the medial aspect of both feet, running from the uterus reflex

Practical tip
If your client is pregnant, avoid deep pressure on both the uterus and ovaries reflexes.

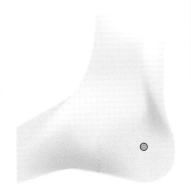

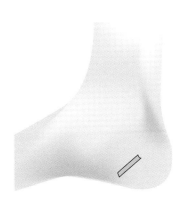

to the bladder reflex. This reflex is usually too small to locate on the hands and is worked through the reflexes of the uterus and bladder.

How do you work the vagina reflex?
Thumb-walk down this reflex from the uterus reflex to the bladder reflex.

Why/When do you work the vagina reflex?
Work the vagina reflex if your client has any problems with this area, such as inflammation, infection or incontinence. This is also an important reflex to work when a woman is in labour.

The mammary glands (Breasts)

The mammary glands, or breasts, are two modified sudoriferous glands. They are located over the pectoralis major muscles and are attached to them by a layer of dense irregular connective tissue. The breasts synthesise and secrete milk through the process of lactation. Milk production is stimulated by the hormone prolactin (with smaller contributions from progesterone and oestrogens) and the ejection of milk is stimulated by the hormone oxytocin whose release is stimulated by the baby sucking on the breast.

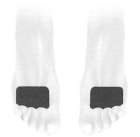

Where are the breast reflexes?
The reflexes for the breasts are located on the dorsal aspects of both feet and hands, in zones 1–4, between the shoulder line and diaphragm line.

How do you work the breast reflexes?
Finger-walk or rotate the breast reflexes.

Why/When do you work the breast reflexes?
The breast reflexes can be worked if they are tender due to premenstrual tension or when a woman is breastfeeding. Working the breast reflexes stimulates lactation so they should not be massaged if a woman is trying to stop breastfeeding.

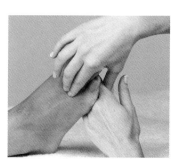

Fingerwalking the breast reflexes

The reproductive system in a nutshell

Main reflexes – testes, vas deferens/spermatic cord, prostate, penis, ovaries, Fallopian tubes, uterus, vagina, breasts/mammary glands. Like many other systems of the body, the health of the reproductive system is closely linked to stress levels and emotions and it is also influenced by diet and nutrition. Look at all these aspects when working with this system and also remember that it is influenced by the endocrine system so this entire system will need to be balanced if there are any problems with the reproductive system.

Associated reflexes
- Solar plexus for relaxation
- Cardiovascular system for hormone distribution
- Hypothalamus and pituitary glands – these produce hormones that control the gonads
- Thyroid gland – this is often called the third ovary and should be worked if there are any fertility issues
- Adrenal glands need to be worked if there is any inflammation or pain (e.g. in premenstrual tension) or if a client is struggling to conceive.

The Special Senses

The sense of touch: the skin

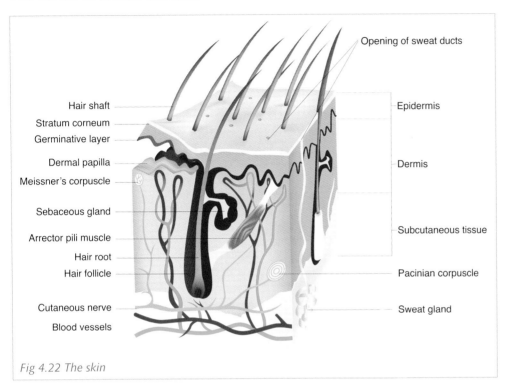

Hair shaft
Stratum corneum
Germinative layer
Dermal papilla
Meissner's corpuscle
Sebaceous gland
Arrector pili muscle
Hair root
Hair follicle
Cutaneous nerve
Blood vessels

Opening of sweat ducts
Epidermis
Dermis
Subcutaneous tissue
Pacinian corpuscle
Sweat gland

Fig 4.22 The skin

The skin is the organ of touch and together with the hair and nails it forms the integumentary system. Although there are no direct reflexes for the skin, it is important to have a basic knowledge of the anatomy and physiology of it and know how to help a client suffering with any skin disorders.

The skin is a cutaneous membrane made of two distinct layers, the epidermis and the dermis. The epidermis is a tough, waterproof outer layer that is continuously being worn away. The dermis lies beneath it and is a thicker layer that contains nerves, blood vessels, sweat glands and hair roots. The functions of the skin include:

- **Heat regulation** – cools the body through sweating and vasodilation. It warms the body through decreased sweat production, vasoconstriction, contraction of the arrector pili muscles, and shivering.
- **Sensation** – contains cutaneous sensory receptors that are sensitive to touch, temperature, pressure and pain.
- **Protection** – protects against trauma, bacteria, dehydration, ultraviolet radiation, chemical damage and thermal damage.
- **Absorption** – absorbs certain substances.
- **Excretion** – excretes wastes.
- **Secretion** – secretes sebum which keeps the skin supple and waterproof.
- **Vitamin D synthesis** – synthesises vitamin D, which helps regulate the calcium levels of the body and is necessary for the growth and maintenance of bones.

Practical tip

Encouraging sweating through either exercise or saunas will help the skin eliminate waste and improve its appearance and texture.

How do you work the skin?

If your client has a skin problem, such as eczema or acne, always work the reflex for the area that is affected. For example, if the eczema is on the arms then work the arm reflexes or if the acne is on the face then work the face reflex. In addition, because the skin is a major excretory organ, work the reflexes for the other organs of elimination to help the skin. These include the lungs, liver, kidneys and large intestine. The adrenal reflexes are also important in helping with any skin problems as inflammation is often associated with a skin disorder. Finally, disorders of the skin often cause a great deal of emotional stress and can have a traumatic effect on a person's confidence so be sure to work their solar plexus reflex to help relax them.

The senses of sight and sound: the eyes and ears

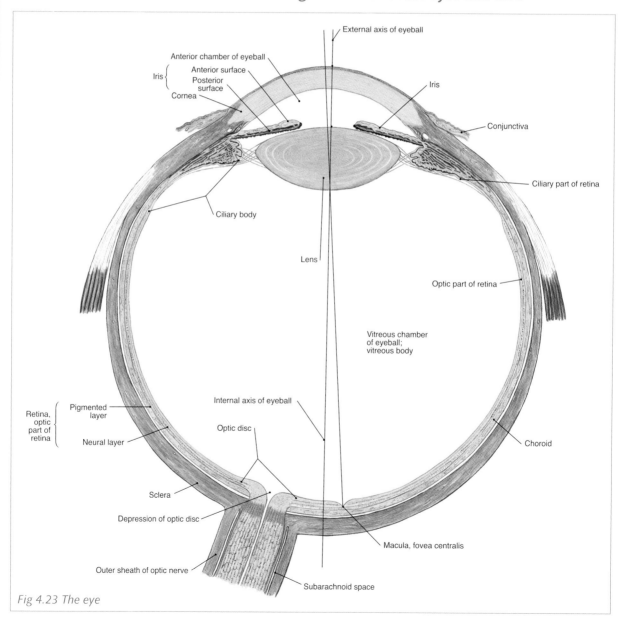

External axis of eyeball

Anterior chamber of eyeball
Iris {
Anterior surface
Posterior surface
Cornea

Iris

Conjunctiva

Ciliary part of retina

Ciliary body

Lens

Optic part of retina

Vitreous chamber of eyeball; vitreous body

Retina, optic part of retina {
Pigmented layer
Neural layer

Internal axis of eyeball

Optic disc

Choroid

Sclera

Depression of optic disc

Macula, fovea centralis

Outer sheath of optic nerve

Subarachnoid space

Fig 4.23 The eye

Our eyes are our organs of sight and contain over a million nerve fibres and more than 70% of the body's total sensory receptors. They convert light into nerve impulses which are then transported to the brain via the optic nerve.

The eyeball is approximately 2½ cm in diameter. However, we only see ⅙th of it as the rest is protected by the orbit into which it fits. The eyeball consists of a strong, protective wall made up of three layers – an outer fibrous tunic, a middle vascular tunic and an inner nervous tunic, the retina. The retina contains specialised cells, called photoreceptors, which convert light into nerve impulses. The interior of the eyeball is a large space that is divided into two cavities by the lens. The anterior cavity of the eyeball is filled with aqueous humour, a watery fluid that nourishes the lens and cornea and helps produce intraocular pressure. The posterior cavity contains a jelly-like substance called vitreous humour, which helps maintain the shape of the eyeball.

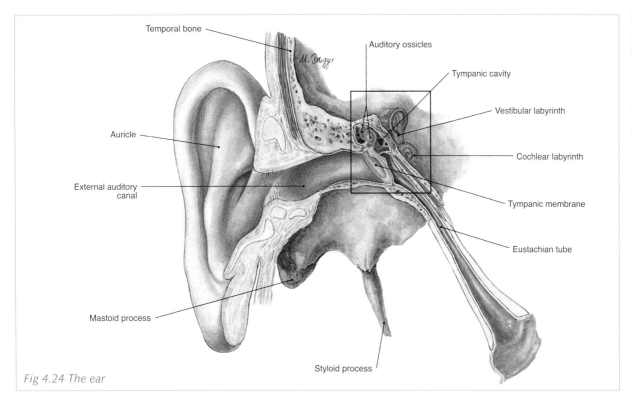

Fig 4.24 The ear

Our ears are our organs of hearing and balance. They can be divided into the outer, middle and inner ear and they convert sound waves into nerve impulses which are transported by the vestibulocochlear nerve to the brain.

The outer ear collects and channels sound waves inwards. It is composed of the auricle, external auditory canal and eardrum. The middle ear is a small air-filled cavity found between the outer ear and the inner ear. It is partitioned from the outer ear by the eardrum and from the inner ear by a bony partition containing two windows – the oval window and the round window. It contains the three auditory ossicles (hammer, anvil and stirrup) and is connected to the throat via the Eustachian tube. The Eustachian tube connects the middle ear with the upper portion of the throat and it equalises

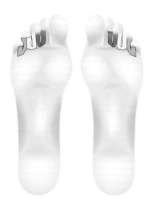

the middle ear cavity pressure with the external atmospheric pressure. The inner, or internal, ear is sometimes called the labyrinth. It consists of a bony labyrinth filled with a fluid called perilymph enclosing a membranous labyrinth filled with a fluid called endolymph. This labyrinth is divided into the vestibule, three semicircular canals and the cochlea. Inside the cochlea lies the actual organ of hearing itself – the organ of Corti.

Where are the eye and ear reflexes?

In reflexology, the eyes and ears are always worked together because anatomically the inner ear lies directly behind the eye and so their reflexes overlap one another. The reflexes for the eyes are found on both feet and hands beneath the pads of toes/fingers 2 and 3. The reflexes for the ears are found on both feet and hands beneath the pads of toes/fingers 3, 4 and 5. The inner ear is on toe/finger 3 (anatomically it lies behind the eye) while the outer ear is on toes/fingers 4 and 5. The shelf or ridge at the base of toes/fingers 2–5 is known as the eye and ear helper reflex and is worked for any chronic eye or ear conditions. In addition to the direct eye/ear reflexes, the reflex for the Eustachian tube is located on the lateral edge of the big toe and thumb and it extends into the eye and ear helper reflex.

How do you work the eye and ear reflexes?

The eye and ear reflexes can be worked in a number of different ways so experiment and see which is best for you. You can:

- thumb-walk the plantar aspect of each toe or finger. Be sure to place your support hand on the dorsal aspect of the toes/fingers so that as you thumb-walk up and down them they are supported from behind.
- grip each toe or finger between the fingers of your support hand and do small thumb-rotations up them.
- work the eye and ear helper reflex by applying a downward pressure, either with a thumb or fingertip, onto the shelf at the base of the toes/fingers and then thumb-walk back and forth repeatedly.

Why/When do you work the eye and ear reflexes?

The eye and ear reflexes should be worked for any problems related to these sense organs, including the sense of balance.

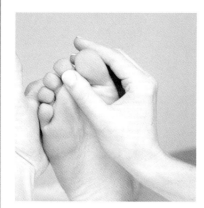

Thumb-walking the eye reflex

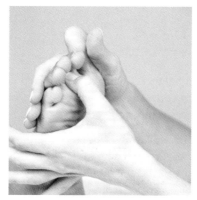

Working the eye and ear helper reflex by applying pressure on the shelf at the base of the toes

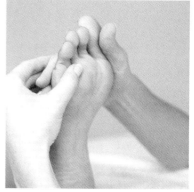

Thumb-walking the eye and ear helper reflex

Practical tip

If your client has any disorder of the eyes or ears, as well as working the reflexes for these organs, also work the reflexes for the Eustachian tubes and the cervical vertebrae. This will deepen and strengthen the effects of your treatment. In addition, when dealing with eye disorders, it has been found that thumb-walking zone 3 is extremely beneficial, as is working the kidney reflex. The eyes and kidneys both lie in the same zone and a disorder of the one is often reflected as a sensitivity of the other.

Reflexions

A person's eyes can tell you a lot about their health. In Chinese facial diagnosis, the eyes and liver are referred to as brother and sister and people with liver meridian imbalances often wear glasses or have scratchy or light-sensitive eyes. Dark bags under the eyes are associated with the kidneys, chronic tiredness and fear. People with eye bags may live against their natural rhythms by having abnormal sleep patterns, overworking themselves or having a poor diet. By learning more about your client's lifestyle and habits and helping them to change them, you can enhance your reflexology treatments.

The senses of smell and taste: the nose and mouth

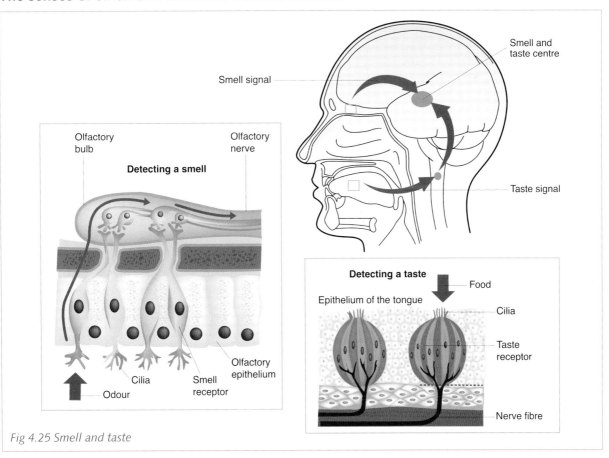

Fig 4.25 Smell and taste

The senses of smell and taste are closely linked because odours from food pass into the nasopharynx and nasal cavity. This is why you often cannot taste foods if you have a blocked nose from a cold and it is also the reason that wine tasters always smell the bouquet of the wine first before tasting it.

At the top of the nasal cavity (nose) is a small patch no larger than the size of a postage stamp that contains olfactory receptors. Olfactory receptors are neurones that have many hair-like projections extending from their dendrites. In the connective tissue that supports the olfactory epithelium are olfactory glands (Bowman's glands) that produce mucous. When you breathe in, airborne particles dissolve in this mucous and come into contact with the hair-like cilia of the olfactory receptors. The olfactory cells are chemoreceptors and convert the chemical stimulus found dissolved in the mucous into nerve impulses. These impulses are then sent to the frontal lobe via the limbic system of the brain.

The mouth houses the receptors of taste. These are called gustatory receptors and are found in taste buds which are located mainly on the tongue, the back of the roof of the mouth and in the pharynx and larynx.

A taste bud is an oval body that contains gustatory receptor cells. Each of these cells has a single hair-like projection that projects from the receptor cell and through a small opening in the taste bud called the taste pore.

Once inside the mouth, food is dissolved in saliva and the hairs of gustatory receptors dip into this saliva and are stimulated by the taste chemical within it. Thus, gustatory receptors are chemoreceptors. The taste receptors then send messages to the areas of the brain responsible for taste, appetite and saliva production.

On the tongue, taste buds are found in elevations called papillae. These elevations give the tongue its rough surface. The reflexes for the nose and mouth are discussed in more detail on pages 173 and 193.

The special senses in a nutshell

Main reflexes – skin (work the area affected), eyes, ears, Eustachian tube, nose, mouth. The special senses are part of the nervous system and if there are any problems with them ensure you work the entire nervous system.

Associated reflexes
- Cranial nerves for their innervations
- Entire nervous system (brain, cranial nerves, spine) if there is a loss of sensation
- Adrenals if there is any inflammation
- Brain if there is any pain
- Lymphatics, liver and spleen if there is any infection
- Cardiovascular system to improve circulation
- Solar plexus to relax your client
- All organs of elimination (lungs, liver, kidneys, large intestine and lymphatics) if there is a problem with the skin.

Study outline

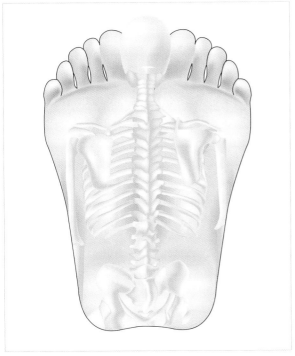

Reflexes of the skeletal system

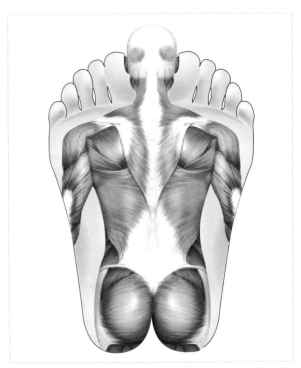

Reflexes of the muscular system

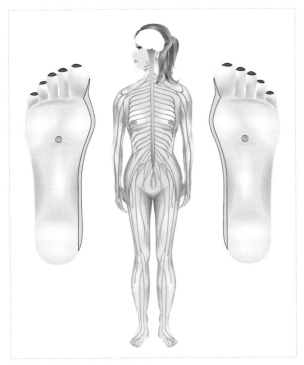

Reflexes of the nervous system

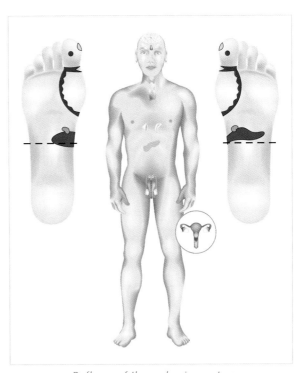

Reflexes of the endocrine system

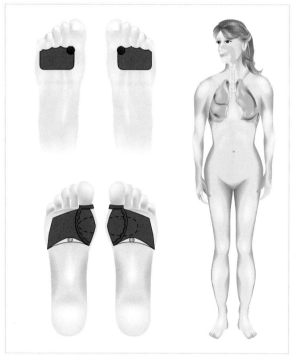

Reflexes of the respiratory system

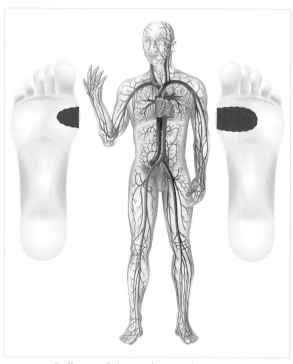

Reflexes of the cardiovascular system

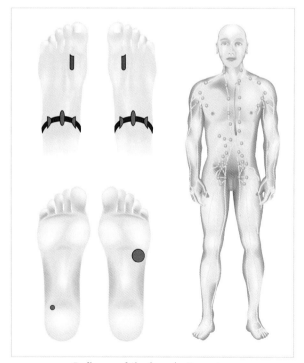

Reflexes of the lymphatic system

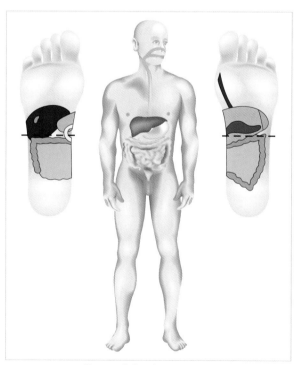

Reflexes of the digestive system

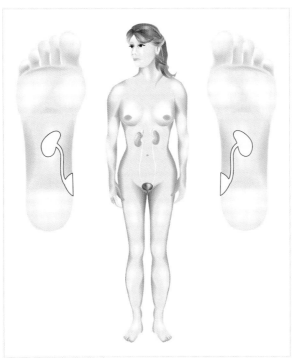

Reflexes of the urinary system

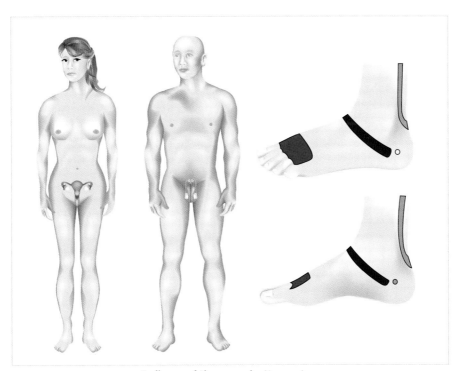

Reflexes of the reproductive system

Multiple choice questions

1. **The reflex area for the heart is found:**
    a. On the right foot only, between the waistline and diaphragm line
    b. Mainly on the left foot, between the shoulder line and diaphragm line
    c. In the centre of the diaphragm line
    d. In the centre of the waistline.

2. **The direct reflex for arthritis in the knees is the:**
    a. Elbows
    b. Hands
    c. Knees
    d. Feet.

3. **Which of the following is not a reason for working the kidneys?**
    a. To help with blood pressure problems
    b. To help with breathing problems
    c. To help with fluid retention
    d. To help with urinary tract infections.

4. **If your client presents with an infection, which of the following reflexes will encourage the body to fight that infection?**
    a. Liver and spleen
    b. Kidneys and adrenals
    c. Brain and solar plexus
    d. Thymus and bladder.

5. **Where on the feet will you find the reflexes for the sinuses?**
    a. The tips of all the toes
    b. The tips of the big toes only
    c. The webbing between all the toes
    d. The webbing between the first and second toes only.

6. **The reflex for the liver is found in:**
    a. Zones 1–5
    b. Zones 1–3
    c. Zones 1–2
    d. Zone 1 only.

7. **Why do you work the lung reflex?**
    a. To improve the circulation of the blood
    b. To encourage digestion
    c. To improve the exchange of oxygen and carbon dioxide
    d. To relieve stress.

8. **The reflex area for the solar plexus is found:**
    a. In the centre of the diaphragm line
    b. In the centre of the waistline
    c. In the centre of the big toe
    d. In the centre of the foot.

9. **If your client presents with a headache, which of the following would be an associated reflex?**
    a. The head
    b. The brain
    c. The neck
    d. The thymus.

10. **If your client suffers from excess mucous, for example they have a runny nose, which of the following reflexes will benefit them if worked on?**
    a. Thyroid
    b. Kidneys
    c. Ovaries
    d. Ileocaecal valve.

5 Meridian therapy

*'Much of what we think is extraordinary in another place is
just the ordinary not understood or experienced'*
Ted J. Kaptchuk

Reflexology has its roots in Traditional Chinese Medicine (TCM) which is a
vast system covering acupuncture, massage, diet, herbalism and exercise.
There is much to learn about TCM and practitioners train for many years
before they can practise it safely. However, having a basic understanding of
some of the concepts of TCM can greatly enhance your reflexology
treatment.

Student objectives

By the end of this chapter you will be able to:

- Explain the concepts of yin and yang
- Describe the five elements
- Define Qi and the fundamental substances of the body
- Recognise the meridian pathways of the body and use them to enhance
  your reflexology treatments.

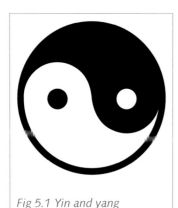

Fig 5.1 Yin and yang

Yin/Yang

*'The principle of yin and yang is the basis of the entire
universe. It is the principle of everything in creation…
Heaven was created by an accumulation of yang;
the Earth was created by an accumulation of yin…
Yin and yang are the source of power and the beginning
of everything in creation.' Nei Ching[1]*

The ancient Chinese based their philosophies on nature and the world in which they lived. An understanding of TCM always begins with the concepts of yin and yang and these are best described through looking at a mountain with the sun shining on one side of it. The sunny side of the mountain is warm, light and dry. It is yang. The shady side of the mountain is cold, dark and damp. It is yin. Taking this idea further, the Chinese looked to the heavens, warm and bright, as yang and the earth, cool and damp, as yin.

Yin and yang are two interdependent forces of nature which are constantly transforming each other. One cannot exist without the other and the presence of each defines the other. For example, without the concept of cold we cannot understand the concept of hot. Hot cannot exist without cold. Yin cannot exist without yang. Everything in nature can be separated into yin and yang and for there to be harmony there needs to be equilibrium between the two.

*'Being and non-being produce each other;
Difficult and easy complete each other;
Long and short contrast each other;
High and low distinguish each other;
Sound and voice harmonise each other;
Front and back follow each other.' Lao Tzu[2]*

YIN	YANG
The shady side of the mountain	**The sunny side of the mountain**
Cold, dark, wet	Heat, light, dry
Rest	Active
Night	Day
Female	Male
Earth	Heaven

People can also be separated into yin or yang types, however every person has yin and yang within them and ideally these should be in balance. Too much of either will cause imbalance and disease. Putting yin and yang into human physical terms:

YIN	YANG
Slender, weak, listless, soft and dense body, enjoys quiet and calm environments, desires regular periods of rest without constant social interaction, conservative, efficient. • Becomes sick progressively and symptoms linger. • Exaggerated yin: depressed and introverted.	Well-made, strong, active, tough and wiry body, tense, great capacity for food and activity, require little time for rest, constant need for stimulation, impulsive. • Become ill very quickly and suffer greatly. • Exaggerated yang: can't relax, hysteria.

The Five Elements

The ancient Chinese studied the cycles of nature and saw how the seasons are reflected in man so they subdivided yin and yang into five elements. These elements interact in a creative cycle to form all other substances, conditions and states. Each element is produced by and produces another and one cannot exist without the others.

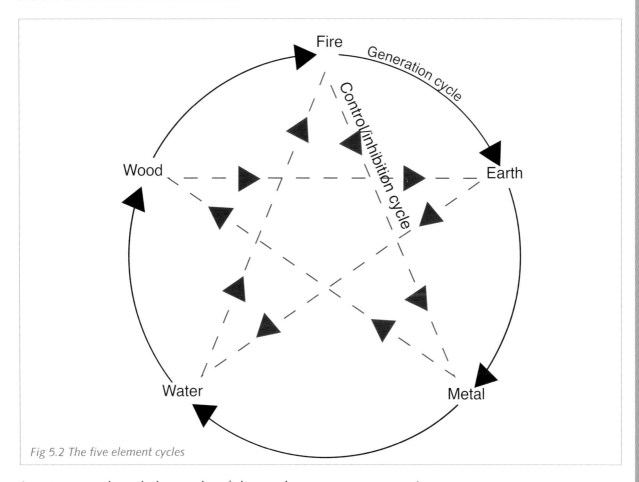

Fig 5.2 The five element cycles

As nature goes through these cycles of change, the same patterns occur in man and these patterns can be used to help us understand a person's condition. A person will always be made up of all five elements but they will be controlled by a more dominant element. The five elements define us as individuals and the way we respond, physically or emotionally, to external forces depends on the balance of the elements within us.

ELEMENT	PERSONALITY	IMBALANCES
Fire Heart (yin) Small intestine (yang) Summer Red	Joyful, confident, dynamic, vibrant, changing, warm, caring, enthusiastic.	Hysteria, unhappiness. Lack of enthusiasm, coldness, difficulty in forgiving, fever, frigidity, perspiration.
Earth Spleen (yin) Stomach (yang) Late summer Yellow	Nurturing, understanding, compassionate, sense of being grounded/rooted.	Over-thinking. Overly sentimental or sympathetic, obsessive, self-pitying, cynical, poor sleep, mouth problems, nervousness.
Metal Lung (yin) Large intestine (yang) Autumn White	Strength, structure, substance, good communication, respects authority, ability to let go of unnecessary emotions.	Grief. Lethargy, depression, grieving, inability to let go of things, low resistance to colds, flu or bronchial problems.
Water Kidney (yin) Bladder (yang) Winter White	Self-confidence, fluidity, vitality, intelligence, understanding, courage.	Fear. Lack of self-confidence, tiredness, lack of will and energy, fatigue, debilitating diseases.
Wood Liver (yin) Gallbladder (yang) Spring Green	Decision makers, planners, patience, active, competitive.	Anger. Intolerance, demanding, unstable, extremist, may abuse stimulants or sedatives, liver problems, muscle spasms.

Qi and The Fundamental Substances of the Body

'Qi is the root of all human beings'. (Nei Ching)

In Chinese medicine there are five fundamental substances found within the body: Qi, Blood, Jing, Shen and the Fluids. In his book *The Web That Has No Weaver*, Ted Kaptchuk wrote that Qi, Jing and Shen are known as the three treasures:

- Qi is responsible for the physical integrity of any entity, and for the changes that entity undergoes
- Jing, best translated as Essence, is the Substance that underlies all organic life … (It) is supportive and nutritive, and is the basis of reproduction and development
- Shen is best translated as Spirit … it is the Substance unique to human life … Shen is the awareness that shines out of our eyes when we are truly awake.

On the remaining two substances, blood circulates continuously through the body, nourishing, maintaining, and to some extent moistening its various parts and Fluids are bodily liquids which moisten and nourish the body.[3]

In reflexology we are concerned mainly with Qi (sometimes written as Chi Ch'i or Ki). Qi is our life force, our life energy. It is essential for the functioning of all the organs and processes in our body from the beating of our hearts to the assimilation of our food. We initially receive our Qi from our mothers and then gain additional Qi through our mouths and noses. Diet, lifestyle and attitude all affect our Qi.

Qi circulates through our bodies via one continuous meridian or channel. This meridian traverses the entire body and is divided into fourteen sections (twelve major meridians and two extraordinary vessels) which are described according to their positions and functions. For total health, Qi must flow through all the meridians freely and evenly. A blockage in a meridian leads to disharmony and disease in the body.

The Meridians

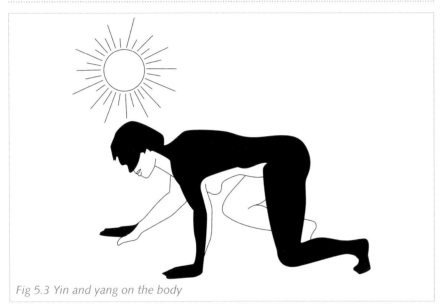

Fig 5.3 Yin and yang on the body

The meridians work in pairs and are categorised according to the element with which they are associated and whether they are yin or yang. The yin meridians flow along the inner aspect of the body and are the heart, lungs, spleen, liver and kidneys (the pericardium is sometimes also considered yin) and these organs produce, transform, regulate and store the fundamental substances in the body. The yang organs flow along the lateral aspect of the body and are the gallbladder, stomach, small intestine, large intestine, bladder and triple burner and they receive, break down and absorb the foods that will be transformed into the fundamental substances. They also transport and excrete any unused food.

The meridian pairs

As mentioned earlier, the 12 meridians are actually part of one meridian through which Qi flows continuously. It flows through this meridian in one direction only and from one specific meridian into another in a cycle that

YIN	ELEMENT	YANG
Heart	Fire	Small intestine
Pericardium	Fire	Triple burner
Spleen	Earth	Stomach
Lungs	Metal	Large intestine
Kidneys	Water	Bladder
Liver	Wood	Gallbladder

spans a 24 hour period. This 24 hour cycle is known as the Chinese clock and each meridian has a two hour period in which it is full of energy. At the opposite time of the day its energy is at a minimum. The Chinese prefer to stimulate the meridian and its organ at the time that it is its most full and to sedate it at its quietest time. For example, the kidney meridian is at its maximum between 5 and 7 pm so this is the best time to stimulate it. It is at its emptiest between 5 and 7 am and this is the time to sedate it.

Using meridians in reflexology

The aim of reflexology is to encourage and balance the flow of Qi. If Qi does not flow easily through the body and is impeded or congested in any way, or if it flows excessively, the body will be thrown out of balance and illness can result. Reflexology aims at balancing the flow of Qi through the meridians. According to the Nei Ching, the meridians move Qi and blood, regulate yin and yang, moisten the tendons and bones and benefit the joints[4] (Dougans). When working with 'energy' conditions such as headaches, nerve pain, muscular aches and pains, or disorders that do not improve with normal reflexology treatments then you can work on a deeper level by including the meridians in your treatment.

Firstly, look for physical signs along the meridian that will indicate congestion. These signs include skin conditions, rashes, infections, warts, birthmarks, lumps, moles or muscular stiffness found along a meridian pathway. Secondly, look specifically at the fingers and toes. Pain, stiffness, arthritis, loss of function, skin blemishes and nail problems on the fingers or toes can be related directly to a specific meridian. Fig 5.4 on the next page shows which toes and fingers are related to which meridian.

The twelve major meridians either begin or end on the fingers and toes and the acupoints found here are easily accessible and have a great influence on the quality and quantity of the Qi in a meridian. You can work them by applying a deep, direct pressure to the point with the tip of either your finger or thumb. Do not jab into the point. Instead, work with your client's breathing and as they breathe out apply the pressure slowly and carefully and go down until you feel a resistance or your client indicates they can feel a slight pain. Do not go further than this pain barrier. When your client breathes in release the pressure and apply it again when they breathe out. Repeat this process six to eight times.

*'The image I often have in my mind when I apply pressure is
that of pressing down through layer upon layer until I find
some solid ground. It is not dissimilar to walking on mud,
where initially you sink but after a short while you meet with
some resistance and then although you are still descending you
find somewhere where your feet settle on terra firma.'*
Jon Sandifer[5]

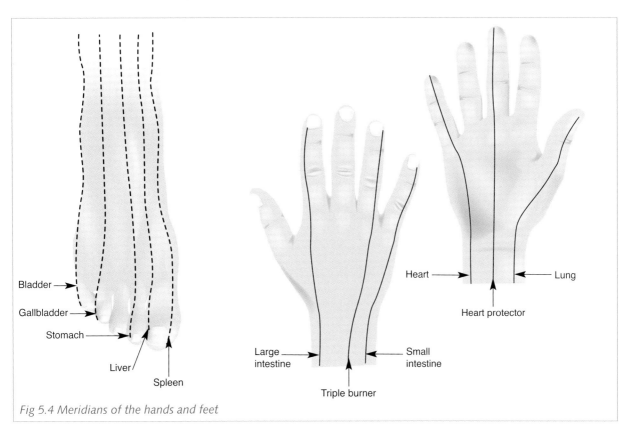

Bladder
Gallbladder
Stomach
Liver
Spleen

Large intestine
Small intestine
Triple burner

Heart
Lung
Heart protector

Fig 5.4 Meridians of the hands and feet

Once you have assessed which meridian is out of balance and worked the
relevant acupoint, you now need to work the reflex for the corresponding
organ. Work this reflex with your normal reflexology techniques.

Case study

Take a look again at the photos of Martin's hands on page 119 and you can
see that his thumb has deep ridges and cracks on the skin and his thumbnail
also has longitudinal ridges and white spots. In addition, his chest and lung
reflexes are discoloured. You may recall that Martin has had a very ill child,
moved homes and jobs a number of times, struggled financially and
separated from his partner all in the last few years. Two months ago he also
tore the deltoid muscles in his left arm and, despite having physiotherapy,
they are not healing. Understandably, he is suffering from depression.

All of the above suggest disharmony in the lung meridian. The lung
meridian runs from the clavicle, down the arm (through the deltoid
muscles) to the thumb and is associated with grief and sadness.

When Martin came for his reflexology treatments, I gave him full treatments that worked his entire body. In addition, I spent time working the different reflexes that showed themselves as unbalanced (these differed over the weeks). Before ending each treatment I would spend some time working the lung acupoints on his thumbs and also spent extra time working his lung reflexes. Note that I referred Martin to a counsellor for his depression and contacted his doctor before beginning a course of reflexology treatments.

How to use the following diagrams

Over the next few pages you will find a brief introduction to the different meridians of the body and the focus of this information will be on using the meridians as part of your reflexology treatment. The diagrams show the meridians on the body. The solid lines are the meridians that are found on the body and the broken lines are the meridians inside the body. Some of the diagrams include triangles and these show where the meridian being depicted passes through other meridians. To make it easier, the diagrams show the meridian on one side of the body only. Please be aware that, except for the Governing and Conception vessels which go through the centre of the body, the meridians are actually bilateral and what is shown on one side of the body will be the same on the other.

The two extraordinary vessels

The two extraordinary vessels act as reservoirs of Qi for the twelve major meridians, filling and emptying as required. They form a central circuit along the midline of the body and influence the twelve major meridians.

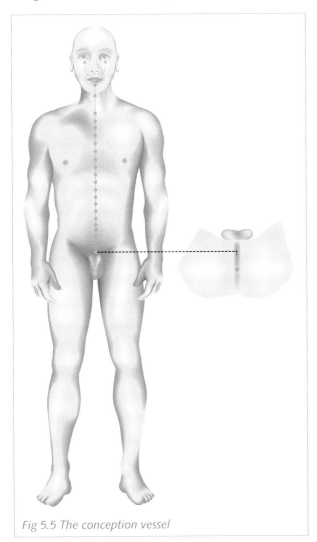

Fig 5.5 The conception vessel

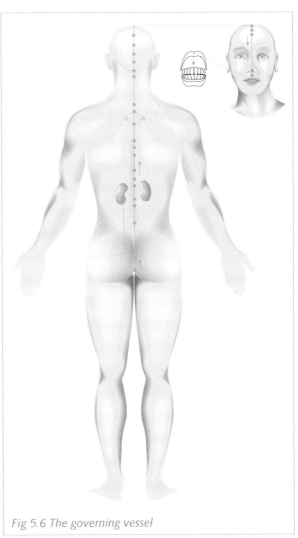

Fig 5.6 The governing vessel

The two extraordinary vessels are the:

- **Conception Vessel, yin** – this starts midway between the anus and the genitals, runs in a straight line up the front of the body and ends at the midline below the lower lip. It plays a vital role in one's ability to reproduce and influences the yin meridians of the body.
- **Governing Vessel, yang** – this starts midway between the coccyx and the anus and runs straight up the midline of the back, over the head and ends on the inside of the mouth at the junction of the gum and upper lip. It governs the yang meridians of the body.

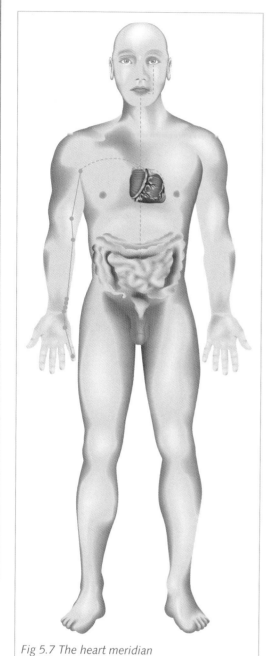

Fig 5.7 The heart meridian

The fire element

The heart meridian
Yin (11am–1pm)

'The Heart rules the Blood and Blood Vessels'[6] (Kaptchuk) and disharmony in this meridian can show as heart disease and palpitations. In addition, 'The Heart stores the Shen (Spirit)'[7] (Kaptchuk) and disharmony can result in fatigue, insomnia, forgetfulness, excessive dreaming, nervous tension and chronic stress. A person suffering from weak heart Qi may tire easily, suffer from mental fatigue and have a poor appetite. Excessive heart Qi, on the other hand, can show as tension in the heart/chest region or a tightness in the solar plexus region, sweaty palms and an overall stiffness in the body. 'The person with excess heart energy is always doing something with his or her hands – adjusting the pants or shirt, touching the face, playing with the hair'[8] (Ohashi).

'The Heart opens into the tongue'[9] (Kaptchuk) and inflammation or ulcers of the tongue or a discolouration of the face (very pale or unusually purple face) reflect disharmony in the heart meridian. The heart is also associated with the emotion of joy and a lack of heart Qi results in a sense of disappointment, lack of will and a poor appetite for life while excessive heart Qi can be seen in 'bouts of hysteria, laughing or crying wildly'[10] (Ohashi).

The heart meridian starts in the centre of the armpit, passes down the inside of the arm and ends on the base of the little finger, on the inside edge. When assessing this meridian, in addition to visible skin conditions, also be aware of swollen glands or pain in the armpits, forearm stiffness, weak wrists and problems with the little finger. The muscle connected to the heart meridian is the subscapularis.

Study tip

Some heart conditions are contra-indicated to reflexology so double-check your contraindications before treating someone with a heart problem.

The small intestine meridian
Yang (1pm–3pm)

The small intestine separates the pure from the impure. On a physical level, it is responsible for absorbing nutrients from the food while on a psychological level it separates the necessary emotions and thoughts from the unnecessary.

Disharmony in the small intestine can result in digestive problems such as abdominal pain, intestinal rumblings, diarrhoea or constipation. Weak small intestine Qi can show itself as malnutrition, anaemia, lower back ache, chronic fatigue, headaches/migraines or chronic menstrual problems in women. Excessive small-intestine Qi can result in poor circulation to the extremities or bladder problems.

In the words of the Shiatsu practitioner Ohashi, 'There is no more important role in our lives than to see what is of value in our environment and make use of it.'[11] People suffering with weak small intestine Qi tend to think too much, suffer from anxiety and are often deeply sad. On the other hand, people with excessive small intestine Qi work too long and have trouble relaxing.

The small intestine meridian starts at the outer edge of the little finger at the base of the nail, runs up the outside of the arm, zig-zags up the back of the shoulder, ascends up the side of the neck, onto the cheek, to the outer corner of the eye and ends in front of the small piece of cartilage which forms the front part of the ear. Assess this meridian for any stiffness and pain or skin conditions along the meridian pathway and pay particular attention to problems with the little finger, tennis elbow, shoulder tension, swollen glands in the throat, trigeminal neuralgia in the face and ear problems.

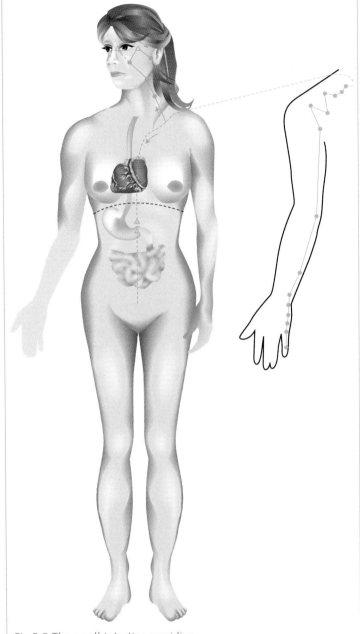

Fig 5.8 The small intestine meridian

The muscles associated with the small intestine meridian are the quadriceps and abdominals. Note that the fire element actually has four meridians while the other elements have only two meridians each.

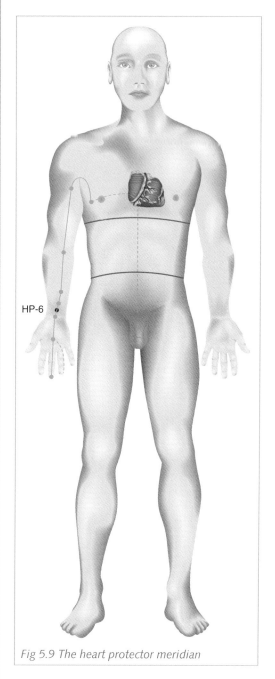

HP-6

Fig 5.9 The heart protector meridian

The heart protector meridian (heart constrictor, pericardium or circulation meridian)
Yin (7pm–9pm)

The heart protector meridian is the 'outer protective shield of the Heart'[12] (Kaptchuk) and has a similar function to the heart meridian. Problems related to this meridian are similar to those of the heart meridian.

The heart protector meridian starts on the chest on the lateral side of the nipple in the space between the 4th and 5th ribs, ascends into the armpit and then runs down the medial aspect of the arm to end at the centre on the tip of the middle finger. Assess the pathway of this meridian for any skin conditions, muscular weakness, tension or pain and be particularly aware of problems in the armpits or elbow crease, carpal tunnel syndrome, hot palms or problems with the middle finger or its nail.

The muscles related to the heart protector meridian are the gluteus minimus and maximus, the adductors and the piriformis.

Practical tip

The sea-sickness bands commonly used for nausea actually work on a point on the heart protector meridian. This point is called HP-6 or PE-6 (Heart Protector/Pericardium 6) and is located on the inside of the wrist, two thumb-widths above the wrist crease. Applying pressure to this point can help with nausea as well as heart, liver, stomach or menstrual disorders. In addition, it is a vital point for calming the mind in times of shock or stress.

The triple burner meridian (triple heater/warmer or endocrine meridian)
Yang (9pm–11pm)

'The triple burner is not exactly an organ, but a relationship between various organs … This meridian governs activities involving all the organs and unites the respiratory, digestive and excretory systems'[13] (Dougans). Disharmony in this meridian results in sensitivity to changes in temperature and humidity and a person with insufficient triple burner Qi will catch colds easily, have tired eyes, low blood pressure and sensitive skin and be prone to allergies. Excessive triple burner Qi shows itself as poor circulation, lymphatic problems and excess mucous.

Psychologically, people with disharmony in the triple heater meridian tend to be obsessive and highly sensitive.

The triple burner meridian starts at the outside of the fourth (ring) finger at the base of the nail, runs up the lateral aspect of the arm, over the shoulder to the ear and then ends on the outside tip of the eyebrow. When reading this meridian be aware of disorders of the fourth finger and its nail, shoulder problems, ear problems and pain in the corner of the eye as well as any skin disorders or muscular stiffness along the meridian pathway.

The muscles associated with the triple burner meridian are the teres minor, sartorius, gracilis, soleus and gastrocnemius.

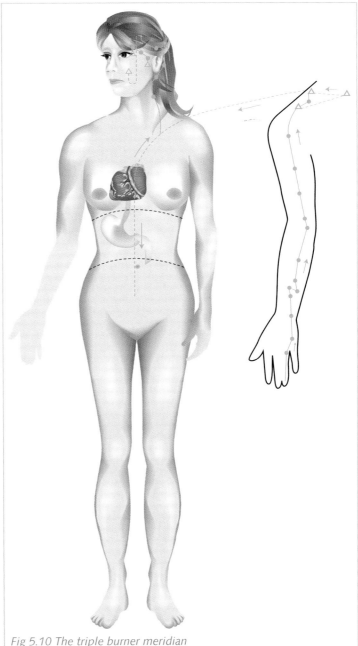

Fig 5.10 The triple burner meridian

The fire element: Self-help
Avoid spicy foods, excess fat in the diet, too much salt and the excessive consumption of animal products (including red meats, dairy food and eggs). 'The heart and small intestine function are further enhanced by an optimistic attitude about life. Faith and gratitude stimulate joy.'[14] (Ohashi)

237

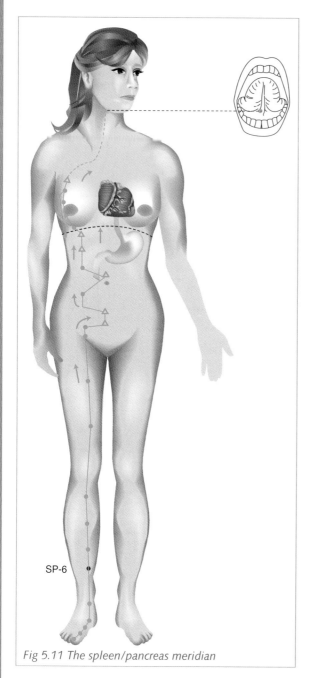

Fig 5.11 The spleen/pancreas meridian

SP-6

The earth element

The spleen/pancreas meridian
Yin (9am–11am)

The spleen meridian plays a central role in transformation and transportation. It is the source of sufficient Blood and Qi in the body and, 'for the Chinese, it is the primary organ of digestion' [15] (Kaptchuk). Disharmony in the spleen meridian can result in digestive disorders such as abdominal bloating, pain, diarrhoea or eating disorders. The spleen also governs the blood and disharmony in this meridian can result in bleeding disorders such as blood in the stool, vomiting blood, severe bruising and abnormally heavy menstrual bleeding. In addition, 'The spleen rules the muscles, flesh, and the four limbs' [16] (Kaptchuk). Thus, disharmony can manifest as problems with the muscles. The spleen also opens into the mouth and disorders of the mouth, such as pale lips, a lack of saliva or an insensitivity to taste, can be due to an imbalance in this meridian.

Insufficient spleen Qi manifests itself in poor digestion, susceptibility to colds, pain along the spine and poor circulation in the feet while excessive spleen Qi can result in a chronic craving for sweets and the subsequent mood and energy fluctuations that accompany excessive sweet eating. Compassion and sympathy are the emotions connected to the spleen.

The spleen meridian starts on the medial side of the big toe at the base of the nail, ascends up the leg, through the reproductive organs and abdomen, and through the chest where it ends 6 thumb widths below the armpit, between the 6th and 7th ribs. In addition to looking for skin disorders and muscular stiffness or pain along the pathway of this meridian, pay particular attention to the big toe. Bunions, fungal infections, ingrown toenails and stiffness all suggest disharmony in this meridian. The muscles connected to the spleen meridian are the latissimus dorsi, trapezius, extensor pollicis longus and triceps.

Practical tip

There is a vital point on the spleen meridian that helps with gynaecological problems and lower abdominal pain. It is also an important point for calming the mind. This point is called SP-6 and is where all three yin meridians of the legs (the spleen, liver and kidney meridian) coincide. SP-6 is found four finger-widths above the medial malleolus on the posterior edge of the tibia. Work this point for any menstrual or reproductive disorders and also if a woman is struggling to conceive. **NB** SP-6 is also used for uterine contractions and so is **contraindicated during pregnancy**.

The stomach meridian
Yang (7am–9am)

'I believe disharmony in the stomach to be the root cause of all disease in the body. The quality of the food ingested goes hand in hand with the quality of life you enjoy. If the fuel is faulty, the functions of the organs will be faulty and disease will be the ultimate result.' Inge Dougans[17]

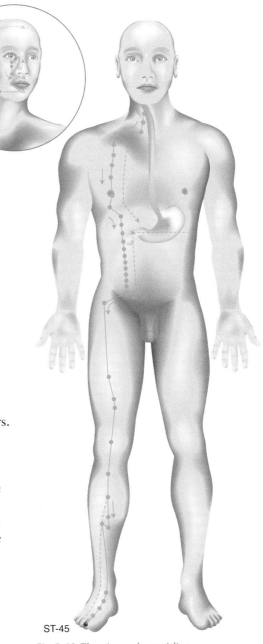

'The Stomach is responsible for 'receiving' and 'ripening' ingested food and fluids'[18] (Kaptchuk) and disharmony with this meridian reflects as stomach problems such as nausea, stomach ache, bloating and belching. According to Ohashi, 'The stomach is one of those organs that we cannot ignore. Any stomach problem tends to disturb us, and chronic stomach ills disturb us throughout the day.'[19]

A person with weak stomach Qi can suffer from fatigue, heavy legs, lack of appetite, gastric discomfort and digestive problems such as constipation or diarrhoea. On the other hand, a person with excessive stomach Qi may overeat, or sometimes have minimal appetite, suffer with shoulder tension, poor circulation, dry skin and reproductive disorders.

Disharmony in the stomach meridian also results in over-thinking, moodiness, frustration and emotional extremes.

The stomach meridian penetrates all the major organs of the body. It starts just above the lower edge of the eye socket in line with the pupil and traverses the nose, jaw and forehead. A branch then descends through the abdomen and down the front of the leg before ending on the outside edge of the second toe at the base of the nail. Assess this meridian for birthmarks, skin conditions, muscular stiffness or pain and disorders of the organs it passes through. In addition, pay particular attention to the second toe, looking for toenail problems, fungal infections and bent or misshapen toes. Because this meridian traverses the nose, jaw and forehead be aware of any mouth or facial problems as well.

The muscles related to the stomach meridian are the pectoralis major, levator scapulae, the anterior neck flexors and the brachioradialis.

ST-45

Fig 5.12 The stomach meridian

The earth element: Self-help
The earth element is negatively affected by refined sugar and acidic foods while it is positively influenced by all vegetables. The way in which we eat our food is very important for this element – food should be eaten slowly and chewed well.

Practical tip
Acupoint ST-45 is known as the 'sick mouth'[20] and working this point will help with any problems of the mouth. ST-45 is located on the lateral side of the second toe at the base of the nail bed.

Meridian therapy

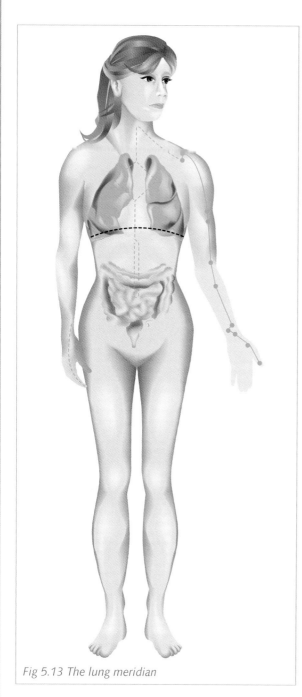

Fig 5.13 The lung meridian

The metal element

The lung meridian
Yin (3am–5am)

'In Oriental medicine, we say that the inhalation of oxygen is the taking in of ki, or life force ... When the lungs are not working properly, therefore, our ability to take in life is diminished.' Ohashi[21]

'The Lungs rule Qi'[22] (Kaptchuk) and govern the intake and elimination of pure Qi. In addition, 'The lungs rule the exterior of the body'[23] (Kaptchuk), specifically the skin, hair and sweat glands. A person with disharmony in the lungs may suffer from constant coughs and colds, respiratory disorders, excessive or inefficient sweating and may lack lustre in their hair and skin. If lung energy is depleted, the person tends to be overweight, have poor circulation, suffer from constant coughs and colds and from anxiety, depression or hypersensitivity. If lung energy is excessive, the person will tend to suffer from respiratory problems such as bronchitis or asthma, nasal congestion and hard coughing that brings up mucous. They may also tend to be obsessive and anxious over small details. Many common nose and throat disorders can also be linked to the lungs as can the emotions of grief and sadness.

The lung meridian starts in the space between the first and second rib near the shoulder and runs along the inside of the arm to the edge of the thumb where it ends at the base of the nail, close to the index finger. Visible disorders such as discolouration, a rash, infection, mole or blemish along this meridian may suggest a lung imbalance. Also be aware of a stiff forearm, wrist disorders such as carpal tunnel syndrome and problems with the thumb or thumbnail.

Muscles associated with the lungs are the serratus anterior, coracobrachialis, deltoids and diaphragm.

The large intestine meridian
Yang (5am–7am)

The large intestine eliminates waste from the body, both physical and mental/emotional. It also absorbs water. Disharmony in this meridian reflects as diarrhoea, constipation and abdominal pain or, emotionally, as the inability to let go of unnecessary emotions. The large intestine is coupled with the lungs and if they are not healthy there is a tendency to hold on to grief and sadness. In addition, disharmony in the large intestine reflects in lung and sinus problems.

The large intestine meridian starts on the outer edge of the index finger at the base of the nail and runs along the outer part of the arm to the face, ending at the outside edge of the nostril. Look for visible disorders along this meridian and also take note of any arthritis or pain in the index finger, a stiff forearm, tennis elbow, frozen shoulder, pain in the trapezius muscle, cold sores on the lips or problems with the nose. Muscles associated with the large intestine are the tensor fasciae latae, hamstrings and quadratus lumborum.

The metal element: Self-help
Aerobic exercise is vital to the health of the lungs and large intestine and diet also needs to be examined. Foods rich in vitamin C, such as citrus fruits and green peppers, have been found to be particularly beneficial for the muscles associated with the lung and large intestine meridians. Fibre, in the form of brown rice, wholegrains and vegetables, benefits the metal element and supports the functioning of the large intestine. Red meat is difficult to digest for people with large intestine imbalances and dairy products and fried foods should also be avoided if there is a lung imbalance.

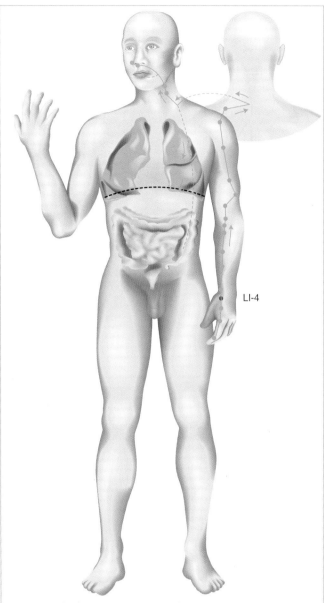

Fig 5.14 The large intestine meridian

Practical tip
The 'Great Eliminator' is probably one of the best-known acupoints in the West. It is called LI-4 and is found on the hands high up in the valley formed between the thumb and forefinger and is commonly used to relieve a headache. Working this point strengthens the digestive system and 'eliminates' waste from the body. It is, therefore, useful for constipation, diarrhoea, headaches, allergies and colds. Note that this point is **contraindicated during pregnancy**.

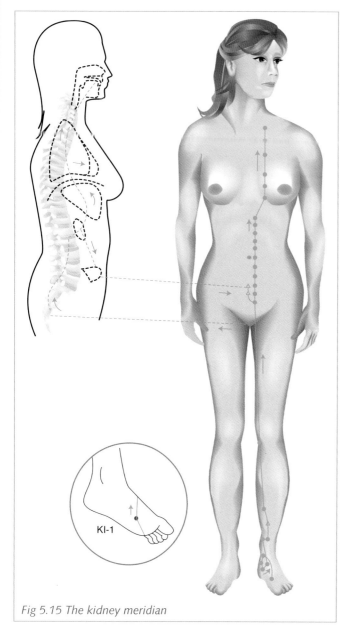

Fig 5.15 The kidney meridian

The water element

The kidney meridian

Yin (5pm–7pm)

The kidneys are vital to the health of the entire body, especially the processes of reproduction, development and maturation. Thus, disharmony in the kidney meridian can be reflected in reproductive problems such as infertility or impotence as well as developmental disorders such as a lack of maturation or premature ageing. The kidneys help regulate water in the body and a kidney imbalance can show itself as oedema or water retention. They are also the 'root of Qi'[24] and influence the respiratory system so problems such as chronic asthma can be linked to disharmony in this meridian. In addition, the kidneys rule the bones and problems with the development and repair of bones, including weak or brittle bones, or stiffness along the spine are associated with disharmony in the meridian. The kidneys also influence the ears and the hair and hearing problems and balding can be linked to them. The kidneys are also associated with fear and courage.

The kidney meridian starts at the inferior aspect of the small toe, runs through the sole of the foot (at the solar plexus reflex), then up the medial side of the leg and through the abdomen. It ends in the depression on the lower edge of the collarbone, two thumb widths from the midline. Look for visible disorders along this meridian such as skin conditions, burning/ painful sensations in the soles of the feet, varicose veins, eczema and fungal infections as well as muscular aches and pains. The muscles associated with the kidney meridian are the psoas, upper trapezius and iliacus.

The water element: Self-help

The water element is enhanced through the consumption of beans, barley and buckwheat as well as small amounts of salt. Excess salt, however, can have a negative effect on the kidneys and bladder.

Practical tip

The first point on the kidney meridian, KI-1, is known as 'the bubbling spring' and is one of the most vital points in acupressure. It is located in the same place as the solar plexus reflex and it helps with acute problems such as shock or palpitations. It is also an essential point to work if a woman is trying to conceive or if a client suffers from fatigue. This point needs to be worked firmly as it is located deep within the foot.

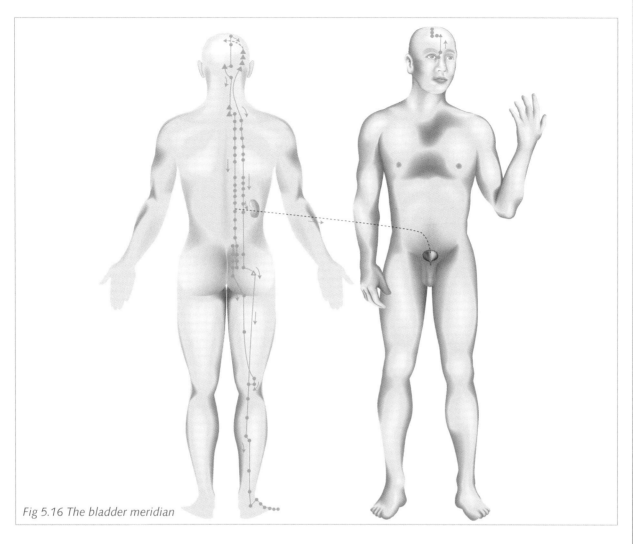

Fig 5.16 The bladder meridian

The bladder meridian
Yang (3pm–5pm)

The bladder receives and excretes urine and helps to maintain normal fluid levels within the body. In addition to affecting the urinary tract, it also influences the autonomic nervous system, hormonal system and sex organs. Depleted bladder energy can result in urinary problems such as incontinence, burning urination or difficulty urinating as well as poor circulation, problems with the sex organs and night sweats. On the other hand, excessive energy in this meridian can be seen in neck stiffness, migraine headaches, heaviness in the eyes and head, frequent urination or an inflamed prostate gland. This meridian is associated with fear and imbalances can reflect as timidity, nervousness and over-sensitivity.

The bladder meridian is the longest meridian in the body. It starts on the inner corner of the eye and ascends over the forehead, down the back running parallel to the spine, then down the back of the leg and ending at the outer edge of the little toe. Assess this meridian by starting with the eyes, looking for eye problems, redness or itchiness. Then work down the meridian looking for headaches and sinus pain (specifically in the forehead), hair loss, neck tension, pain and stiffness along the spine, coolness along the spine and buttocks, haemorrhoids, tightness in the back of the legs, sciatica, varicose veins, weak ankles, athlete's foot (between toes 4 and 5) and problems with the little toes or their nails. The muscles associated with the bladder meridian are the peroneus, sacrospinalis and tibialis anterior.

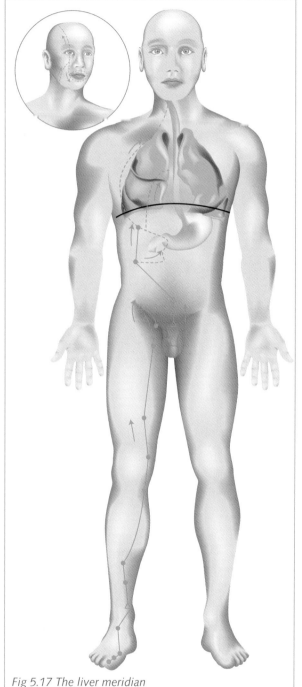

Fig 5.17 The liver meridian

The wood element

The liver meridian
Yin (1am–3am)

'In the Orient, we say that the liver is the seat of the soul.' Ohashi[25]

The liver 'maintains evenness and harmony of movement throughout the body. Words such as soft, subtle, light, and gentle begin to characterise the desirable state of the Liver.' Ted J. Kaptchuk[26]

The liver meridian is responsible for the smooth movement of Qi and blood in the body and affects many systems and structures, especially the digestive system, the muscles and tendons, the eyes and the nails. It is also a meridian that is easily prone to stagnation. Disharmony in this meridian can be seen in digestive problems such as loss of appetite, abdominal pain, bloating, nausea, belching, flatulence and diarrhoea. Disorders related to bile, for example, a bitter taste in the mouth and jaundice, can also be related to the liver meridian. The liver meridian opens into the eyes and so is implicated in many eye disorders such as dry eyes. This meridian also 'rules the tendons and is manifest in the nails'[27] (Kaptchuk) and disharmony in the liver can be reflected in thin, brittle, pale nails or muscular spasms, numbness and a difficulty in bending and stretching. In addition, the liver meridian encircles the genitals and disorders in this region, such as premenstrual tension, ovarian cysts, impotence or prostate problems, can sometimes also be related to this meridian.

The liver is related to the emotion of anger. If liver Qi is weak, a person may tire easily, suffer from dizzy spells and become irritable, inconsistent and anger easily. However, if liver Qi is excessive, a person may become a workaholic and obsessive. Such people tend to drink alcohol excessively, to be stubborn, aggressive, hyper-sensitive and prone to anger and emotional outbursts.

The liver meridian starts on the lateral edge of the big toe at the base of the nail, ascends up the medial aspect of the leg, encircles the genitals, ascends through the abdomen and ends between the 6th and 7th ribs, just below the nipple. Look for visible signs along this meridian such as an ingrown toenail or fungal nail infection on the big toe, muscular pain or skin disorders along the meridian, genital/reproductive problems or digestive disorders. Also be aware of any emotional outbursts, uncontrolled anger, aggression or hypersensitivity in your client. The muscles associated with the liver meridian are the pectoralis major and rhomboids.

The gallbladder meridian
Yang (11pm–1am)

The gallbladder stores and secretes bile and is closely linked to the liver meridian – disharmony in one meridian will affect the other. Bile plays an important role in the digestion of fats and disharmony in the gallbladder meridian results in poor digestion. Weak energy in this meridian can lead to poor sleep, dizziness, mucous in the eyes and an acid stomach. Excessive energy can reflect in a bitter taste in the mouth, yellowing eyes, migraines, constipation or stiff muscles.

The gallbladder rules decision-making and a person with weak gallbladder Qi can tend to suffer from repressed anger, nervous tension, timidity and an inability to make decisions. On the other hand, a person suffering from excessive gallbladder Qi can push themselves too hard, over-think and over-plan things and be impatient.

The gallbladder affects the tendons. It starts in the small depression at the outer corner of the eye. It traverses 'almost the entire body except the arms. It zig-zags throughout the head in a pattern which, in times of stress and tension, becomes like a vice and is therefore important in cases of headaches, neck tension and 'uptightness"[28] (Dougans). It then descends through the chest and abdomen, down the lateral side of the leg and ends at the outer edge of toe 4 at the base of the nail. When assessing this meridian, be aware of eye disorders, headaches/migraines, jaw problems, a bitter taste in the mouth, and shoulder tension as well as any visible disorders along the meridian pathway. Also look for athlete's foot, fungal toenail infections, corns or hammer toe of the fourth toe in particular.

The muscles related to the gallbladder meridian are the anterior fibres of the deltoid muscle and the popliteus.

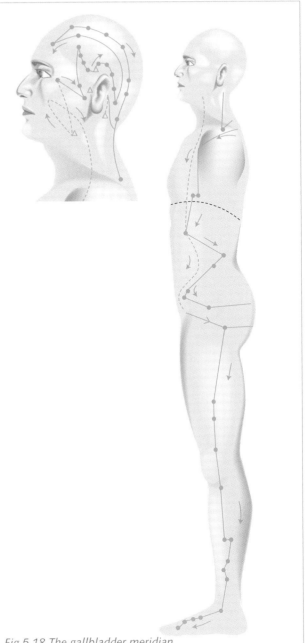

Fig 5.18 The gallbladder meridian

The wood element: Self-help
It is very important to look after the liver and gallbladder by avoiding greasy foods, excess fat, caffeine and alcohol. Vegetable-based sources of vitamin A such as carrots, parsley and yellow or green vegetables, are thought to help with the muscles related to the wood element.

Study Outline

Yin and Yang
- Yin and yang are two interdependent forces of nature that form the basis of all existence.
- Yin is the earth, night, female, cold, dark, wet and inactive.
- Yang is the heaven, day, male, warm, light, dry and active.

The Five Elements
- Yin and yang can be subdivided into the five elements as reflected in nature. These elements interact in a creative cycle.
- The five elements are fire, earth, metal, water and wood.

Qi and The Fundamental Substances of the Body
- Qi is our life force or life energy.
- Jing is the essence/substance that underlies all life.
- Shen is the spirit within a person.
- Blood and the Fluids moisten and nourish all parts of the body.

The meridians
- Qi circulates throughout the body in 12 major meridians and two extraordinary vessels.
- Each of these meridians is aligned to a specific element, paired with a partner meridian and is either yin or yang:

YIN	ELEMENT	YANG
Heart	Fire	Small intestine
Heart protector	Fire	Triple burner
Spleen	Earth	Stomach
Lungs	Metal	Large intestine
Kidneys	Water	Bladder
Liver	Wood	Gallbladder

- Please review the diagrams on pages 233–245 when learning the meridians.

Multiple choice questions

1. A male client comes to you with gout in his big toe, impotence and digestive disorders. When taking a consultation you learn that he drinks alcohol excessively and eats a diet of mainly red meats and fried foods. You also notice that he is quite an irritable person and after chatting to him for a while you learn that he struggles to control his temper and is prone to outbursts of uncontrollable anger. Which of the following reflexes do you think would most benefit your client if it were worked on in addition to your normal reflexology treatment?
   a. The kidneys
   b. The large intestine
   c. The liver
   d. The spleen.

2. When assessing a meridian pathway, which of the following visible signs would you look for?
   a. Moles
   b. Eczema
   c. Fungal infections
   d. All of the above.

3. A pregnant woman comes to you for reflexology treatments. Which of the following acupoints is contraindicated?
   a. Spleen 6
   b. Pericardium 6
   c. Liver 1
   d. None of the above.

4. On which of the following would you find the kidney meridian?
   a. Big toe
   b. Thumb
   c. Little finger
   d. Little toe.

5. On which of the following would you find the lung meridian?
   a. Thumb
   b. Middle finger
   c. Fourth toe
   d. Little toe.

6. Which of the following meridians is related to the wood element?
   a. Lungs
   b. Spleen
   c. Liver
   d. Pericardium.

7. Which of the following meridians is yin?
   a. Small intestine
   b. Heart
   c. Triple burner
   d. Stomach.

8. The acupoint KI-1, or bubbling spring, is located on which reflexology reflex?
   a. Bladder
   b. Kidney
   c. Solar plexus
   d. Pituitary.

9. Which meridian is the lung meridian partnered with?
   a. Liver
   b. Large intestine
   c. Bladder
   d. Heart.

10. What is the Chinese term for 'life force'?
    a. Qi
    b. Shen
    c. Jing
    d. Blood.

6 Diseases and disorders

Reflexology is a holistic therapy that treats a person rather than a disease and every treatment should involve a thorough working of all the reflexes of the body as well as the reworking of any reflexes that are found to be out of balance or congested.

However, sometimes it helps to have a basic understanding of certain diseases and disorders so that you can, in addition to giving a full treatment, spend some extra time focusing on reflexes that will deepen the effects of your treatment. In this chapter you will find suggestions for reflexes that can be worked for some specific diseases and disorders. Please be aware that these are only suggestions and that there are many different approaches to treatments.

Please also be aware that this chapter should not, in any way, be used to diagnose a condition. Reflexologists are not medically trained and should not diagnose conditions or attempt to treat them in the place of conventional medical treatment.

Study tip

If you forget everything else, try to remember the following:

- If there is pain, work the brain
- If there is inflammation, work the adrenals
- If there is mucous, work the ileocaecal valve
- If there is stress, work the solar plexus and diaphragm
- If there are toxins or waste, work the organs of elimination (lungs, liver, kidneys, large intestine, lymphatics and skin)
- If there is infection, work the lymphatics, liver and spleen

Diseases and disorders of the musculo-skeletal system

Arthritis – Osteoarthritis

Degenerative joint disease caused by ageing and wear-and-tear. Characterised by deterioration of articular cartilage and formation of spurs in joint cavity. Symptoms include pain, swelling and limited range of movement. Common in the elderly and often in weight-bearing joints such as the knees and hips.

Direct reflex
Reflex of area affected. For example, if osteoarthritis is in the client's right knee then the right knee will be the direct reflex.

Associated reflexes
- Adrenals
- Brain
- Thyroid/Parathyroids
- Solar plexus
- Organs of elimination and lymphatics
- Relaxation techniques to improve circulation

Comment
Be aware of any arthritis in client's feet or hands and adjust your pressure and techniques so that you do not hurt them. If client is on anti-inflammatory medication treat the stomach reflex as well.

Arthritis – Rheumatoid

Autoimmune disease in which the body attacks its own cartilage and joint lining. Synovial membrane becomes inflamed, thickens and produces abnormal granulation tissue that erodes joint's cartilage, thus exposing bone ends. Exposed bone ends are then joined by fibrous tissue which ossifies and renders joint immovable. Symptoms include inflammation, pain and loss of function. Thought to be hereditary and can affect any age group. Often in smaller joints of the hands and feet and always bilateral.

Reflexes
As for osteoarthritis

Bursitis

Inflammation of a bursa. Can be caused by overuse, irritation, injury, gout, arthritis or infection. Symptoms include inflammation, pain and limited movement.

Direct reflexes
Reflex of area affected

Associated reflexes
- Adrenals
- Organs of elimination and lymphatics
- Relaxation techniques to improve circulation

Cramp

Sudden, painful contraction of muscle or group of muscles. Can result from low blood levels of electrolytes, muscular fatigue, poor posture, stress or exercising immediately after eating.

Direct reflex
Reflex of area affected

Associated reflexes
- Thyroid/Parathyroids
- Adrenals
- Brain
- Solar plexus
- Diaphragm
- Relaxation techniques to improve circulation

Frozen Shoulder

Inflammation of shoulder joint. Characterised by chronic, painful stiffness. Can be caused by injury, a stroke or can develop slowly for no apparent reason.

Direct reflex
Shoulder

Associated reflexes
- Neck
- Spine (especially cervical spine)
- Adrenals
- Brain
- Relaxation techniques to improve circulation

Ganglion Cyst

Fluid-filled growth that usually develops near joints or tendon sheaths on hands or feet. Cause unknown.

Direct reflex
Reflex of area affected

Associated reflexes
Relaxation techniques to improve circulation

Comment
Ganglion cysts can be removed surgically or sometimes disappear over time. Reflexology is not known to affect them.

Golfer's Elbow (Medial Epicondylitis/Forehand Tennis Elbow)

Damage to tendons that bend the wrist toward the palm, located on inside of elbow. Symptoms include pain on palmar side of forearm. Can be caused by movements that bend wrist towards palm with excessive force. For example, certain golf swings, tennis swerves, javelin throws or carrying heavy suitcases.

Direct reflex
Elbow

Associated reflexes
- Shoulder
- Arm and hand
- Neck
- Cervical spine
- Adrenals
- Brain
- Relaxation techniques to improve circulation

Gout

Build-up of uric acid and its salts in blood and joints. Crystals accumulate in, irritate and erode cartilage of joints causing bones to fuse and become immovable. Symptoms include inflammation, pain, tenderness and loss of mobility. Occurs mainly in middle-aged and older males and can be caused by diet, abnormal genes or environmental factors such as stress.

Direct reflex
Reflex of area affected. Note, if the big toe is affected then work the corresponding thumb reflex and do not apply direct pressure to the toe itself.

Associated reflexes
- Adrenals
- Brain
- Kidneys (and other organs of elimination)
- Thyroid/Parathyroids
- Lymphatics
- Relaxation techniques to improve circulation

Housemaid's Knee (Prepatellar Bursitis)

Bursitis of the knee often due to frequent kneeling – see *Bursitis* for more details.

Direct reflex
Knee

Associated reflexes
- Adrenals
- Kidneys
- Lymphatics
- Relaxation techniques to improve circulation

Kyphosis

Exaggerated curvature of thoracic spine. Characterised by hunched back, rounded shoulders and mild, persistent back pain. Common in the elderly or can be a result of rickets, osteoporosis or poor posture.

Direct reflex
Thoracic spine

Associated reflexes
- Entire spine
- Shoulders
- Neck
- Chest
- Diaphragm
- Adrenals
- Brain
- Relaxation techniques to improve circulation
- Thyroid/Parathyroids if caused by rickets or osteoporosis

Lordosis

Exaggerated curvature of lumbar spine. Characterised by sway back and lower back ache. Can be result of excess weight around abdomen, pregnancy, poor posture or rickets.

Direct reflex
Lumbar spine

Associated reflexes
- Entire spine
- Adrenals
- Brain
- Sciatic nerve
- Relaxation techniques to improve circulation
- Thyroid/Parathyroids if caused by rickets

Osteogenesis Imperfecta (Brittle Bone Disease)

Genetic disease of abnormally brittle bones. Characterised by frequent fracturing of bones, bone deformity, discolouration of sclera of eyes, translucent skin, possible deafness and thin dental enamel.

Direct reflex
Entire skeletal system

Associated reflexes
Full, general treatment

Comment
A person with osteogenesis imperfecta should be under the care of a doctor and be made aware that reflexology cannot cure or change the disorder. Its main benefit will be in relaxing the client and helping them cope with it.

Osteoporosis

Progressive disease in which bones lose their density and become brittle and prone to fractures. Common in elderly and post-menopausal women or women whose bodies produce inadequate levels of oestrogen.

Direct reflex
Entire skeletal system

Associated reflexes
- Thyroid/Parathyroids
- All endocrine and reproductive glands
- Relaxation techniques to improve circulation

Comment
Adapt pressure and techniques as person will have fragile bones.

Poliomyelitis

Contagious, viral infection of nervous system resulting in muscle weakness and sometimes paralysis.

Reflexology is contraindicated during the infectious stage. When a person is no longer infectious and is recovering from poliomyelitis, a full and general treatment is recommended.

Prolapsed (Slipped/Herniated) Intervertebral Disc (PID)

Tearing or rupture of covering of intervertebral disc. Results in disc's soft interior bulging out and compressing the accompanying spinal nerve. Often occurs if ligaments surrounding disc are injured or weakened. Symptoms include pain, numbness and weakness along affected nerve's pathway.

Direct reflex
Spine

Associated reflexes
- Entire musculo-skeletal system
- Adrenals
- Brain
- Relaxation techniques to improve circulation

Rheumatism

General term for aches and pains of muscles and joints. Can be caused by disorders such as arthritis or gout.

Direct reflex
Reflex of areas affected

Associated reflexes
- Entire musculo-skeletal system
- Adrenals
- Brain
- Lymphatics
- Organs of elimination
- Relaxation techniques to improve circulation

Scoliosis

Lateral curvature of the spine. Symptoms can include backache after sitting or standing for a long time. Can be hereditary or caused by poor posture, having one leg shorter than the other, paralysis of one side of the body or chronic sciatica.

Direct reflex
Spine

Associated reflexes
- Adrenals
- Brain
- Sciatic nerve
- Relaxation techniques to improve circulation

Synovitis

Inflammation of synovial membrane of joint. Symptoms include pain and swelling. Can be caused by rheumatic disease such as arthritis or injury or infection.

Direct reflex
Reflex of area affected

Associated reflexes
- Adrenals
- Brain
- Organs of elimination
- Relaxation techniques to improve circulation

Tendonitis

Inflammation of tendon. Symptoms include inflammation, pain and tenderness when moved or touched. Can be result of overuse or repetitive use, infection or another musculo-skeletal disorder.

Direct reflex
Reflex of area affected

Associated reflexes
- Entire musculo-skeletal system
- Adrenals
- Brain
- Relaxation techniques to improve circulation

Tennis Elbow (Lateral Epicondylitis/Backhand Tennis Elbow)

Damage to tendons of lateral, or outer border, of elbow. Symptoms include pain in elbow and on outer, back side of forearm. Can be caused by improper backhand tennis techniques, weak shoulder or wrist muscles or repetitive extension of wrist.

Direct reflex
Elbow

Associated reflexes
- Shoulder
- Arm and hand
- Neck
- Cervical spine
- Adrenals
- Brain
- Relaxation techniques to improve circulation

Tetanus (Lockjaw)

Infectious bacterial disease characterised by muscle stiffness, spasms and rigidity in jaw and neck. A person with tetanus needs to be treated by a doctor.

Whiplash

Damage to ligaments, vertebrae and occasionally spinal cord of neck. Usually caused by sudden jerking back of head and neck, for example in car accidents. Symptoms include pain and stiffness in neck and shoulder region.

Direct reflex
Neck and shoulders

Associated reflexes
- Whiplash helper reflex (see page 143)
- Entire musculo-skeletal system
- Adrenals
- Brain
- Relaxation techniques to improve circulation

Diseases and disorders of the nervous system

For disorders of the ears, eyes and skin please see Diseases and Disorders of the Special Senses and Integumentary System on page 270.

Alzheimer's Disease

Progressive degeneration of brain tissue. Symptoms vary but can include forgetfulness, confusion, disorientation, paranoia, hallucination and mood changes. Cause is unknown but usually affects the elderly and is a common cause of dementia.

Direct reflex
- Brain
- Spinal nerves

Associated reflexes
- Solar plexus
- Diaphragm

Comment
A full, general treatment will help with any minor problems associated with Alzheimer's Disease

Bell's Palsy

Sudden weakness or paralysis of muscles on one side of face due to malfunctioning of the facial nerve (cranial nerve VII). Symptoms include pain behind ear, weakening or paralysis of facial muscles on one side of face and sense of numbness. Cause can be unknown or result of infection.

Direct reflex
Face

Associated reflexes
- Cranial nerves
- Neck
- Cervical spine
- Solar plexus
- Diaphragm

Depression

Excessive feeling of sadness that can affect sleeping patterns, appetite and ability to concentrate. Causes vary but can include illness, side-effects of medication or traumatic events such as the loss of friends or loved ones.

Direct reflex
- Brain
- Spinal nerves

Associated reflexes
- Solar plexus
- Diaphragm
- All endocrine glands
- Full, general treatment with emphasis on any problematic areas

Epilepsy

Group of disorders of the brain characterised by seizures. These are short, recurrent, periodic attacks of motor, sensory or psychological malfunction. Cause is unknown but can result from head injury, brain tumour, stroke or can be triggered by stress, drugs, infections, fever, low blood sugar or physical or emotional stresses.

Direct reflex
Brain

Associated reflexes
- Cranial nerves
- Entire spine
- Solar plexus
- Diaphragm

Comment
Recommend therapist is trained in First Aid in case client has seizure.

Fainting (Syncope)

Sudden, temporary loss of consciousness. Caused by inadequate supply of oxygen and nutrients to the brain.

If a person faints regularly the cause of this fainting should be diagnosed by a doctor before they receive a reflexology treatment. The reflexes to be worked will then depend on this diagnosis.

Headache

Pain felt within the skull. Can vary in intensity, frequency and cause.

Direct reflex
Head/brain

Associated reflexes
- Sinuses
- Cranial nerves
- Neck
- Shoulders
- Spine
- Adrenal glands
- Solar plexus
- Diaphragm
- LI4 (The Great Eliminator) acupoint on hand

Insomnia

Disorder in which a person either cannot fall asleep, or cannot stay asleep for an adequate amount of time. May be a symptom of many different disorders including stress.

Direct reflex
Pineal

Associated reflexes
- All endocrine glands
- Brain
- Spine
- Solar plexus
- Diaphragm

Meningitis

Inflammation of the meninges that cover the brain and spinal cord. Symptoms include fever, headache, vomiting, weakness and stiff neck. Usually caused by bacterial or viral infection or can be allergic reaction to certain drugs.

A person with meningitis should be under the care of a doctor and should only receive reflexology when they are in the recovery stages of the disease.

Migraine

Severe, throbbing headache that usually affects one side of head and can last from a few hours to a few days. Symptoms include throbbing pain, nausea, vomiting, mood and behaviour changes. Often worsened by movement, light, sounds and smells.

Direct reflex
Head/brain

Associated reflexes
Work the same reflexes as for a headache and also:
- Eyes
- Liver
- Stomach
- Large intestine
- Pituitary

Motor Neurone Disease (MND)

Degeneration of the motor system. Characterised by progressive weakness and wasting away of muscles and eventual paralysis. Affects both skeletal and smooth muscles but does not affect the senses.

Direct reflex
- Brain
- Spine

Associated reflexes
- Entire musculo-skeletal system
- All endocrine glands
- Solar plexus

Multiple Sclerosis (MS)

Autoimmune disorder in which patches of myelin sheaths and underlying nerve fibres of the eyes, brain and spinal cord are damaged or destroyed. Nerve transmission is disrupted and symptoms include weakness, numbness, tremors, loss of vision, pain, fatigue, paralysis, loss of balance and loss of bladder and bowel function. Occurs in periods of relapses and remissions.

Direct reflex
- Brain
- Spine

Associated reflexes
- Entire musculo-skeletal system
- Thymus
- Adrenals
- Solar plexus
- Reflexes of areas affected (e.g. eyes, bladder or bowels)

Muscular Dystrophies

Group of inherited muscle-destroying diseases that lead to muscular weakness. Characterised by progressive atrophy of skeletal muscle due to degeneration of individual muscle fibres.

Direct reflex
Entire musculo-skeletal system

Associated reflexes
- Brain
- Spine
- Solar plexus
- Sciatic nerve
- Relaxation techniques to improve circulation

Neuralgia

Severe pain along nerve pathway. Generally characterised by stabbing or burning pains.

Direct reflex
Reflex area for nerve affected (e.g. work sciatic nerve if neuralgia is in legs or feet, arm reflex if it is in arms or hands, face reflex if it is in face, etc)

Associated reflexes
- Brain
- Spine
- Entire musculo-skeletal system
- Relaxation techniques to improve circulation

Pain and Referred Pain (Synalgia)

Pain is an unpleasant bodily sensation and is a reaction to injury, illness or harmful bodily contact such as heat. Referred pain is pain that is felt in a different part of the body to where it is produced. It arises because sensory nerves from different parts of the body often share nerve pathways in the spinal cord.

Direct reflex
Reflex for area affected

Associated reflexes
- Brain
- Adrenals
- Solar plexus

Comment
Refer your client to a doctor for a medical diagnosis of their pain.

Paralysis

Impairment or loss of motor nerve function. Symptoms vary from muscle weakness, spasticity or flaccidity to complete loss of function. Has many different causes.

Direct reflex
Reflex for area affected

Associated reflexes
- Brain
- Cranial nerve
- Spine
- Sciatic nerve if legs affected
- Relaxation techniques to improve circulation

Parkinson's Disease (PD)

Progressive disorder of the CNS thought to be due to an imbalance in neurotransmitter activity. Symptoms include tremors, rigidity, impaired motor performance and slow muscular movements.

Direct reflex
Brain

Associated reflexes
- Cranial nerves
- Spinal cord
- Entire musculo-skeletal system
- All endocrine glands
- Solar plexus
- Diaphragm

Sciatica

Inflammation of the sciatic nerve. Symptoms include pain, numbness or pins-and-needles down back of leg. Can be caused by lower back tension, herniated disc, osteoarthritis, diabetes or pregnancy.

Direct reflex
Sciatic nerve

Associated reflexes
- Brain
- Spine (especially lumbar and sacral)
- Entire musculo-skeletal system
- Relaxation techniques to improve circulation

Stress and tension

State caused by physical or mental demands which becomes problematic when people fail to manage it adequately. Stress can break down the body's defences, making it more susceptible to illness.

Direct reflex
Solar plexus

Associated reflexes
- Diaphragm
- Brain
- Cranial nerves
- Spine
- All endocrine glands
- Entire musculo-skeletal system
- HP-6 acupoint on wrist

Stroke (Cerebrovascular Accident/CVA)

Occurs when the arteries to the brain become blocked or rupture and brain tissue dies. Symptoms can include sudden weakness or paralysis of face and leg on one side of body, slurred speech, confusion, loss of balance and co-ordination and sudden severe headaches. Risk factors include old age, narrowing of arteries (artherosclerosis), high blood pressure, diabetes and smoking.

Direct reflex
Brain

Associated reflexes
- Cranial Nerves
- Spine
- Reflexes to areas affected
- Entire musculo-skeletal system
- Relaxation techniques to improve circulation

Diseases and disorders of the endocrine system

Addison's Disease

Disorder caused by hyposecretion of hormones by adrenal cortex. Symptoms include pigmentation, low blood pressure, weakness, tiredness and dizziness on standing. Thought to be an autoimmune disorder or caused by destruction of adrenal cortex by cancer or infection.

Direct reflex
Adrenals

Associated reflexes
- All endocrine glands
- Relaxation techniques to improve circulation of hormones

Cushing's Syndrome

Disorder caused by hypersecretion of hormones by adrenal cortex. Symptoms include fatigue and excessive fat deposits on face, torso and back. Face is usually large and round and skin bruises or tears easily. Causes include problems with either adrenal glands or pituitary gland.

Direct reflex
- Adrenals
- Pituitary

Associated reflexes
- All endocrine glands
- Relaxation techniques to improve circulation of hormones

Diabetes Insipidus

Excessive production of large amounts of very dilute urine. Characterised by excessive thirst and urination which can lead quickly to dehydration. Caused by lack of antidiuretic hormone produced by pituitary gland.

Direct reflex
Pituitary

Associated reflexes
- All endocrine glands
- Kidneys
- Relaxation techniques to improve circulation of hormones

Diabetes Mellitus

Disorder of high levels of glucose in blood. Symptoms include increased thirst and urination, weight loss, fatigue, nausea, vomiting, frequent infections and blurred vision. There are 2 types: **Type I Diabetes** (insulin dependent diabetes mellitus) is a hereditary autoimmune disorder in which the body destroys its own insulin producing cells. **Type II Diabetes** (non insulin dependent diabetes mellitus) is more common in overweight people or those who eat unhealthily. They may have normal insulin levels but their body cells are resistant or less sensitive to the insulin and their metabolism is therefore affected.

Direct reflex
Pancreas

Associated reflexes
- All endocrine glands
- Liver
- Relaxation techniques to improve circulation of hormones

Comment
Use only light pressure and do not give treatments longer than 20 minutes. Remember to work closely with your client's doctor.

Goitre

Enlarged thyroid gland caused by lack of dietary iodine. Note that goitre is often a symptom of other thyroid disorders.

Direct reflex
- Thyroid
- Thyroid helper

Associated reflexes
- Neck
- All endocrine glands
- Relaxation techniques to improve circulation of hormones

Myxoedema (Hypothyroidism)

Hyposecretion of thyroid hormones in adults. Characterised by swollen and puffy face, slow heart rate, low body temperature, sensitivity to cold, dry hair and dry skin, lethargy and weight gain. Causes vary.

Direct reflex
- Thyroid
- Thyroid helper

Associated reflexes
- All endocrine glands (especially pituitary)
- Relaxation techniques to improve circulation of hormones

Comment
Work with the client's doctor as their medication may need to be monitored and/or adjusted.

Seasonal Affective Disorder (SAD)

Increased secretion of melatonin by pineal gland that causes depression, lack of interest in one's usual activities, oversleeping and overeating. Usually occurs at onset of winter and thought to be caused by lack of sunlight.

Direct reflex
Pineal

Associated reflexes
- All endocrine glands
- Solar plexus
- Diaphragm
- Brain
- Cranial nerves
- Spine
- Relaxation techniques to improve circulation of hormones

Thyrotoxicosis (Hyperthyroidism)

Hypersecretion of thyroid hormones that causes a speeding up of vital body functions. Symptoms include rapid heartbeat, sweating, loss of weight, anxiety and intolerance to heat. Causes vary.

Direct reflex
- Thyroid
- Thyroid helper

Associated reflexes
- All endocrine glands (especially pituitary)
- Relaxation techniques to improve circulation of hormones

Comment
Work with the client's doctor as their medication may need to be monitored and/or adjusted.

Diseases and disorders of the respiratory system

Asthma

Chronic inflammatory disorder of respiratory system. Airways narrow in response to stimuli, resulting in coughing, difficulty breathing, wheezing and inability to exhale easily. Stimuli range from pollen and house dust mites to cold air and emotional upsets.

Direct reflex
- Lungs
- Trachea/bronchi

Associated reflexes
- Chest/intercostal reflexes on dorsum of foot
- Diaphragm
- Adrenals
- Ileocaecal valve
- Liver
- Spleen
- Lymphatics

Bronchitis

Inflammation of bronchi. Characterised by excessive mucous secretion, productive cough with sputum, wheezing and difficulty breathing. Causes vary from infection to exposure to irritants.

Direct reflex
- Lungs
- Trachea/bronchi

Associated reflexes
- Chest/intercostal reflexes on dorsum of foot
- Diaphragm
- Adrenals
- Ileocaecal valve
- Liver
- Spleen
- Lymphatics

Emphysema

Disintegration of alveolar walls that leaves large spaces in lungs which fill with air. Person is unable to exhale this air and is constantly exhausted from breathing out. Irreversible condition caused by cigarette smoke, air pollution or occupational exposure to industrial dust.

Direct reflex
Lungs

Associated reflexes
- Chest/intercostal reflexes on dorsum of foot
- Solar plexus
- Diaphragm
- Adrenals
- Liver
- Spleen
- Lymphatics

Hay fever

Seasonal allergy resulting from exposure to pollens and other airborne substances. Characterised by sneezing and itching of eyes, nose, roof of mouth and back of throat.

Direct reflex
Head (including face, nose, sinuses, mouth)

Associated reflexes
- Adrenals
- Ileocaecal valve
- Lungs
- Liver
- Spleen
- Lymphatics

Hyperventilation

Abnormally fast breathing when body is at rest. Characterised by dizziness, tingling sensations and tightness across chest.

Direct reflex
Solar plexus (on both hands and feet)

Associated reflexes
- Diaphragm
- Lungs
- Adrenals
- Brain
- HP-6 acupoint on wrist

Pharyngitis (Throat infection)

Infection of the pharynx (throat). Symptoms include sore throat, pain on swallowing and occasional earache. Can be caused by bacteria or virus and often accompanies common cold.

Direct reflex
Throat

Associated reflexes
- Thymus
- Liver
- Spleen
- Lymphatics

Pleurisy

Inflammation of pleura. Symptoms include chest pain, rapid and shallow breathing and referred pain to neck and shoulder. Causes vary and include bacterial or viral infection, injury, cancer, irritants, drug reactions or other diseases.

Direct reflex
Lungs

Associated reflexes
- Adrenals
- Solar plexus
- Diaphragm

- Liver
- Spleen
- Lymphatics

Pneumonia

Inflammation of lungs due to infection and inflammation of alveoli. Symptoms include sputum-producing cough, chest pain, chills, fever and shortness of breath. Can be caused by bacteria, viruses or fungi.

Direct reflex
Lungs

Associated reflexes
- Adrenals
- Solar plexus
- Diaphragm
- Liver
- Spleen
- Lymphatics

Pulmonary embolism

Blockage of pulmonary artery by embolus (material carried in blood, e.g. blood clot). Symptoms vary but generally characterised by sudden shortness of breath, rapid breathing and extreme anxiety. Usually caused by blood clot formed in a person who has kept still for a long time, such as due to prolonged bed rest or long aeroplane flight. A person with a pulmonary embolism should be under the care of a doctor.

Sinusitis

Inflammation of sinuses. Characterised by pain, tenderness and swelling over affected sinus as well as nasal congestion and post-nasal drip. Usually caused by allergy or infection.

Direct reflex
Sinuses

Associated reflexes
- Head (including face and nose)
- Ileocaecal valve
- Adrenals
- Chest/lung
- Lymphatics
- Liver
- Spleen

Tuberculosis (TB)

Contagious infectious disease caused by airborne bacteria. Can affect any organ of the body but usually affects the lungs. Bacteria destroy parts of lung tissue which is then replaced by fibrous connective tissue or nodular lesions called tubercles. Symptoms include coughing, night sweats, sense of malaise, decreased energy, loss of appetite and weight loss.

Reflexology is contraindicated during the infectious stage. When a person is no longer infectious and is recovering from tuberculosis, a full and general treatment is recommended with emphasis on the lungs, lymphatics, liver, thymus and spleen.

Whooping cough (Pertussis)

Contagious bacterial infection. Begins with mild cold-like symptoms and develops into severe coughing fits characterised by prolonged, high-pitched indrawn breath or whoop at end of them. Coughs also produce large amounts of thick mucous.

Reflexology is contraindicated during the infectious stage. When a person is no longer infectious and is recovering from whooping cough, a full and general treatment is recommended with emphasis on the ileocaecal valve, lungs, lymphatics, liver, thymus and spleen.

Diseases and disorders of the cardiovascular system

Anaemia

Reduction in oxygen-carrying capacity of blood characterised by reduced number of red blood cells or reduction of haemoglobin. Symptoms include fatigue, paleness, breathlessness on exertion, lowered resistance to infection, intolerance to cold. Causes include loss of blood, lack of iron or insufficient number of red blood cells. There are many different types of anaemia, the most common being iron-deficiency anaemia and pernicious anaemia. Iron-deficiency anaemia is due to loss of blood or lack of/malabsorption of dietary iron. Common in menstruating or pregnant women, infants and the elderly. Pernicious anaemia results from low levels of vitamin B12 (folic acid) due to low dietary levels of B12 or inability of stomach to produce instrinsic factor necessary for absorption of B12.

Direct reflex
- Spleen
- Liver

Associated reflexes
- All digestive reflexes
- Relaxation techniques to improve circulation

Aneurysm

Balloon-like swelling in wall of an artery. May be congenital or result of injury or infection. The Core Curriculum for Reflexology in the United Kingdom states: '*Reflexology improves, not increases, circulation. There are no recordings of an aneurysm being precipitated, or immediately preceded, by reflexology, whereas many treatments will have been given, in retrospect, to patients unknowingly having an aneurysm.*'[1]

Angina pectoris

Temporary sensation of chest pain that spreads to arms or jaw. Sometimes includes sensation of suffocating. Caused by lack of oxygen to heart muscle (usually due to coronary artery disease) and generally induced by exercise or emotional stress and relieved by rest.

A person with angina pectoris should be under the care of a doctor and treatment should only be given under their supervision. A full, general treatment may be given with emphasis on the heart reflex.

Arteriosclerosis

Hardening of arteries. Can be related to many different diseases.

Direct reflex
Heart

Associated reflexes
- Relaxation techniques to improve circulation
- Liver

Atheroma

Formation of fatty plaques and scar tissue in walls of arteries. Results in obstruction of blood flow and also increases risk of thrombosis.

Direct reflex
Heart

Associated reflexes

- Relaxation techniques to improve circulation
- Liver

Gangrene

Death and decay of tissue due to lack of blood supply. Can be caused by many conditions including diseases such as diabetes mellitus, injury, frostbite or severe burns.

Reflexology is contraindicated if a person has gangrene. He or she should be under the care of a doctor.

Heart Attack (Myocardial infarction)

Death of area of heart muscle due to interruption of blood supply to heart. Commonly caused by blood clot in coronary artery. Main symptom is severe pain in middle of chest, back, jaw or left arm. Pain is not alleviated by rest. Note that pain is not always felt. Other symptoms include sweating, nausea, shortness of breath, faintness and heavily pounding heart.

Person should be under the care of a doctor and treatment should only be given once their condition has stabilised. A full, general treatment may then be given with emphasis on the heart reflex, chest area, solar plexus, diaphragm, brain and spine.

Heart with artificial pacemaker fitted

Artificial pacemakers are small electronic devices that replace the heart's own, natural pacemaker. They are surgically implanted beneath the skin, usually below the collarbone, and connected to the heart by wires. They send small electrical currents into the heart to set its pace.

A full, general treatment may be given under the supervision of the client's doctor.

Hole in heart (Septal defect)

Congenital condition in which there is a hole in the partition between the left and right sides of the heart (septum). Results in abnormal blood flow with excessive amounts of blood flowing through the lungs. May lead to pulmonary hypertension or heart failure.

A person with a septal defect needs to be under the care of a doctor.

Hypertension

Abnormally high blood pressure (systolic higher than 140mm Hg and diastolic higher than 90 mm Hg or both). Risk factors include old age, obesity, poor diet, lack of exercise, stress, metabolic defects and genetics.

Direct reflex

Heart

Associated reflexes

- Kidneys
- Adrenals
- Brain
- Solar plexus

Comment

If person is on medication for hypertension then reflexology should be given with the doctor's consent and their medication should be monitored.

Hypotension

Abnormally low blood pressure causing dizziness and fainting. Other symptoms include shortness of breath and chest pain. Causes include heart disease, infections and excess fluid or blood loss.

Direct reflex

Heart

Associated reflexes

- Kidneys
- Adrenals
- Brain
- Solar plexus

Nosebleeds (Epistaxis)

Bleeding through the nose. Can be caused by nose picking, injury, as a side effect of aspirin or anticoagulant drugs, fever, high blood pressure or blood disorders. If person suffers with regular or unusually heavy nosebleeds they should see their doctor for a medical diagnosis.

Palpitations

Awareness of the heart beating. Causes include strenuous exercise or extremely emotional experiences.

Direct reflex

Heart

Associated reflexes

- Solar plexus
- Diaphragm
- HP-6 acupoint on wrist

Comment

If person is on medication for palpitations then doctor's consent is required.

Panic attack

Episode occurring during anxiety disorders. Symptoms include palpitations, chest pain, dizziness, chills, nausea and feelings of unreality.

Direct reflex

- Solar plexus
- Diaphragm

Associated reflexes

- Heart
- Brain
- Adrenals
- Spinal cord
- HP-6 acupoint on wrist

Phlebitis

Inflammation of walls of vein. Characterised by localised pain, tenderness, redness and heat. Can occur as complication of varicose veins and can lead to development of thrombosis.

Direct reflex

Reflex for area affected

Associated reflexes

- Heart
- Adrenals
- Relaxation techniques to improve circulation

Comment

If phlebitis is on person's leg work their hand instead and vice versa.

Raynaud's Disease

Abnormal constriction of arterioles of fingers and toes. Triggered by exposure to cold or strong emotions. Symptoms include numbness, tingling or pins-and-needles sensations in fingers and toes. Ends of fingers or toes become pale and bluish. Cause not always known but may accompany other disorders.

Direct reflex

Fingers and toes (work these gently to improve circulation to them)

Associated reflexes

- Heart
- Relaxation techniques to improve circulation

Thrombosis

Condition in which a blood clot, or thrombus, is produced. If large enough, clot may obstruct flow of blood to an organ. In coronary thrombosis blood clot forms in the coronary artery and may obstruct flow of blood to heart. In Deep Vein Thrombosis (DVT) clot forms in deep veins such as those of legs. Leg becomes swollen and tender and clot may become detached and cause pulmonary embolism. Risk factors for DVT include thrombophilia, prolonged bed rest, pregnancy and surgery.

If person has thrombosis reflexology should only be performed under medical supervision. If thrombosis is on person's leg work their hand instead and vice versa.

Varicose Veins (Varices)

Abnormally enlarged veins in which veins lengthen, widen and valve cusps within them separate. Results in backflow of blood which in turn causes veins to become larger and more distended. Symptoms include pain, itchiness, phlebitis and varicose ulcers.

Direct reflex

Reflex for area affected (e.g. legs)

Associated reflexes

- Heart
- Adrenals
- Large intestine
- Relaxation techniques to improve circulation

Comment

Do not perform reflexology on the foot of the affected leg. Work the hands instead.

Diseases and disorders of the lymphatic and immune system

Allergy (Hypersensitivity)

Over-reaction to substance that is normally harmless to most people. Occurs if person has been previously exposed to allergen and so developed antibodies to it. Symptoms range from running nose and streaming eyes to anaphylactic shock. Any substance can be an allergen and common allergens are milk, peanuts, shellfish, eggs, pollens, dusts and moulds.

Direct reflex
Reflex for area affected (e.g. nose if running nose, eyes if streaming eyes, arms if eczema on hands)

Associated reflexes
- Adrenals
- Liver
- Ileocaecal valve
- Large intestine
- Lymphatics

Breast lumps

Lumps in the breast can be non-cancerous cysts, hardened glandular tissue or scar tissue. However, because breast lumps can also be cancerous they need to be checked by a doctor.

Direct reflex
Breast

Associated reflexes
- Lymphatics
- All endocrine glands
- Uterus
- Adrenals

Comment
Always refer client to doctor for a medical diagnosis.

Cancer

Uncontrolled division of cells. Can develop within any tissue in the body and can replicate to form a mass known as a tumour. Cancer can spread from its origin to other sites via a process called metastasis which occurs across body cavities, via the bloodstream or via the lymphatic system.

Continuing professional development (CPD) training is recommended.

Fever

Abnormally high temperature in response to infection. Reflexology is contraindicated if client has a fever.

HIV and AIDS

AIDS is acquired immunodeficiency syndrome and is a syndrome caused by the virus HIV. HIV is human immunodeficiency virus and it destroys certain lymphocytes, resulting in a lowered T4 lymphocyte count. This makes a person susceptible to opportunistic infections which their immune system cannot fight. HIV is transmitted through bodily fluids such as blood, semen, vaginal secretions and breast milk.

Direct reflex
- Lymphatics
- Spleen
- Liver
- Thymus

Associated reflexes
- Solar plexus
- Diaphragm
- Relaxation techniques to improve circulation

Continuing professional development (CPD) training can help you understand this disease and training in counselling will be helpful. Be aware of standard hygiene procedures.

Influenza (Flu)

Contagious viral infection of respiratory system. Symptoms include runny nose, sore throat, cough, headache, fever and muscular aches and pains. Reflexology is contraindicated if there is a fever or infection.

Lymphoedema

Accumulation of lymph in tissues. Results in swelling and most often affects legs. Can be caused by congenital defect, surgery, parasites, tumours or injuries.

Direct reflex
Lymphatics

Associated reflexes
- All organs of elimination
- Kidneys
- Adrenals
- Heart
- Relaxation techniques to improve circulation

It is recommended that reflexology is given under the supervision of a medical practitioner or lymphoedema specialist nurse. Reflexologists should not work on the affected limb. For example, if client's right leg is affected the reflexologist should perform reflexology on their right hand instead.

Lymphomas

Cancer of lymphocytes. Can remain confined to a lymph node or spread to other lymphatic tissues or organs of the body. Hodgkin's disease/lymphoma is a malignant lymphoma characterised by progressive, painless enlargement of lymph nodes of neck, armpits, groin, chest or abdomen. Can be accompanied by fever, night sweats, weight loss, itching and fatigue and cause is unknown. Non-Hodgkin's Lymphoma is a diverse group of lymphomas common in elderly people and those whose immune systems are not functioning normally. Characterised by painless enlargement of lymph nodes. Continuing professional development (CPD) training is recommended.

Myalgic encephalomyelitis (ME, Chronic fatigue)

Syndrome characterised by extreme, debilitating fatigue that is not relieved by rest. Often accompanied by poor memory, reduced concentration, sore throats, muscle and joint pain, headaches and persistent feeling of illness after exercise. Cause is not always known.

Reflexes
Full gentle treatment.

Comment
Light pressure is often recommended.

Oedema

Excessive accumulation of interstitial fluid in body tissues resulting in swelling and puffiness. Causes can range from local injuries to heart or kidney disorders.

Direct reflex
Reflex for area affected

Associated reflexes
- Kidneys
- Adrenals
- Lymphatics
- All organs of elimination
- Relaxation techniques to improve circulation

Comment
If oedema is severe refer client to doctor for medical diagnosis.

Thrush (Candidiasis, Candidosis, Yeast infection)

Infection by the yeast *candida*. Candida is normally found in mouth, digestive tract and vagina but can infect other areas of body if allowed to grow. Risk factors include pregnancy, diabetes, obesity and frequent use of antibiotics.

Direct reflex
Reflex for area affected (e.g. mouth, colon, vagina)

Associated reflexes
- Large intestine
- Lymphatics
- All organs of elimination
- Liver
- Thymus
- Spleen
- All endocrine glands

Comment
Diet must be addressed and probiotics recommended.

Diseases and disorders of the digestive system

Cholecystitis (Inflammation of gallbladder)

Inflammation of gallbladder. Characterised by severe abdominal pain. Usually accompanies gallstones. A person with cholecystitis should be seen by a doctor.

Cirrhosis of liver

Destruction of liver tissue and replacement of it by scar tissue. Symptoms include weakness, nausea, lack of appetite and weight loss. Bile flow can be obstructed leading to jaundice and itchiness. Commonly caused by alcohol abuse or chronic hepatitis.

Direct reflex
Liver

Associated reflexes
- All organs of elimination
- All endocrine glands

Comment
Person should be under the care of a doctor.

Colitis

Inflammation of colon. Characterised by abdominal pain, diarrhoea and sometimes presence of blood or mucous in stools. Ulcerative colitis is condition in which rectum and part of colon become inflamed and ulcerated. It is thought to be genetic or linked to overactive immune system.

Direct reflex
Colon/large intestine

Associated reflexes
- Adrenals
- All organs of elimination (especially liver)
- Lymphatics

Constipation

Condition in which bowel movements are infrequent or uncomfortable with stools that are hard and difficult to pass. May be caused by medication, lack of physical exercise, dehydration, low-fibre diet, ageing, depression or obstruction of large intestine.

Direct reflex
Large intestine

Associated reflexes
- All organs of elimination
- Solar plexus
- Diaphragm
- Chest/Lungs
- Relaxation techniques to improve circulation

Crohn's Disease

Chronic inflammation of wall of gastrointestinal tract, most often affecting small and large intestines. Characterised by irregular flare-ups of abdominal cramping, chronic diarrhoea, fever, loss of appetite and weight loss. Blood can also be present in stools. Cause is unknown but thought to be genetic or autoimmune.

Direct reflex
Small and large intestines

Associated reflexes
- Adrenals
- All digestive organs
- All organs of elimination (especially liver)
- Solar plexus
- Thymus
- Lymphatics

Diarrhoea

Frequent passing of abnormally soft or liquid stools. Can be accompanied by abdominal cramping, large amounts of gas or nausea. Causes include infection, inflammation, stress or irritable bowel syndrome.

If diarrhoea is acute and due to infection client should not be treated until they are in recovery. If diarrhoea is due to stress or irritable bowel syndrome then work the large intestine, stomach, all organs of elimination, solar plexus and diaphragm.

Diverticulosis and Diverticulitis

Diverticula are small sac-like pouches that protrude through weak areas of the muscular layer of gastrointestinal tract, usually the large intestine. Development of diverticula is called diverticulosis. Inflammation or infection of diverticula is called diverticulitis. Symptoms include lower abdominal pain, tenderness and fever. Can be accompanied by either diarrhoea or constipation. Causes often linked to low-fibre diet or inadequate fluid intake.

Direct reflex
Large intestine

Associated reflexes
- Adrenals
- All digestive organs
- All organs of elimination (especially liver)
- Solar plexus
- Thymus
- Lymphatics

Flatulence

Presence of excess gas in gastrointestinal tract that is expelled via mouth (belching) or anus (flatulence). Can be accompanied by abdominal pain and bloating. Causes include swallowing air while eating, production of gas by bacteria in large intestine or deficiencies of certain digestive enzymes.

Direct reflex
Sigmoid reflex

Associated reflexes
- Large intestine
- All digestive organs
- All organs of elimination
- Solar plexus

Gallstones

Hard masses of bile pigments, cholesterol and calcium salts formed in gallbladder. Do not always have symptoms but if they pass into bile duct can obstruct flow of bile, leading to nausea, vomiting and sometimes infection.

Direct reflex
Gallbladder

Associated reflexes
- Liver
- Thyroid/Parathyroids
- Solar plexus

Comment
Client should be seen by a doctor

Gastroenteritis (Food poisoning)

Inflammation of stomach and small intestine. Characterised by diarrhoea, cramping, vomiting, nausea and loss of appetite. Causes can be viral or bacterial. A person with gastroenteritis should not receive reflexology until they are recovering. Then, a full and general treatment is recommended.

Haemorrhoids (Piles)

Enlarged, dilated and often twisted veins located in rectum and anus. Characterised by small amounts of bleeding after bowel movements. Can be caused by repeated straining during defecation (usually due to constipation), frequent heavy lifting or pregnancy.

Direct reflex
Rectum/anus

Associated reflexes
- Large intestine
- Solar plexus
- Diaphragm
- Adrenals
- All organs of elimination (especially liver)

Hepatitis

Inflammation of liver. Symptoms can include loss of appetite, nausea, diarrhoea, fever, and jaundice. Can be caused by viruses (infectious Hepatitis A, B and C), chemicals, excessive alcohol intake or use of certain drugs. If the client has infectious hepatitis they should not receive treatment until they are in the recovery stages. Reflexes to then be worked

include the liver, adrenals, all organs of elimination, gallbladder, lymphatics and spleen.

Hiatus hernia

Protrusion of stomach from abdominal cavity, through diaphragm, into thoracic cavity. Can be asymptomatic or accompanied by gastro-oesophageal reflux or indigestion. Cause unknown.

Direct reflexes
- Stomach
- Diaphragm

Associated reflexes
- Oesophagus
- Adrenals
- Solar plexus

Indigestion (Dyspepsia)

Pain or discomfort in lower chest or upper abdomen after eating. May be accompanied by nausea or vomiting. Causes range from anxiety to gastritis or ulcers.

Direct reflex
Oesophagus

Associated reflexes
- Stomach
- Entire upper abdominal area
- Adrenals
- Solar plexus

Irritable Bowel Syndrome (IBS, Spastic Colon)

Characterised by recurring flare-ups of abdominal pain, constipation and diarrhoea in otherwise healthy person. Symptoms can also include fatigue, nausea, headaches, depression, anxiety, difficulty concentrating, abdominal bloating and gas. Flare-ups usually triggered by eating too quickly or too much, stress, diet, hormones, drugs or minor irritants such as wheat, dairy, tea, coffee or citrus fruit.

Direct reflex
Large intestine

Associated reflexes
- All digestive reflexes
- Solar plexus
- Diaphragm
- Adrenals
- All organs of elimination (especially liver)

Jaundice

Yellowing of skin and whites of eyes due to high levels of bilirubin in bloodstream. Can result from liver disease, blockage of bile ducts or excessive breakdown of red blood cells.

A person suffering with jaundice should be seen by a doctor for a medical diagnosis. Once diagnosed a full treatment can usually be given with emphasis on the liver and gallbladder.

Peptic ulcers

Breaks in mucous lining of gastrointestinal tract due to combined action of pepsin and hydrochloric acid. Symptoms include feelings of gnawing, burning, aching, emptiness or hunger. Can be caused by bacterial infection or drugs that irritate lining of stomach. Apthous ulcers occur in the mouth, duodenal ulcers in the duodenum, gastric ulcers in the stomach.

Direct reflexes
- Stomach
- Duodenum (mouth if apthous ulcer)

Associated reflexes
- Solar plexus
- Adrenals
- Brain
- Diaphragm

Diseases and disorders of the urinary system

Cystitis

Inflammation of the bladder. Characterised by frequent, burning urination.

Direct reflex
Bladder

Associated reflexes
- Kidneys
- Adrenals
- Liver
- Spleen
- Lymphatics
- All organs of elimination

Comment
If client is pregnant and suffering with cystitis refer them to their doctor or gynaecologist immediately.

Incontinence

Involuntary passing of urine. Can be caused by weakened pelvic floor muscles after childbirth or pelvic surgery, menopause, enlarged prostate, prostate surgery, obesity, constipation or psychological factors.

Direct reflexes
- Bladder
- Vagina/Penis

Associated reflexes
- Entire pelvic region (including kidneys and ureters)
- Solar plexus
- Brain
- Spine (especially lumbar and sacral)

Kidney Stones (Calculi)

Hard masses of calcium salts located in kidneys. Symptoms include renal colic, back pain, nausea, vomiting, fever and blood in urine. Can form from excess salts in urine or lack of stone inhibitors in urine. More common in men, the elderly or those who eat high protein diets or have low water intake.

Direct reflexes
- Kidneys
- Ureters
- Bladder

Associated reflexes
- Adrenals
- Thyroid/Parathyroids
- Diaphragm

Nephritis (Bright's Disease)

Inflammation of kidneys. Characterised by impaired kidney function, fluid and urea retention and blood in urine. Causes include bacterial infection, exposure to toxins or immune reactions. A person with nephritis should be under the care of a doctor.

Renal Colic

Severe cramping pain occurring in lower back region or radiating from groin. Is a symptom of many kidney or urinary tract disorders. A person with renal colic should be referred to their doctor for a medical diagnosis.

Urethritis

Inflammation of urethra. Characterised by painful or difficult urination.

Direct reflex
Urethra

Associated reflexes
- Kidneys
- Bladder
- Vagina/Penis
- Adrenals
- Liver
- Spleen

Urinary tract infections (UTI)

Urinary tract infections are any infections along the urinary tract, including cystitis and urethritis. Usually caused by microbes and tend to be more common in women than men.

Reflexes
See Cystitis and Urethritis.

Diseases and disorders of the reproductive system

Endometriosis

Development of endometrial tissue (usually only found lining the uterus) outside of the uterus. Symptoms include lower abdominal and pelvic pain, irregular menstrual cycle and severe bleeding and cramping during menstruation. Cause unknown.

Direct reflex
Entire pelvic region

Associated reflexes
- All reproductive organs
- All endocrine glands
- Adrenals
- Solar plexus

Fibroid

Non-cancerous tumour consisting of muscle and fibrous tissue. Can develop in wall of uterus and cause pain, sense of pressure or heaviness in pelvic area and excessive menstrual bleeding.

Direct reflex
Uterus

Associated reflexes
- All reproductive organs
- All endocrine glands
- Adrenals

Impotence (Erectile dysfunction)

Inability to either achieve or maintain erection. Causes include diseases affecting circulation, nerve damage, illness, fatigue or stress.

Direct reflex
All reproductive organs

Associated reflexes
- All endocrine glands
- Brain
- Spine
- Solar plexus
- Diaphragm

Infertility

Inability for couple to conceive a baby after trying for at least one year. There are many causes, including problems with ovulation, sperm or Fallopian tubes.

Direct reflexes
- All reproductive organs
- All endocrine glands (especially thyroid)

Associated reflexes
- Brain
- Spine
- Solar plexus
- Diaphragm

Mastitis

Inflammation of breast. Symptoms include swelling, redness, warmth and tenderness. Can be caused by bacterial infection, usually around time of childbirth or after injury or surgery to breast. A woman with mastitis should be treated by a doctor.

Menstrual problems – Amenorrhoea

Absence of menstrual period. Causes include obesity, extreme weight loss, or abnormal levels of oestrogens.

Direct reflex
Uterus and ovaries

Associated reflexes

- Entire pelvic region
- All endocrine glands
- Solar plexus
- Relaxation techniques to improve circulation
- Parasympathetic nervous system (see page 160 on how to relax this system)

Menstrual problems – Dysmenorrhoea

Severe pain associated with menstruation. Symptoms include headaches, nausea, diarrhoea or constipation and the urge to urinate frequently. Often caused by another disorder such as pelvic inflammatory disease, endometriosis or fibroids.

Direct reflex

Uterus and ovaries

Associated reflexes

- Entire pelvic region
- All endocrine glands
- Solar plexus
- Relaxation techniques to improve circulation
- Parasympathetic nervous system (see page 160 on how to relax this system)

Menstrual problems – Menorrhagia

Abnormally heavy bleeding during menstruation. Often caused by another disorder such as pelvic inflammatory disease, endometriosis or fibroids.

Direct reflex

Ovaries and uterus

Associated reflexes

- Entire pelvic region
- All endocrine glands
- Solar plexus
- Relaxation techniques to improve circulation
- Parasympathetic nervous system (see page 160 on how to relax this system)

Comment

Use only light pressure over the ovaries and uterus reflexes during menstruation.

Pelvic inflammatory disease (PID)

Collective term for any infection of pelvic organs. More common in sexually active women and characterised by cyclical symptoms usually occurring around the end of menstruation and including fever, abdominal pain, irregular vaginal bleeding and foul-smelling vaginal discharge. Cause is generally bacterial infection. A client with PID should be under the care of a doctor.

Post-natal depression (postpartum depression)

Depression occurring in first few weeks or months after childbirth. Characterised by feeling of extreme sadness that lasts for weeks or even months. Causes unknown but linked to sudden changes in hormone levels, lack of sleep and stresses of having to care for new-born baby. A woman with post-natal depression should be under the care of a doctor and/or counsellor. Reflexology can be given and should be a full, general treatment.

Pre-menstrual syndrome (PMS)

Physical and emotional distress occurring late in postovulatory phase of menstrual cycle. Symptoms include oedema, weight gain, breast swelling and tenderness, abdominal distension, backache, joint pain, constipation, skin eruptions, fatigue and lethargy, depression or anxiety, irritability, mood swings, food cravings, headaches, poor co-ordination and clumsiness.

Direct reflex

Ovaries and uterus

Associated reflexes

- Entire pelvic region
- All endocrine glands
- Solar plexus
- Relaxation techniques to improve circulation
- Parasympathetic nervous system (see page 160 on how to relax this system)

Prostate disorders

Group of disorders more common in elderly men and generally characterised by difficulty in urinating, incomplete urination and need to urinate frequently. Benign prostatic hyperplasia (BPH) is the benign enlargement of the prostate gland and is thought to be linked to changes in testosterone levels. Prostate cancer is a slow growing cancer that begins as a small bump on the prostate gland and may have no other symptoms until it is in its advanced stages. Causes unknown. Prostatitis is inflammation of the prostate gland and symptoms include lower back pain, muscular spasms of the bladder and pelvis and painful urination. Usually caused by bacterial infection.

Direct reflex
Prostate

Associated reflexes
- Entire pelvic region
- Adrenals
- All endocrine glands
- All reproductive organs
- Solar plexus
- Relaxation techniques to improve circulation

Diseases and disorders of the special senses and integumentary system (the skin)

Boil (Furuncle)

Pus-filled pocket of infection beneath skin. Bacterial infection common in people with poor hygiene or weakened immune system.

Direct reflex
Reflex of area affected

Associated reflexes
- Lymphatics
- All organs of elimination
- Liver
- Spleen

NB: Do not touch the boil itself.

Cataract

Clouding-over of lens of eye. Leads to opacity of eye and loss of vision. Common in elderly people or can be congenital or result of disease or injury to lens. A person with a cataract should be referred to a medical professional or eye specialist.

Corneal Ulcer

Sore on cornea of eye. Symptoms include pain, sense of something being in eye, sensitivity to bright light and increased tear production. Causes include injury or irritation to cornea.

A person with a corneal ulcer should be referred to a medical professional or eye specialist. Reflexology can be given and emphasis should be on the eye reflex, head area and brain.

Cyst

Semi-solid or fluid-filled lump above and below skin. Cysts should be diagnosed by a doctor.

Deafness

Partial or total loss of hearing. Can affect one or both ears and causes include mechanical problems related to the ears, injury or infection. A person suffering from loss of hearing should be referred to a medical professional. Reflexology can be given and emphasis should be on the ear reflex, head area and brain.

Dermatitis

Inflammation of upper layers of skin (includes contact dermatitis and eczema). Symptoms range from itching, blistering, redness and swelling to more severe oozing, scabbing and scaling. Causes can include allergens, irritants, dryness, scratching or fungi.

Direct reflex
Reflex of area affected

Associated reflexes
- Adrenals
- Liver
- Lymphatics
- All organs of elimination
- Solar plexus

Earache

Pain thought to originate in ear. Causes include infection or blocked Eustachian tube. Can also be referred pain from infection in nose, throat, sinuses or mouth. A person with earache should be referred to their doctor for a medical diagnosis. Reflexology can be given and emphasis should be on the ear reflex, head area, brain, adrenals, liver and lymphatics.

Eczema

Form of dermatitis caused by either internal or external factors. Characterised by itchiness, redness and blistering. Can be either dry or weeping and can cause scaly and thickened skin.

Direct reflex
Reflex of area affected

Associated reflexes
- Adrenals
- Liver
- Large intestine
- Lungs
- Solar plexus
- Lymphatics
- All organs of elimination

Glaucoma

Loss of vision due to abnormally high pressure in eye. Results from eye's inability to drain aqueous humour as quickly as it produces it. People most at risk are those whose relatives have glaucoma, those who have very far or near sightedness, diabetics or those who have had an eye injury.

A person with glaucoma should be referred to a doctor. Reflexology may be given and emphasis should be on the eye reflexes.

Glue Ear (Secretory or Serous Otitis Media)

Accumulation of fluid in middle ear. Symptoms include feeling of fullness in ear or popping/crackling sound on swallowing and often temporary hearing loss. Usually caused by otitis media or blocked Eustachian tube.

A person suffering with glue ear should be referred to their doctor for a medical diagnosis. Reflexology can be given and emphasis should be on the ear reflex, head area, brain, adrenals, liver and lymphatics.

Hyperhidrosis (Hyperidrosis)

Excessive or almost constant sweating. Can affect entire surface of skin but usually limited to armpits, genitals, palms and soles. Can be caused by illness, medical condition or after use of certain drugs.

A person suffering with hyperhidrosis should be referred to their doctor for a medical diagnosis. Reflexology can be given and emphasis should be on the endocrine glands, lymphatics, organs of elimination and solar plexus.

Melanoma

Cancer originating in melanocytes of skin. Develops in sun-exposed areas or on moles and can metastasise. A person with a melanoma or suspected melanoma must be referred to their doctor.

Shingles (Herpes Zoster)

Re-emergence of chicken pox virus usually occurring when a person's immune system is weakened. Develops as painful eruption of blisters limited to area served by infected nerves. Symptoms include feeling of being unwell, fever, pain, tingling and itching.

Direct reflex
Reflex for area affected

Associated reflexes
- Brain
- Cranial nerves
- Spine
- Sciatic nerve
- Solar plexus
- Diaphragm
- Liver
- Thymus
- Spleen
- Lymphatics

Tinnitus

Sensation of hearing sounds in the ear that have not originated from external environment. Common in elderly. Can also be symptom of other ear disorders.

Direct reflex
Ear

Associated reflexes
- Brain
- Cranial nerves
- Spine
- Neck

Comment
A person with tinnitus should be referred to a doctor for a diagnosis of the cause.

Vertigo

Sensation of you or your surroundings constantly moving or spinning. Usually accompanied by nausea or loss of balance. May be symptom of another disease or caused by disorder of inner ear or vestibular nerve.

Direct reflexes
- Ear
- Eustachian tube

Associated reflexes
- Brain
- Cranial nerves
- Spine
- Neck

Comment
A person with vertigo should be referred to a doctor for a diagnosis of the cause.

Wart

Small, firm growth that has rough surface and can grow in clusters or as isolated growth. Generally painless. Caused by virus.

A person with a wart should be made aware that reflexology cannot change this condition and the treatment will be for relaxation purposes only. The reflexologist must not touch the wart.

Note: For disorders and diseases of the hands, feet and nails please see Chapters 2 and 3.

7 Clinical practice

Now that you know the theory of reflexology, it is time to put it all into practice.

Student objectives

This chapter covers the logistics of clinical practice and by the end of it you should be able to:

- Prepare yourself as a therapist
- Prepare a therapeutic environment in which to work
- Take a consultation with a client
- Decide on a treatment plan for your client and give them home care advice
- Adapt your treatment for specific client groups
- Write up treatment notes for a client
- Carry out reflective practice on yourself and your treatment.

Included at the end of this chapter is a sample of a completed client consultation and treatment record.

Preparing Yourself As A Therapist

'To foster ideas of positive health in our clients we need to live them in our own lives. To lead clients to find their balance we need to have awareness of our own balance.'
Vicki Pitman[1]

A good reflexology treatment is based on much more than simply theory or technique. It is an experience that begins when a client walks through the door and it relies on the preparation, focus and intention of the therapist.

In order to give a good treatment you need to be in good health yourself – you need to practise what you preach. Invest in yourself by living a positive lifestyle, eating well, exercising well and ensuring you get enough rest and relaxation. Do not treat a client if you are exhausted or feeling ill. You will not be able to give a good treatment and you will also be more susceptible to any negativity in your client.

Practical tip: Grounding yourself

Many new students find that after giving a treatment they feel drained or tired. To avoid this it is important to ground yourself properly. There are many different ways to do this and prevent yourself from picking up your client's negative energy or allowing them to drain your own energy. Here are a few suggestions for you to explore:

- If you follow a religion, you can say a prayer before your client arrives. This will help you to be aware of your own energies and will ground and protect you.
- Before a treatment, spend some time doing deep-breathing exercises in which you focus on inhaling deep into your abdomen. Your abdomen is not only the centre of gravity in your body, it is also the energy centre of your body (known as your hara) and through focusing on it and breathing deeply into it, you are grounding your own energies and nourishing and developing this vital centre.
- When working with a client try to distance yourself from the outcome of the treatment. It sounds odd, but don't try too hard. Don't try to cure your client or make them better. Simply relax into the treatment and do the best you possibly can. Distance yourself from the outcome of the treatment and let your client's body heal itself. You are simply a facilitator for the healing, you are not responsible for the actual healing process.
- Many therapists like to ground themselves with visualisation techniques. Some therapists imagine the roots of a tree encircling their feet and holding them firmly in the ground, others visualise themselves inside a white ball/egg that encircles and protects them, others imagine building a brick wall between themselves and their clients.
- After a treatment it is important to wash your hands, not only for hygiene reasons, but also to 'wash off' any negative energy you may have picked up. Place your hands under cold running water for a few minutes and visualise any negative energy being washed away.

In his book *Reading the Body*, Ohashi talks of how when diagnosing and working one's hara, or energy centre, his teacher always told him 'we must become a mother with a samurai's mind. That means that while we are eminently gentle, we are at the same time focused, directed and alert.'[2] There is no better way to describe the attitude and presence needed by a therapist to give a good reflexology treatment.

It is also important to develop yourself as a therapist. There are many post-graduate or continuing professional development (CPD) courses available as well as literature, conferences, workshops, research projects and volunteer work. Take part in these and continually explore yourself and develop your abilities.

Professionalism and ethics

As a practitioner of a professional therapy, you need to maintain a professional image at all times. This means that you must maintain high standards of hygiene, and comply with a professional code of practice and ethics. Codes of practice differ with each examining or professional body but they all generally cover the following. The therapist needs to:

- Always put the client first
- Treat the client with respect, regardless of class, colour or creed
- Keep accurate, confidential treatment records
- Maintain the client's confidentiality at all times
- Refer when necessary, but never diagnose
- Ask the client's doctor for permission to treat their patient if necessary
- Explain reflexology to the client prior to the treatment
- Perform only one therapy at a time
- Maintain high standards of hygiene and safety at all times
- Advertise correctly
- Be registered with a professional body
- Not poach another therapist's clients.

Another element of professionalism is looking after the client and showing interest in them. This includes:

- Listening to the client when they talk
- Maintaining their confidence
- Helping the client on and off the treatment couch or reflexology chair
- Ensuring they are warm or cool enough
- Providing the client with a glass of water after the treatment
- Always showing a genuine interest in their condition
- Giving the client your full attention
- Not bringing your personal problems to the treatment
- Listening to, rather than gossiping with, the client
- Avoiding sexual misconduct.

Study tip
Ask your examining or professional body to provide you with its own code of practice which you can learn.

Preparing Your Environment

No matter where you give your reflexology treatment, always spend some time creating a therapeutic environment and a positive ambience. The room in which you work should be:

- Quiet, secure and private
- Clean
- Well ventilated
- Warm
- Have relaxing lighting and music.

> **Reflexions**
> Not everyone has the same taste in music, decor and aromas so be careful when considering these aspects of a treatment. It is important to create a relaxing and positive atmosphere, but don't overwhelm a client with loud music that they may not like, or with esoteric decor they may find off-putting, or with aromas that may have negative associations for them.

In general, the following equipment and products are recommended in order to carry out a reflexology treatment:

- A reflexology couch or reflexology chair
- Fresh linen – never use the same linen for two clients
- Pillows/Bolsters to support your client under their knees, in the small of their back and behind their head and neck
- Reflexology medium (cream or talc)
- Disposable gloves in case of an emergency
- A lined waste bin with a lid
- Antiseptic solution and cotton wool, wipes (or similar) to clean your client's feet before you begin the treatment
- A blanket in case they get cold during the treatment
- A glass of water to give your client after the treatment
- A consultation sheet and pen
- A box of tissues for you or your client
- A comfortable chair or stool for you to sit on.

You also need to be aware of the safety aspects of the room in which you are working and ensure they meet the health and safety, as well as the fire regulations of your country.

In the classroom
Laws and regulations differ from country to country so spend some time finding out those of your country. Look into any Health & Safety at Work, Fire, Electricity and Trading legislature.

Hygiene

> *'Hygiene is not so much a set of rules as an attitude of mind.'*
> *Menna Buckland Kleine*[3]

It is vital that the room in which you work is clean and that you maintain high levels of hygiene at all times. As a therapist, you need to be aware of your own personal cleanliness and hygiene and you also need to ensure you take all necessary precautions to avoid contracting a contagious disease from a client or cross-infecting one client with another's disease.

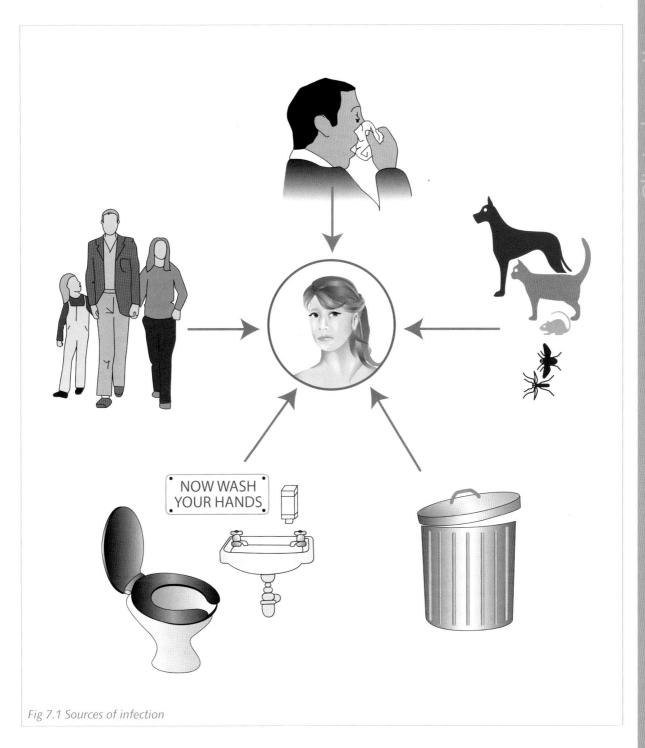

Fig 7.1 Sources of infection

You need to:

- Have bathed/showered, deodorised, brushed your teeth, washed your hair and tied it off your face if it is long
- Keep your nails short and clean and do not wear jewellery or perfume
- Always wear clean clothes
- Wash your hands before and after each treatment.

In addition:

- Always use fresh linen for every client
- Clean your client's hands or feet before working on them
- Do not touch any contraindicated areas on your client
- Dispose of any waste properly.

> **Study tip**
>
> Here is a quick reminder of some vocabulary you will need to know when considering hygiene:
>
> - **Hygiene** – the science and practice of preserving health
> - **Micro-organism/Microbe** – an organism too small to be visible to the naked eye (includes bacteria, viruses and fungi)
> - **Pathogenic** – disease-causing
> - **Sanitation** – a process in which conditions are rendered and maintained clean and healthy
> - **Sterilisation** – a process in which all living micro-organisms are destroyed.

Disease-causing micro-organisms

There are three different groups of organisms that you need to be aware of during a reflexology treatment. These are:

- **Bacteria** (**sing. bacterium**) are a group of unicellular micro-organisms that lack organelles and an organised nucleus. They are generally classified according to their shape – *coccus* are round, *bacillus* are rod-shaped and *spirillum* are spiral-shaped. Not all bacteria are pathogenic. Paronychia (bacterial infection of the nail wall or cuticle) is a common bacterial infection that you may encounter when doing reflexology.
- **Fungi** (**sing. fungus**) are simple organisms that lack chlorophyll and they are not always micro-organisms. For example, mushrooms and yeasts are fungi. Some fungi can infect the body and often thrive in moist areas of the skin. Tinea pedis (athlete's foot) and candidiasis (thrush) are examples of fungal infections you may see when doing reflexology.
- **Viruses** are pathogenic micro-organisms that consist mainly of nucleic acid in a protein coat that can only multiply when inside another living cell. Many diseases, such as the common cold, influenza, chickenpox and AIDS are all caused by viruses. In reflexology, you will often encounter verrucae (plantar warts) which are viral infections.

The most common infections of the hands and feet are discussed in Chapters 2 and 3. You will need to be able to recognise these in a client.

As a reflexologist you also need to be aware of any infestations of parasites on the body, such as scabies, head lice or fleas. These are easily transmitted from person to person and a client who presents with such an infestation is contraindicated for treatment.

There are many ways in which disease-causing micro-organisms can enter the body. For example, they can enter via the nose, mouth, eyes, ears, skin or genito-urinary tract. Once inside us, our bodies deal with them in a number of different ways and this is discussed in more detail in Chapter 4.

Putting your knowledge of hygiene into practice

In clinical practice, clients have a right to expect high levels of hygiene and it is of the utmost importance that you, as a therapist, develop good sanitation procedures that become second nature to you:

- Do not treat a client who has an infectious disease that you may contract
- Always wash your hands before and after every treatment
- If you have a cut or sore on your hands ensure you cover it with a plaster
- Always wash your client's hands or feet before working on them
- Do not touch any open wounds, sores or infected areas of skin on a client
- Always use clean linen for every client
- Put down fresh couch roll for each client and dispose of it immediately after use
- Always dispose of waste properly
- Do not let your client walk around barefoot and provide disposable slippers if necessary
- Ensure your treatment room is always clean, that all surfaces (walls, ceiling, doors, shelves, flooring, furniture) and products are clean and that any products or equipment you use are clean and sterile. Also ensure the toilet, bathroom and reception areas are clean.
- There are many different cleaning products on the market but when buying some for your clinic, be aware of the following terminology:
  - **Antiseptics** destroy or inhibit micro-organisms on living tissue. They are often used to clean wounds.
  - **Bactericides** kill bacteria only.
  - **Disinfectants** destroy or inhibit micro-organisms and are used to clean instruments and equipment.

Laws and legislation

Because different areas and countries have different laws regarding the practice of reflexology, it is important that you contact your local authority to obtain their legislation. You must:

- Be qualified to practise reflexology
- Be registered with a professional body such as a reflexology association
- Adhere to your professional body's code of ethics
- Be insured to practise as a reflexologist
- Carry out correct hygiene procedures according to health and safety legislation
- Keep up-to-date confidential client records
  - ensure that all clients sign an informed client consent form
  - keep all records securely. You must not show your records to anyone, or discuss them without your client's consent. All records should be written clearly and legibly in case they are needed for legal proceedings
  - ensure that any computer records comply with the Data Protection Act
- Adhere to health and safety at work regulations regarding accidents or injuries to clients and staff, storage of products and equipment, dealing with any spillages or breakages and fire regulations
- Adhere to the Child Protection Act
- Only work within the limitations of your qualification.

Informed client consent

After you have completed the consultation form and developed a treatment plan you need to explain exactly what the treatment does and does not involve so that your client does not have the wrong expectations. You also need to explain the effects of reflexology to them. Once you have done this, your client must sign to confirm that they understand the treatment and its effects and that they have given you all necessary medical information. If your client is unable to sign due to age or illness, their legal guardian or carer must sign on their behalf.

Working With A Client

When a client first calls to book a reflexology appointment take some time to get to know them. Find out why they are coming for reflexology, what they hope to gain from the treatment and whether or not it is safe for them to receive a treatment (refer to page 28 for contraindications). If they then book an appointment, you can begin to establish a therapeutic relationship with them by completing a consultation form at the beginning of their first appointment.

The consultation

The initial consultation will always take about 15 minutes longer than a normal consultation so ensure you have booked enough time. The consultation is the time in which you:

- Get to know your client
- Reassure them that everything you discuss will be confidential
- Take their personal details and medical history
- Find out about any contraindications they may have
- Find out why they are coming for the treatment
- Find out exactly what they want from the treatment
- Discuss their lifestyle and give them advice on nutrition, etc (if you are qualified to do so)
- Refer them to another practitioner if necessary.

The consultation is also the time in which your client can:

- Openly and confidentially discuss their health and lifestyle.
- Learn what a reflexology treatment involves and what its limitations are.
- Learn about any possible reactions (contra-actions) they may have during and after the treatment.
- Ask any questions they may have.

When to refer

If your client has any of the following symptoms with no obvious explanation then you should refer them to their doctor for a diagnosis before they can have a treatment:

- Severe mood alterations
- Unusual changes in appetite
- Nausea, vomiting, diarrhoea

- Infection
- High temperature
- Extreme fatigue
- Persistent hoarseness or cough
- Chronic indigestion
- Change in bowel or bladder function
- Chronic oedema
- Undiagnosed inflammation, pain, bleeding or bruising
- Sores that are not healing
- An unusual or unidentifiable lump.

In addition, if your client has contraindications such as diabetes (see page 28 for contraindications) advise them to discuss their reflexology treatment with their doctor.

There will be times when you can give a client a reflexology treatment and still refer them to another professional who is better equipped or qualified to help them in other ways. For example, you may want to refer your client to a dietician or nutritionist for help with their diet, a chiropodist or podiatrist to help with foot problems, an osteopath, chiropractor or massage therapist to help with musculo-skeletal disorders, or a counsellor if you feel your client would benefit from professional counselling. You may also refer them to other complementary practitioners such as acupuncturists or herbalists if you feel your client would benefit from that.

Occasionally you may find you cannot work with a particular client. You may have a personality clash or you may feel inadequately equipped to deal with them. At times like this it is best to refer them to another reflexologist. Remember, you always need to put your client's wellbeing first.

Communication skills

> 'When a client arrives, greet him or her warmly and be grateful
> that he or she has come. The person must sense your openness;
> he or she must recognise your lack of prejudice. You make no
> judgements or criticisms. Your only desire is to help in your
> limited way. Together you and this person will find a way
> towards better health.' (Ohashi)[4]

The concept of communication can be defined as 'the transmitting and receiving of information'[5] (O'Hara) and good communication skills are integral to reflexology. Communication begins when your client books their treatment. At this early stage you are already forming a picture of each other.

From the moment your client walks through the door you are communicating with them. You as the therapist can begin to assess them by taking in their appearance, posture, movements and expressions. The way in which a person dresses and cares for themselves says a lot about their self-esteem and who they are. Remember that just as you are assessing your client, so they will be assessing you. Be aware of how you are dressed, how you greet and welcome them and how comfortable you make them feel. Be aware of both the tone and pitch of their voice and of your own. Be aware of their body odour and of yours – poor personal hygiene or the body's

Practical tip

Make a list of voluntary and statutory support services that you may need to refer a client to. For example, support or advice services for elderly people, people who are being abused or struggling with addictions, etc. In this list also include organisations that support and educate people with certain diseases such as HIV, cancer, lupus, etc. Sometimes just giving a client the number of an organisation you feel may help them can make a big difference.

inability to eliminate waste properly can often be 'smelled' on a person before it is seen. Be aware of how your client shakes your hand and you theirs – 'Whenever we shake another person's hand, we sense his or her character, we 'feel' the inner nature, and we try to communicate our own. A subtle yet profound exchange of information takes place when we shake another person's hand.' (Ohashi)[6]

Listening skills are a vital part of your role as a therapist and a good listener encourages clients to help themselves and find their own solutions. Remember that as a reflexologist you are not there to advise or judge your client. You are there simply to listen. Listening skills include the following:

- Listening quietly and not talking about yourself or your own problems
- Asking open questions. An open question encourages your client to talk, for example 'Tell me about any medication you are on' as opposed to a closed question which usually elicits a yes or no answer, for example, 'Are you on any medication?'
- Not giving advice, but offering different options so your client can make their own decisions
- Not judging
- Allowing your client to lead the conversation.

Being aware of body language is also vital and many researchers believe that nonverbal communication forms about 50% of all communication. When taking your client's consultation be aware of their body language and of yours. Remember to:

- Sit close to your client (but not too close) when taking the consultation. Avoid sitting at a desk as this creates a barrier between you
- Avoid crossing your legs or arms as this creates a barrier
- Avoid fidgeting or playing with anything in your hands
- Maintain eye contact
- Be confident. Relax and smile!

Completing the consultation form

Have a set consultation form that you use with every client (an example is given on page 289). This form should include areas for you to write notes on why your client has come for the treatment, their health, details of any medication, their medical history, their family's medical history, their lifestyle and psychology. The form should also include an area where you can write or draw your reading of their feet and note down a treatment plan. Once you have completed your consultation form, give it to your client to check and then ask them to sign an informed consent agreement.

Formulating a treatment plan

After taking the consultation, you need to formulate a treatment plan to ensure that you give your client the best possible treatment. You will need to discuss the following with your client:

- Client's objectives – what do they want to gain from the treatment?
- Therapist's objectives – what do you want to achieve from the treatment?
- Primary problems to be addressed – what are your client's main concerns?

- Medium to be used – cream, talc or no lubricant?
- Length of treatment?
- Frequency of treatments – how many treatments will your client need and how often?

How do you decide on the length and frequency of treatments?

There are no set rules when it comes to reflexology as each treatment should be unique and tailored to the individual receiving them. However, some basic guidelines are:

- In general a 45 minute treatment can be given once or twice a week. After 4–6 regular treatments, clients can then reduce their treatments to once a month or come only when they need to.
- If a client comes for 4–6 treatments and has had no reactions or sees no benefits whatsoever, then recommend that they try a different type of therapy.
- If a client is elderly, frail, very sick or a child then the treatment time should be limited to 20 minutes. Babies should only receive very short treatments. Please see page 287 for how to adapt your treatments to suit specific groups of clients.

When formulating a treatment plan, also take into account the following:

- How much time does your client have?
- What can they afford?
- How long has your client been suffering from the condition? The longer they have had a condition the more treatments they will need.
- What time can they come for treatments? If they come during their lunch break they need a stimulating treatment while if they come in the evening after work they can have a more relaxing one.

The use of instruments in a reflexology treatment

As you begin to practise reflexology, you will become more aware of the many different tools or instruments available to reflexologists. Think twice before using any of these in your treatment as they may have the potential to damage a client's skin, cross-infect or hurt them through lack of sensitivity and control. Remember that in reflexology your thumbs and fingers become your eyes and ears and it is through the power of touch that you explore both your client's body and their mind. Nothing can replace the controlled, refined movements of a sensitive and caring practitioner.

Aftercare and homecare advice

Your client's treatment does not end when you have finished doing the reflexology, only when they leave the room. Likewise, the effects of the treatment should not end when they stand up. Instead they should last for at least a few days. The best way to achieve this is to advise your client on what they can do to prolong the effects of the treatment.

After the treatment allow your client to relax for a few minutes before helping them off the couch. Then give them a glass of water and spend a few minutes discussing the treatment and any possible reactions they may have. Recommend that they:

- Drink some water
- Rest
- Avoid drugs, alcohol or excessive exercise.

Also, try to encourage your clients to take responsibility for their own health by discussing topics such as:

- Diet
- Water intake
- Exercise
- Relaxation
- Posture
- Working environment.

However, remember this is a reflexology treatment and not a session in which your client receives nutritional prescriptions or specific advice on exercise.

Scope of practice

Remember to work within the limitations of your qualification. Reflexologists are not medically qualified and so cannot diagnose or claim to cure any disorders. Neither can they practise any other therapies in which they are not formally qualified. Be careful not to give specific advice on subjects such as diet or exercise. If you think your client needs help in these areas then refer them to someone qualified in that discipline.

Reactions (Contra-actions) to reflexology

During a treatment your client could react in a number of different ways which are normal reactions to neural stimulation. Your client could:

- Become hot or cold
- Change facial expressions
- Change mood – cry, laugh, sigh or groan
- Gesture pain or contract certain muscles
- Sweat on their palms or feet
- Become light-headed or dizzy
- Become hungry or thirsty
- Develop a headache
- Become nauseous
- Shake
- Experience referred sensitivity
- Develop a rumbling stomach
- Experience a warmth or tingling
- Get cramp.

Although these are normal reactions during a treatment, they can be alarming for both therapist and client. If your client has a reaction try to keep calm, ensure your voice is calm and soothing, and deal with the reaction in one of the following ways depending on the situation:

- Stop any deep pressure techniques you may be doing and instead do gentle relaxation techniques on the foot. Or
- Stop and hold the foot and encourage your client to focus on their breathing. Or

- Gently effleurage the foot and massage the solar plexus. Or
- Repeatedly zone-walk the feet until they have calmed down.

There are also reactions unrelated to reflexology that a client may develop during a treatment, for example they could have an asthma attack. As a reflexologist you need to be prepared to deal with all types of reactions.

Reactions after a treatment are also common but can sometimes be alarming for clients. Let them know that the following reactions are completely normal and do not usually recur after subsequent treatments:

- Temporary discomfort or pain
- Increased urination
- A change in bowel movements and flatulence
- Increased mucous secretions (nasal or vaginal)
- Toothache (usually due to tooth decay or gum infections)
- Tiredness, fatigue or sleepiness
- A sense of feeling wonderful
- Digestive or appetite changes
- Headaches
- Skin changes
- Emotional changes – old problems could resurface
- Changes in dreams and sleeping patterns
- A healing crisis – a latent disorder may be brought to the surface before the body can improve.

Your client should feel free to phone you at any time if they are concerned about any reactions they may be experiencing.

A healing crisis

A healing crisis is quite a common reaction to a person's first reflexology treatment, especially if they are ill or their body is out of balance. After the treatment they may feel very tired or nauseous, have diarrhoea or a headache. Or they may have an emotional reaction in which they have bad dreams and are tearful or upset. These are normal reactions and should not last longer than 48 hours.

It is important for the therapist to try and avoid a healing crisis in their client as it is not a pleasant experience and may put the client off reflexology. Therefore, during the first treatment do not work too hard on the client and use a lot of relaxation techniques and zone-walking. Ensure you work the organs of elimination well and do not do any deep, prolonged work on the endocrine glands. Remember, reflexology is a very powerful therapy and true healing happens slowly and gently.

Encourage your client to drink plenty of water after the treatment and to feel free to contact you if they are concerned about any reactions they may have.

Self-help

'Ultimately, the power for healing lies in the client's own hands.'[7] (Vicki Pitman)

No matter how hard you try to help your client they are ultimately responsible for their own healing and if they are not involved in the process they will not heal. The home care advice mentioned on pages 283–284 is extremely important and another way to encourage their involvement is to recommend simple self-help techniques that they can use at home.

Depending on your client's condition, try to teach them one or two reflexes that they can work themselves to improve their condition. Don't show them too many reflexes as they may feel overwhelmed. Common disorders that clients can work on at home are:

- **Back problems** – clients can use their thumb to work up and down their spine reflex on either their hand or foot.
- **Digestive disorders/Constipation** – if your client suffers with chronic digestive disorders teach them to knuckle the digestive area on their hands and feet. Also show them how to work the Great Eliminator (LI-4) acupoint discussed on page 241.
- **Headaches** – clients can knuckle their thumb or big toe regularly to help with headaches. You can also show them how to work the Great Eliminator (LI-4) acupoint discussed on page 241, as well as their neck and spinal reflexes which will help with the headaches.
- **Sinus problems** – clients can either knuckle the tips of all their fingers or firmly press the tips of the fingers of both hands together for a few minutes each day.
- **Stress, tension, anxiety** – the solar plexus reflex on the hand is an easy and convenient reflex to work (it can be worked anywhere at any time). Teach your client to work this reflex regularly and to also focus on their breathing as they work it. The heart protector acupoint HP-6 is also a very good point to help calm the mind and can easily be worked by a client. Turn to page 236 to see how to work this point.

Good foot care

As a reflexologist you should be able to appreciate the importance of good foot care and understand the negative impact poor care can have on a person's entire body. Sometimes you need to remind your client about basic foot care. This includes:

- Feet should be washed daily and dried well, especially between the toes.
- To avoid developing ingrowing toenails, nails should be cut straight across and not curved.
- Any foot infections or problems should be seen by a chiropodist.
- In addition, your female clients should be made aware of how very high-heeled, tight or constricting shoes can, over time, deform their feet. On the other hand, wearing completely flat shoes that do not support the arch of the foot can also cause foot problems such as heel spurs or dropped arches.

Adapting your treatments

Reflexology treatments need to be adapted for every individual, but there are certain groups of people who need particular attention.

Reflexology for children

Children respond quickly to reflexology and regular treatments can help with many discomforts. When working with a child always have a parent or guardian in the room and ensure that they have signed the informed consent form on behalf of the child. If they are willing to learn, show the parents how to do the relaxation techniques themselves – children respond better to a parent's touch. Give a child a short, gentle treatment with little pressure and adjust the treatment according to their age, size and symptoms:

- **Babies** – Give a gentle five-minute treatment consisting of gentle stroking from the heel up to the toes along all five zones, followed by light pressure on the reflex points of symptom areas. In order to maintain a lighter pressure use only your index finger and not your thumb.
- **Children under 12** – Give a gentle 20 minute treatment that works the entire body. Use only light pressure.
- **Teenagers** – Give a complete 45 minute treatment on all zones and reflexes, adjusting the pressure according to the client's size and symptoms. Be aware that teenage girls may have issues that they do not wish to discuss in front of their parents, such as eating disorders, menstrual problems or an unwanted pregnancy. As a therapist, you will need to show the utmost sensitivity and professionalism in such cases.

Always refer a child to a doctor if they have any undiagnosed medical condition. This is a legal obligation when dealing with children.

Reflexology for people with disabilities

People with disabilities, whether mental or physical, can benefit greatly from regular reflexology treatments. However, there are a few practical factors that need to be considered before working with a disabled client:

- When working with a disabled client be aware that you may need to adapt your own position to give the treatment. Vertical reflexology (discussed on page 309) is a wonderful type of therapy to use with clients who are in wheelchairs as well as with very elderly clients.
- You may also need to have your room prepared to accommodate a wheelchair or a guide-dog if your client is visually impaired.
- You will need to ensure your treatment room is safe and easy to manoeuvre in. Walk through the room checking for furniture, electrical wires, or anything else a client may trip over or collide with.

In addition to the above, it is important to have the client's carer or guardian in the room with you if they have mental health problems.

You can perform a complete treatment on most clients with disabilities (depending on their health) and if they have a foot missing you can work the corresponding hand or vice versa. Get their guardian's or doctor's consent first where necessary and ensure the treatment is not contraindicated.

Reflexology for the elderly

Elderly clients sometimes need more patience and understanding than the average client, especially if they have hearing difficulties, poor vision or are less mobile. Be careful not to rush an elderly client and give them a slow, gentle treatment with minimum pressure, adjusting it according to their health and frailty. To help improve their circulation gently massage their lower legs as well as their feet. If a client is particularly old or frail, do not work on them for longer than 20 minutes. Also be aware of the following:

- Be careful not to damage or bruise the skin which can be thin and fragile.
- Be careful with manipulation techniques and the ankle boogie as their joints are often weak.
- Remember to help them on and off the couch and with anything else they may need (for example, putting on their shoes). However, do not make them feel incompetent.
- If the client is under medical care, ensure you get their doctor's or guardian's consent first.

Reflexology in cancer care

A person with cancer can benefit greatly from reflexology but it is recommended that the therapist is first trained in cancer care – there are many post-graduate or CPD courses available. Therapists working in cancer care need to have a thorough knowledge of the disease and its effects as well as the different types of treatment available and their effects. In addition, it helps if they are trained in counselling.

Reflexology in pregnancy care

You should undertake post-graduate training in reflexology and pregnancy care before you treat pregnant women. Remember, you will be working with two lives, not one. The information below does not replace proper training in pregnancy care, nor does it teach you how to apply reflexology to benefit a pregnancy or help with specific pregnancy-related disorders. It simply tells you what you should not do if you have a pregnant client.

Always ensure there is no element of risk to the pregnancy and obtain her doctor's permission before treating a pregnant woman. When working with a pregnant woman, take the following into account:

- **Positioning** – when a woman is heavily pregnant she should not lie flat on her back. When giving her reflexology either put her on her side or place some pillows behind her so that she is in a semi-reclining position.
- **Relaxation techniques** – do not do any manipulation techniques that affect the ankle area, for example side-to-side friction and the ankle boogie. To be beneficial these techniques should be done vigorously and this creates too much movement in the pelvic region. Also, do not massage the Achilles tendon and lower leg deeply as these areas contain acupoints used to help with labour.
- **Pressure techniques** – do not do any deep work over the ankle area and also avoid deep pressure on the pituitary gland, uterus and ovaries.
- **Acupoints** – the following acupoints are forbidden in pregnancy care: Large Intestine 4, Spleen 6, Bladder 60 and Bladder 67. In this book you have only been introduced to Large Intestine 4 on the hand and Spleen 6 above the medial malleolus.

Record keeping

At the end of every treatment you need to record what type of treatment you gave your client and any sensitivities or imbalances you found. In addition, take note of any reactions the client may have had during the treatment and note down any homecare advice you gave him or her.

At the start of the following treatment you should then do a mini-consultation in which you discuss any reactions your client had to the previous treatment and how his or her current health is. Note this on your record card. Lock your records away in a private and safe place.

Case study

The case study below demonstrates how to complete a consultation form. Different colleges and examining bodies often have their own consultation and record-keeping procedures so please find out what is expected of you from your college.

Roger is a 34 year-old man who leads a relatively healthy lifestyle and who has not suffered from any major diseases or disorders. However, because he is a manager in a large investment bank he works long hours (average 60 per week) and has a very stressful, pressurised job. He has also just had a baby daughter and so does not get much sleep. Consequently, he is always tired and often struggles to keep awake during the day.

Roger suffers from chronic lower back pain and knee problems (he cannot bend his right knee into a crouching position) due to numerous sports injuries. His main hobby is sport and so he is very depressed that whenever he plays any sport (mainly golf and football) he suffers from chronic lower back and knee pain for the next few days. He has been to a number of specialists with this problem and they have all told him he must give up sport. Roger will come for a weekly treatment for four weeks. After that we will reassess.

Name: Roger			
Age: 34	**DOB:** 07/07/65	**Sex:** Male	**Marital status:** Married
Address: N/A for this case study			**Home phone:** N/A
Occupation: investment banker – manager of large team of traders	**Children:** Daughter – 4 months		**Work phone:** N/A
Height: 5' 11"	**Weight:** 13.5 stone	**Reason for visit:** Knee problems	**Referred by:**
Doctor's name: N/A for this case study	**Address:** N/A for this case study		
Emergency contact details: N/A for this case study			

MEDICAL HISTORY

Medication/Pill/HRT: *none*

Vitamins/Self Prescribed: *none*

Anaemia: No	**German measles:** No	**Chicken pox:** No	**Diphtheria:** No
Measles: No	**Mumps:** No	**Pneumonia:** No	**Whooping cough:** No
Rheumatic fever: No	**Sinuses:** No	**Glandular fever:** No	**Scarlet fever:** No
Shingles: No	**Polio:** No	**Other:** No	

Operations (inc. appendix/tonsils): None	**Accidents/Injuries/Falls (dates)** 1994 – Cricket, broke four fingers and both wrists broken 1985 – Football, fractured big right toe 1997 – Cricket , broke three metatarsals in left hand – still weak

Insertions (metal pins/plates): None	**Back Problems:** 1987 – slipped disc in lumbar region – still suffers with constant, chronic lower back pain	**General state of health:** *Good*
Last visit to the doctor: 1994	**Reason:** Check up	**Result:** Fine

Other therapy: No	**Date of last treatment:** N/A	**X-ray or Hospital tests in last 3 years:** No	**Why/Result:** N/A

Skin problems: Daughter has very bad eczema but he has none	**Infectious Diseases / HIV:** None

Do you or any blood relatives suffer any problems relating to the following?:

Diabetes: No	**Epilepsy:** No	**Blood Pressure (H/L):** No	**Thrombosis:** No
Heart: No	**Chest:** No	**Migraine:** brother has them (stress)	**Kidneys:** No
Bladder: No	**Digestion:** No	**Constipation:** brother suffers with it (stress)	**Varicose veins:** No
Allergies: No	**Hepatitis:** No	**Hay Fever:** No	**Asthma:** No
MS: No	**Cancer:** No	**Arthritis:** mother (legs)	**Colitis:** No
Lupus: No	**Other:** No		

Women's health

Pregnant now?: N/A	**Regular periods:** N/A	**Date of last period:** N/A	**PMT:** N/A
Symptoms of PMT: N/A	**Breast feeding:** N/A	**Hysterectomy (date):** N/A	**Menopause:** N/A

Further comments/Additional information: Always excessively tired and struggles to keep awake. Right knee problems – cannot bend his right knee into a crouching position. Very painful – aches a lot. Lower back pain – frequent and extremely painful.

LIFESTYLE			
Smoke/Day: No	**Alcohol:** No	**Units/Week:** No	**Type:** None
Tea/Day: 2	**Coffee/Day:** 0	**Water/Day:** 4	**Other/day:** 0
Balanced Diet: No. A lot of red meat and very little fruit/veg	**Regular Meals:** Yes	**Eat before bed:** No	**Eat between meals:** No
Exercise/Type/Frequency: Golf, Football once a week – but very painful back and knee afterwards			
Hobbies: Sport	**Work hours:** 60	**Work worries:** Very stressful environment	**Recent Promotion:** No
Take care of children: Only his own daughter	**How many/ages:** New-born – 4 months	**Take care of elderly/sick/handicapped:** No	
Sleep: 5 hours – restless		**Sleep during day:** Always very tired during the day	
Depression: No	**Tension:** Average	**Anxiety:** No	**Stress:** Work – very stressful and long hours
Why: Due to his demanding, stressful job he does not spend much time with his wife and new daughter			
How do any of the above conditions affect you?: Constantly tired			
Optimistic/Pessimistic: Optimistic	**Posture:** Good	**Physical Handicap:** None	**Glasses/Contacts/ Hearing Aid:** None
Confident/Nervous: Confident	**Partner:** Married – very happy	**Bereavement:** None	**Phobias:** None

The information I have given about my general health in this case history is true to the best of my knowledge and belief, and I hereby give my consent to myself/my child being treated with reflexology.

Signed: *Roger*   Date: 08/07/99

Observation	Right foot	Left foot
Colour	Ankle – red, bruised, swollen	Ankle – red, bruised, swollen
Smell	A bit sweet	A bit sweet
Skeletal deformities (bunions)	Mid spine – hard lump. Large toe – deformed (it was fractured)	None
Temperature	Normal	Normal
Muscle tone	Good	Good
Flat foot/High arch	Normal	Normal
Nail condition	Ingrowing toenail Z1	Ingrowing toenail Z1. Nail on little toe is damaged and inflamed
Skin condition (dry,oily, spotty, cracked, lined, crepey)	Neck, Z1 – dry. Shoulder, Z1 – dry	Neck, Z1 – dry
Hard skin build up (zone, area)	Neck, Z1 – dry. Shoulder Z4/5 – callus	Neck, Z1 – dry. Shoulder Z4/5 – callus
Other	Toe, Z4/Z5 – minimal athlete's foot. Bladder – swollen Knee (on top of foot) – very swollen	Toe, Z4/Z5 – minimal athlete's foot. Bladder – swollen Knee (on top of foot) – very swollen

GENERAL OBSERVATIONS OF FEET: 08/07/99

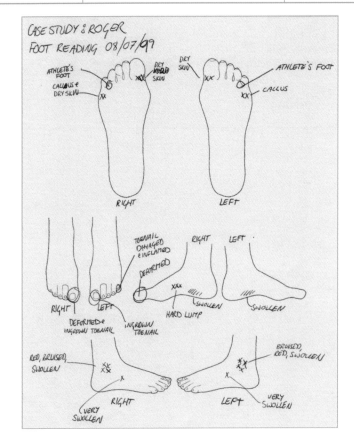

TREATMENT CARD				
C = Crystal S = Sensitivity P = Pain				
Date	Right foot	Left foot	Reactions	Time
08/07/99	Shoulders – S Mid Spine – lump, P Knee helper – swollen, P Bladder – swollen, P	Shoulders – C, S Knee helper – swollen, P Bladder – swollen, P	Very tired/sleepy/struggled to keep awake during treatment but did not want to sleep. Talkative.	18.30
15/07/99	Shoulders – C Knee helper – swollen, P Prostrate – S Lymph/Inguinal walk – blotchy colour, swollen, S	Shoulders – C Bladder – swollen, P Solar Plexus – S Prostrate – S	Did not relax. Talkative.	18.00
04/08/99	Shoulders- C, S Bladder – S Knee – S	Shoulders – C, S Bladder – S Lower abdomen – P Knee – S	Very tired, dozed during the treatment and so did not indicate sensitivities.	18.30
10/09/99	Shoulder – P Thoracic & lumbar spine – P Knee – S Bladder – S	Was asleep therefore did not indicate any sensitivities.	Very tired & stressed. Fell asleep before I finished the right foot.	18.00
03/11/99	Mastoid – S	Pituitary – P	Knee has been giving him a lot of problems. Quite relaxed, not too stressful at work.	18.00
05/12/99	Mastoid – P Temple – P Solar Plexus – S	Solar Plexus – P Mastoid – P Temple – P Back of neck – P Medial lymphatics – P	Last week elbows very sore, knee fine. But hurt knee working in garden. Work very busy.	18.00

Treatment 1

Reading of the feet
See original observations of the feet.

Treatment plan
Full 45 minute treatment to be given. The focus will be on relaxation.

Treatment details, including reactions during the treatment
Roger was very tired and stressed from work today and during the treatment he became sleepier and sleepier, but did not want to fall asleep. He was very talkative. The shoulder reflexes on both feet were sensitive, but not painful, and he said his shoulders were tense from working at a computer all day. There was a painful lump in the middle of his spinal reflex, and the knee reflexes on both feet were swollen and very painful when pressed. His bladder reflexes on both feet were also swollen and painful.

Because it was Roger's first treatment and he was quite sensitive to the pressure, I did not go back to any of the sensitive areas to treat them further after the basic treatment. I felt this might be too much for the first treatment.

Clinical practice

Aftercare advice

Roger was relaxed after the treatment and I gave him a glass of water to drink. We discussed his diet which consists mainly of red meat and minimal fruit or vegetables and he said he will try to make some healthy changes. I suggested that he contact a nutritionist who could guide him through these changes. We also discussed different ways in which he can learn to cope better with his stress and relax more. Unfortunately, there is nothing we can do about his broken sleep at the moment – that is part of having a young baby! I also showed him how to cut his toenails properly to avoid getting ingrowing nails and recommended he use an antifungal cream for his athlete's foot.

Treatment 2

Reactions after last treatment

Roger enjoyed the treatment last week and slept very well after it. However, the following day he was very tired and struggled to keep awake or function properly. For the entire week following the treatment he was extremely tired.

Reading of the feet

The athlete's foot infection on Roger's feet has improved slightly as he has been applying an antifungal cream. Otherwise, the reading of his feet is the same as before.

Treatment plan

Full 45 minute treatment to be given. The focus will be on relaxation and I will also spend some extra time working his back and knee reflexes and associated reflexes that can help with his back and knee problems.

Treatment details, including reactions during the treatment

Today Roger's shoulders were still sensitive and there were a few crystals in these areas. His bladder reflexes on both feet were still swollen and painful. His prostate reflexes on both feet were sensitive. His knee reflex on his right foot only was swollen and painful and the lymphatic/inguinal area on his right foot was blotchy, swollen and sensitive. His solar plexus on his left foot was sensitive. I reworked all these reflexes and also spent some time working the acupoint HP-6 to help calm his mind. Roger was talkative during the treatment, but did not relax.

Homecare advice

Roger has been trying to improve his diet this week and also took my advice on using an antifungal cream on his athlete's foot infection. Unfortunately, he has had a very stressful week at work and says he has not had a chance to teach himself to relax.

Treatment 3

Reactions after last treatment

After the last treatment Roger slept well and found he felt better the next day – he had more energy and felt great. When playing golf on the Sunday, he suddenly noticed that he could crouch down on both knees – although this was still painful, he has not been able to do this for over a year.

Reading of the feet

I noticed that the knee reflexes on Roger's feet arc no longer so swollen. The slightly sweetish odour has also gone and so has his athlete's foot infection. His bladder reflexes were also less swollen than previously. Otherwise, the reading of his feet remains the same.

Treatment plan

Full 45 minute treatment to be given. The focus will be on relaxation as well as working his spine and its associated reflexes.

Treatment details, including reactions during the treatment

Today Roger was very stressed and tired from work and actually slept during the treatment so did not indicate much sensitivity. His shoulder reflexes were sensitive on both feet and there were crystals in these areas. His knee reflex was sensitive but not swollen as previously. His bladder reflexes on both feet were sensitive, but not painful as previously – they were also considerably less swollen. His lower abdomen region on the left foot was painful.

Homecare advice

Roger is doing well with his healthier approach to eating and he says his wife is pleased with his new attitude! His athlete's foot has gone and we discussed basic foot hygiene and ways in which to prevent him contracting it again. With regard to relaxation, he says he is still really struggling to unwind but finds the reflexology treatments very beneficial.

Treatment 4

GENERAL OBSERVATIONS OF FEET: 10/09/99		
Observation	Right foot	Left foot
Colour	Normal	Normal
Smell	Normal	Normal
Skeletal deformities (bunions)	Mid spine – hard lump. Large toe – deformed (it was fractured)	None
Temperature	Normal	Normal
Muscle tone	Good	Good
Flat foot/High arch	Normal	Normal
Nail condition	Ingrowing toenail Z1	Ingrowing toenail Z1
Skin condition (dry, oily, spotty, cracked, lined, crepey)	Neck, Z1 – dry	Neck, Z1 – dry
Hard skin build up (zone, area)	Neck, Z1 – dry. Shoulder Z4/5 - callus	Neck, Z1 – dry. Shoulder Z4/5 – callus
Other	Bladder slightly swollen	Bladder slightly swollen

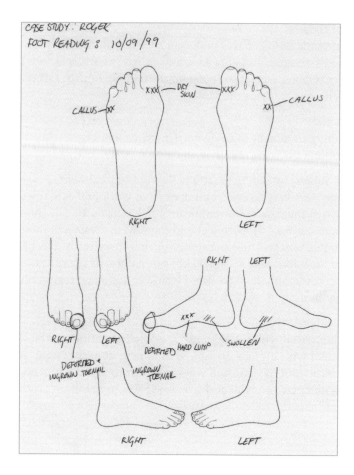

Reactions after last treatment

I have not been able to treat Roger for a month now as he has been very busy at work and has not had the time. Roger found that for the first week after his last treatment he felt very well and energetic and his knee was not at all painful. However, he has since strained his back while moving boxes and he has also been working very long hours, until at least 9pm every night. Consequently, he has been feeling very tired, stressed and has had backache in his lumbar region.

Reading of the feet

Roger's feet have changed quite a lot since we took the first reading of his feet so I have done another complete reading as shown on the previous page.

Treatment plan

Full 45 minute treatment to be given. The focus will be on relaxation as well as working his spine and its associated reflexes.

Treatment details, including reactions during the treatment

I gave Roger a complete treatment and as he was very tired he quickly fell asleep. His shoulder reflexes and his thoracic and lumbar spine reflexes were painful. His knee reflex was sensitive but not swollen as before. His bladder reflex was also still sensitive. I returned to the sensitive areas and treated them with seven pressure circles each.

Homecare advice

I suggested to Roger that he try to leave work earlier if possible and relax more in the evenings. He also needs to get more sleep as he was looking very tired and run down. Despite his exhaustion, he is still trying to eat a healthy diet.

I spoke to Roger the day following the treatment and he said he slept very well and felt energetic and wonderful.

Re-assessment of treatment plan

Roger has been finding it quite difficult to keep to regular times for his reflexology sessions as his job is so demanding and he often does not know what hours he will be working. However, he would like to continue with them as he feels they have really helped him to relax and helped with his knee. We agreed that he would try to come once a month for a treatment. During this time I did stress to him the importance of relaxation and he says he will try to spend a few minutes every morning and evening focusing on his own breathing – he realises the importance of spending some time on himself.

Treatment 5

Reactions after last treatment

It is now a month since I last saw Roger. Although he has had a very stressful month, work has now quietened down a lot and this last week has not been too stressful. Consequently, Roger is feeling quite relaxed today. He feels that since he has begun the treatments his energy levels have improved remarkably and he is not constantly struggling to keep awake. He also says his knees have improved a great deal and he can now crouch down on them. However, his knees and lower back are still uncomfortable.

Reading of the feet

Since his last treatment, I have noticed that the dry skin on Roger's neck and shoulder reflexes is lessening. His toenails on his big toes have also improved greatly.

Treatment plan

Full 45 minute treatment to be given. The focus will be on relaxation as well as working his spine and its associated reflexes.

Treatment details, including reactions during the treatment

Roger's feet were not very sensitive today and only his mastoid and pituitary reflexes showed any reactions. His knee and back reflexes showed no sensitivities at all although I did still spend a great deal of time working these and their associated reflexes.

Homecare advice

Roger has been trying to spend 10 minutes every morning and evening doing some deep breathing exercises and he feels they are really helping him to relax. He finds that he is now calmer at work and feels he can cope better with stressful situations. He also says he is enjoying having the time to himself.

Treatment 6

GENERAL OBSERVATIONS OF FEET: 05/12/99		
Observation	Right foot	Left foot
Colour	Normal	Normal
Smell	Normal	Normal
Skeletal deformities (bunions)	Mid spine – hard lump. Large toe – deformed (it was fractured)	None
Temperature	Normal	Normal
Muscle tone	Good	Good
Flat foot/High arch	Normal	Normal
Nail condition	Good	Good
Skin condition (dry, oily, spotty, cracked, lined, crepey)	Shoulder Z4/5 – dry	Shoulder Z4/5 – dry
Hard skin build up (zone, area)	None	None
Other	None	None

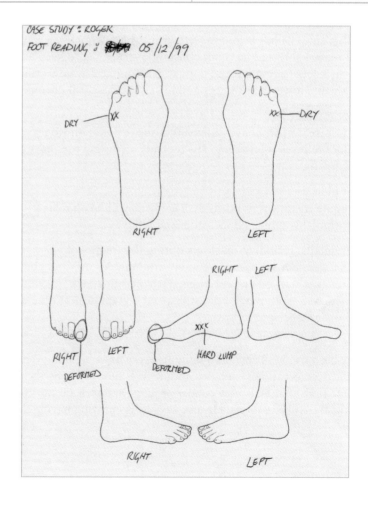

Reactions after last treatment

After the last treatment the pain in Roger's knee went away until he was working in the garden over the weekend and hurt it again. Interestingly, both his elbows ached terribly for the first 2–3 days after last week's treatment. Roger also felt very well during the week and had a lot of energy.

Reading of the feet

There have been slight changes in Roger's feet over the last month as shown below.

Treatment plan

Today Roger's knee is aching and he is quite tired and stressed from work as things are very busy again. He is also in a hurry and so instead of giving him a complete 45 minute treatment, I will reduce the treatment to 30 minutes.

Treatment details, including reactions during the treatment

Roger felt sensitivities in the solar plexus, mastoid, temple and medial inguinal lymphatics. He was very relaxed and dozed during the treatment.

Homecare advice

One area of homecare advice we have not really focused on yet is exercise. Roger feels he simply does not have the time to exercise. However, he agrees that having now made an effort to improve his diet and spend a few minutes doing deep breathing exercises every day he can really see the benefits of looking after himself. Because he has to be careful with his knee, Roger has decided to try swimming twice a week to begin with. He will let me know how this goes when I see him next.

Conclusion

Roger has enjoyed the treatments immensely and found that his knee condition has improved remarkably. He also finds that after the treatments he feels energised and relaxed for 3–4 days. However, he has found it difficult to fit them into his schedule and has had to cancel them a number of times due to his demanding work. Roger would like to continue with the treatments on a monthly basis.

Reflective Practice

Note: The information given here is only intended as an introduction to the topic of reflective practice.

Reflexology is a holistic therapy in which self-awareness and personal growth are fundamental steps to self-healing. As reflexology practitioners, however, we need to acknowledge that this self-awareness and growth is not only for the recipient, but also for the giver. To give a good reflexology treatment you need to be aware of your own attitudes, beliefs and values and develop yourself to the best of your ability. Reflective practice is one way in which you, as a practitioner, can learn to be more self-aware and foster your own personal growth.

What is reflective practice?

Reflective practice is an innovative approach to learning in which we constantly reflect on our experiences and learn from them. Although reflective practice is now an essential part of most reflexology syllabi, it should not be confined to students only. Every practitioner, no matter how experienced, can still develop themselves through analysing and evaluating their treatments and their interactions with their clients. In addition, through attending Continual Professional Development (CPD) workshops, reading journals and literature on reflexology and discussing cases or techniques with other practitioners, we can continue to learn about ourselves and our profession.

In the 1980s, the philosopher Donald Alan Schön identified two types of reflection: reflection-in-action and reflection-on-action. These underlying notions can be used in your daily practice to help you develop yourself:

- **Reflection-in-action** can be described as thinking on your feet because it involves making decisions and acting on them in a situation as it is occurring. For example, while giving a client a treatment she starts to cry uncontrollably. You need to make a decision as to what you will do and how you will continue with the treatment. You can draw on your theoretical knowledge and past experiences, but essentially you need to think on your feet – make a decision quickly and act on it. Often, reflection-in-action is following your natural instincts and letting your intuition take over.
- **Reflection-on-action** can be described as looking back on a situation, analysing and assessing it and learning from it. Continuing with the above example, once your client has gone home you can think back on how you reacted to her crying. You can read up in your text books about reactions to treatments and you can discuss the situation with your peers or perhaps a more experienced reflexologist. In essence, you can use this situation to develop yourself and learn from the experience. Perhaps you might want to improve your counselling skills? Or perhaps you feel good about how you reacted to the situation and you may realise that you are developing into a more intuitive reflexologist.

What are the basic elements of reflective practice?

When you stop to think exactly what reflective practice is, you will realise that it is a process we often do throughout the day without really being aware of it. Most of us take a minute or two to analyse a situation before we make a decision upon which we act. We practise the basic elements of reflection by:

- Being aware of and questioning what, why and how we do things
- Looking for choices, options and possibilities
- Comparing and contrasting possible results and asking 'what if' questions
- Trying to understand the mechanisms or rationale underlying the situation.

In addition, after making a decision and acting on it, we practise reflection again by:

- Looking back on and analysing our decisions and actions
- Getting feedback from other people
- Thinking about what we did right, what we did wrong and what we will do differently next time.

The basic elements of reflective practice are summarised in an educational model called the Learning Cycle. This was developed by an educational theorist called David Kolb who suggested that a person does not learn through simply experiencing something. They need to reflect on that experience, draw conclusions from it and then put these theories into practice.

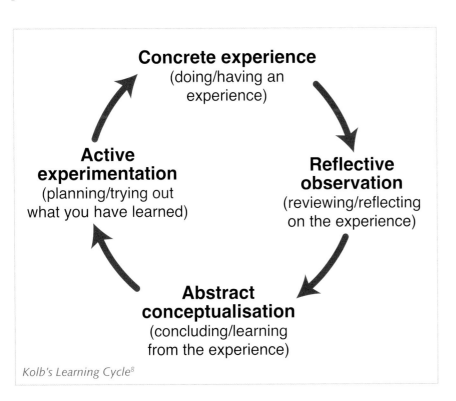

Kolb's Learning Cycle[8]

How can you use reflective practice to develop yourself?

Keep a reflective practice journal

The easiest way to begin developing reflective practice skills is to keep a journal or diary of your experiences and then spend some time reflecting on them. Try using the Reflective Cycle below to help you.

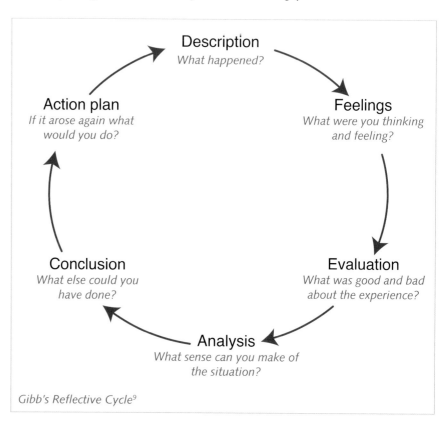

Gibb's Reflective Cycle[9]

You may like to refer to the Reflective Log on the next two pages and use it when assessing a treatment.

Reflective log

How were you feeling before you began the treatment? Looking forward to giving the treatment? Excited to see your client? Tired? Irritated because of something else that had happened that day? Dreading seeing that specific client?

....

....

....

....

....

....

What did you observe in terms of both verbal and non-verbal communication? How did your client communicate with you and how did you communicate with them?

....
....
....
....
....
....

How did you feel after the treatment? Did you feel that you gave a good treatment? Did anything either technical or theoretical come up that you did not know and would like to learn more about? Did you feel relaxed? Tired? Irritated? Drained? Why did you feel like this?

....
....
....
....
....
....

What do you feel you have learned from this treatment?

....
....
....
....
....
....

Considering your responses to the above questions, what would you like to change or do differently next time? How do you think you can improve?

....
....
....
....
....
....

Are there any areas in which you felt inadequate or are there any courses (CPD workshops) you feel could help you give a better treatment next time? Did any topics come up which you would like to research further or ask someone about?

....

....

....

....

....

....

What did you do well? What are your strengths?

....

....

....

....

....

....

Note: Reflective practice should not be used to beat yourself up. It is a time in which you learn about yourself and this includes your strengths as well as the areas in which you would like to develop further.

Ask your clients for feedback

Another way in which you can develop your reflective practice skills is through asking your clients for feedback. Ask them how they found the treatment and if there is anything you can do to improve the experience for them? Being open with your clients will help you develop a trusting relationship which will enhance the effectiveness of your treatment as well as help you develop yourself. Furthermore, establishing a good rapport with your client may encourage them to come back to you more often and recommend you to their friends.

Take part in peer reviews, mentoring programmes or discussions with other therapists

Finally, you can develop yourself further as a reflexologist by working closely with other therapists, asking their advice and discussing different topics with them. Even swopping treatments with your peers and then asking them to review your treatment will enable you to reflect on both your strengths and weaknesses and so foster your personal growth. The more time you spend reflecting on your experiences, assessing and analysing them, the more you will learn from them.

Study Outline

Remember the following when conducting your consultation:

- Private, comfortable area
- Positive body language
- Positioning of the client – no barriers such as a desk between you
- Good communication skills – ask open questions such as 'What do you think the Reflexology treatment will do?' rather than 'Do you think the treatment will relax you?'
- Trust and confidentiality
- Professionalism, confidence, enthusiasm
- Consent – of doctor, guardian, parent
- Contraindications
- Referrals – refer when necessary and work only within the realms of your own expertise and experience. Refer to doctor, counsellor, complementary therapist, social worker, etc.
- Client profile and lifestyle – age, marital status, diet, profession, etc can tell you a lot about their health
- Treatment plan – don't forget their religious, moral and social beliefs
- Determine the client's needs and expectations
- Obtain their agreement to your treatment plan
- Explain any side effects or expected reactions during and after the treatment
- Discuss the treatment plan with carer, parent or guardian if necessary
- Obtain the client's signature
- Client care:
  - Always discuss consultation and treatment plan with them
  - Explain what the treatment is and what it involves
  - Help client on to and off the couch
  - Protect client's modesty at all times
  - Wash your hands before and after each treatment
  - Clean the client's feet
  - Ensure client is comfortable and use supports under head, knees and ankles
  - Adapt techniques to suit each client
- Self-care – don't forget you are just as important as the client! Ensure you are always comfortable, do not touch infected areas and look after your hands.

Multiple choice questions

1. **If a client becomes upset during the consultation, which would be the most appropriate form of behaviour by the therapist?**
   a. The therapist should avert his or her eyes from the client and continue with the consultation as normal
   b. The therapist should stop the consultation and give the client a big hug
   c. The therapist should stop the consultation, give the client a tissue and a glass of water and, when the client is ready, continue with the consultation
   d. The therapist should ask the client to pull themselves together and continue with the consultation.

2. **When is it appropriate for the therapist to share the client's records?**
   a. If the client's husband or wife asks to see them
   b. If the client's friend asks to see them
   c. If the clinic manager asks to see them
   d. None of the above.

3. **Which of the following is a group of unicellular micro-organisms that lack organelles and an organised nucleus?**
   a. Bacteria
   b. Fungi
   c. Virus
   d. Parasite.

4. **What type of infection is tinea pedis?**
   a. Bacterial
   b. Fungal
   c. Viral
   d. None of the above.

5. **If a client presents with an infestation of fleas can they still receive a reflexology treatment?**
   a. Yes
   b. No
   c. Only with their doctor's permission
   d. None of the above.

6. **Which of the following is an example of an open-ended question?**
   a. Tell me about your diet?
   b. Do you eat a lot of sugar?
   c. Do you like junk food?
   d. How many times a week do you eat healthy meals?

7. **Which of the following are not generally discussed when giving homecare advice to a client?**
   a. Diet
   b. Water intake
   c. Sexual habits
   d. Ergonomics.

8. **Which of the following are all normal reactions to a reflexology treatment?**
   a. Changes in body temperature, changes in mood, developing a rumbling stomach
   b. Becoming slightly nauseous, experiencing a tingling sensation, having an asthma attack
   c. Vomiting, developing a headache, becoming sweaty and hot
   d. Feeling good, getting cramp in the foot, having an epileptic fit.

9. **If your client suddenly becomes nauseous during a treatment which of the following should you not do?**
   a. Zone-walking
   b. Holding the solar-plexus
   c. Holding the foot
   d. Deep pressure techniques on the stomach reflex.

10. **How would you adapt your treatment for a 6-month old baby?**
    a. Give a full 45 minute treatment
    b. Give a 30 minute treatment
    c. Give a 20 minute treatment
    d. Give a 5 minute treatment.

8 Exploring reflexology and other complementary therapies

*'As we cannot smile or breathe for another person,
how can we presume to be able to heal him?'*
Gaston Saint Pierre & Debbie Shapiro[1]

What makes complementary therapy so unique and powerful is that it empowers a person to heal themselves. It encourages them to take responsibility for their health and through the use of a variety of techniques, tools or mediums it sets the body's own healing mechanisms into action. This chapter explores the world of complementary therapy by introducing you to some of the different therapies available.

Student objectives

By the end of this chapter you will have a basic understanding of the following therapies:

Reflexology-related therapies
- Auricular Therapy
- The Metamorphic Technique
- Precision Reflexology
- Vertical Reflexology (VRT)

Other complementary therapies
- Acupuncture and Acupressure
- Alexander Technique
- Aromatherapy
- Ayurveda
- Bach Flower Remedies
- Beauty Therapy
- Biochemical Tissue Salts
- Bowen Technique
- Chiropractic
- Herbalism (Herbology)
- Homeopathy
- Hypnotherapy
- Indian Head Massage
- Iridology
- Kinesiology
- Manual Lymphatic Drainage
- Neurolinguistic Programming (NLP)
- Oriental Facial Diagnosis (Chinese Face Reading)
- Osteopathy
- Physiotherapy
- Reiki
- Shiatsu
- Spiritual Healing
- Stone Therapy Massage
- Swedish Massage
- Yoga

Taking Reflexology Further

Once you have an understanding of the basics of reflexology you can start to explore the different types that are available. A few of these are briefly introduced below and if you are interested in any of them you can continue your education with a post-graduate or continuing professional development (CPD) course.

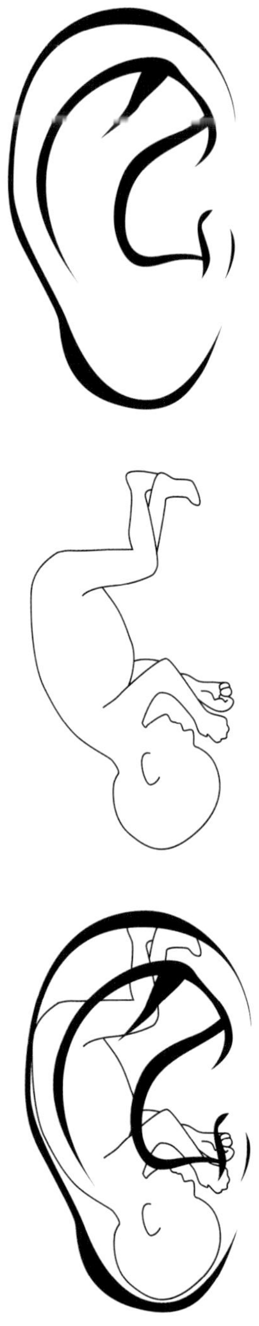

Auricular Therapy

Just as the organs and structures of the body can be mapped onto the hands and feet, so too can they be found on the ears. The ears mirror a foetus as it lies in the womb, with the lobe of the ear being the head.

Auricular therapy has its roots in traditional Chinese medicine and in the 1960s it was developed into a therapy in its own right by a French acupuncturist, Dr Paul Nogier. He took the use of acupuncture further by using very fine needles, light therapy, electrical therapy and magnetically-charged ball bearings on the ears.[2]

Auricular massage can be used to help diagnose a condition. As with the hands and feet, blemishes, puffiness or tenderness on the ears correspond to imbalances in the body. Massage or deep pressure to points on the ears can help with pain relief, activate the flow of Qi through the meridians and improve the circulation of both blood and lymph throughout the body. It is a very gentle, non-invasive therapy which can be used on anyone, even the very ill, elderly or young. The only contraindications to auricular massage are local contraindications such as broken skin on the ears.

The Metamorphic Technique

'In nature the acorn becomes an oak tree and a caterpillar metamorphoses into a butterfly. We ourselves have within us the potential to do and to become far more than we are at present.' Gaston Saint-Pierre & Debbie Shapiro[3]

The metamorphic technique was first developed by Robert St John, a British naturopath and reflexologist who worked mainly with mentally handicapped children. He discovered that people develop a structure of patterns that predispose them to illness or a certain mindset. This structure develops from the moment of conception and is influenced by one's parents, culture and environment. In their book, *The Metamorphic Technique*, Gaston Saint-Pierre and Debbie Shapiro wrote: 'Life starts at conception when the first cell is formed. During the gestation period, the nine months between conception and birth, our physical, mental, emotional and behavioural structures are all established. Our life following birth is rooted in and influenced by this prenatal period, our life before birth'.[4]

This structure is reflected in parts of the hands, feet and head and through very gentle techniques applied to them the structure can be loosened and the body's internal healing activities can be set into action. The outcome of a metamorphic session is that the recipient is able to let go of old patterns and fulfil their life's potential.

Fig 8.1 Auricular therapy

What is vital in St John's revolutionary approach to healing is that a metamorphic practitioner is simply a catalyst that enables the life force within a person to heal them. The practitioner is not a healer, so sessions do not include consultations or diagnoses. The practitioner simply works on the hands, feet and head without imposing any thoughts of their own.

Precision Reflexology

Precision reflexology was developed by a British reflexologist called Prue Miskin and it is a very different method of reflexology to what you have studied in this book as it requires a minimum of pressure.

The main technique in precision reflexology is known as the linking technique and it involves gently holding two to three different reflexes at the same time, applying no pressure to them and simply 'listening' to the energy within them. In her book *A Guide to Precision Reflexology*, Jan Williamson writes: 'The aim of precision reflexology is to connect to a person's energy system, to adjust it and to harmonise it within itself and with the world surrounding that person.'[5] Although it is so gentle, it has very powerful results and can be used safely with the very ill, elderly or young and its techniques can be used to enhance your normal reflexology treatment.

Vertical Reflexology (VRT)

The reflexology techniques you have studied in this book are generally given to a person who is lying down or seated with their feet up. Vertical reflexology therapy is a revolutionary approach in that it is given to a person who is either seated or standing, with their feet down and bearing the weight of their entire body. It is a wonderful way to work the feet of elderly or disabled people who cannot easily put their feet up and it has been found to have very good results.

Vertical reflexology was developed by a British reflexologist called Lynne Booth who spent many years working in a residential nursing home and found she had to adapt her traditional reflexology methods so that she could work with chronically ill clients who were often in wheelchairs. Booth noticed that through working the tops of the feet when they were weight-bearing she got very quick results and in her book *Vertical Reflexology* she writes: 'The upright body appears to be in a position of increased vitality because it is weight-bearing – the muscles are taut, there is pressure on the bones to support the upright skeleton, and the heart is pumping oxygenated blood to the organs, which, in a standing position, will be less impacted by possible posture.'[6]

Vertical reflexology includes working the zones of the feet, the tops of the feet and simultaneously working specific hand and foot reflexology and its techniques can be used to enhance a normal reflexology treatment.

Other Complementary Therapies

Acupuncture and Acupressure

Acupuncture and acupressure form part of traditional Chinese medicine (TCM). The Chinese believe that life is activated by the energy force known as Qi, which is determined by one's constitution and lifestyle. It flows through the body in energy pathways (meridians) and any congestion in a meridian manifests as an imbalance or disorder in the body.

A TCM therapist treats the meridians of an individual to improve their health and encourage the body to heal itself. During a treatment, the therapist determines which points in the body are sluggish or blocked and stimulates these by thumb and finger pressure (acupressure) or by inserting very fine needles (acupuncture). This improves the energy flow, enhances the functions of the body and is also a form of preventative health care.

Alexander Technique

The Alexander Technique is more a form of education than a therapy. Through a series of lessons a pupil is encouraged to increase his or her awareness of posture, movement and balance. As a result, movement becomes easier and balance and co-ordination are improved. Pupils learn to adopt postures of perfect balance and movement with a minimum of tension. Lessons are usually conducted on an individual basis.

Aromatherapy

Aromatherapy is the art and science of using oils extracted from aromatic plants to enhance health, beauty and emotional well-being. These oils represent the 'life force' of the plants – they are essential to the plants' biological processes, as well as being the substance that gives them their scent. Synthetic oils, even if chemically similar, will lack all the natural elements, and this vital life-force. Thus only natural essential oils are therapeutically valuable. Essential oils are extracted from flowers, herbs, spices, fruit, bark, roots, seeds and grasses. They are used in massage, baths, compresses, inhalations, vaporisation and perfumes.

Ayurveda

Ayurveda is a Sanskrit term meaning 'life science' and is a system of preventative medicine that originated in India. It forms an integral part of one's lifestyle, rather than simply being a one-off cure for the symptoms of a disease. It incorporates all aspects of a healthy lifestyle and has medical, spiritual and dietary philosophies.

Central to the philosophies of Ayurveda is the concept prana or energy: everything in our universe, including ourselves, is made up of prana and all we know and all we see has emerged from a blending of ether, air, fire, water and earth. These are known as the five elements and they form the basic concept of Ayurveda. All medical, spiritual and dietary philosophies are based on these elements.

Bach Flower Remedies

Flower Essence Therapy is sometimes called 'soul therapy' and is based on the theory that illness is often a result of a psychological imbalance. Flower essences have a therapeutic effect on the mind and emotions of an individual, and promote the process of personal evolution. They work primarily on the human psyche and, if we compare ourselves to a plant, the flower is the most complex, beautiful and unique part of the plant, as is the human mind of the body.

Beauty Therapy

The aim of beauty therapy is to enhance the natural beauty of an individual and to encourage good health and beauty habits. Beauty therapists are required to have an in-depth knowledge of the anatomy and physiology of the body; skin types, functions, disorders and skin care; eyebrow shaping and tinting; facial massage; makeup; pedicures and manicures; cosmetic chemistry; waxing; body massage; electrotherapy; dietetics and exercise; and UV/infra-red rays. An essential part of beauty therapy is the ability to advise clients on health and well being and recommend the correct products for their individual types.

Biochemical Tissue Salts

Researched, studied and documented by Dr Schuessler in 1890, Tissue/Cell Salts represent the 12 main minerals of the body that are vital to our health. A lack or insufficiency of any essential minerals will lead to an imbalance in our health. Tissue salts simply replace these minerals in small amounts. They have no side-effects.

Bowen Technique

The Bowen Technique was developed in Australia by Thomas Bowen and aims to rebalance the body holistically by using gentle moves on the tissues. A Bowen practitioner can feel whether muscles are stressed or tense and uses light, rolling movements to stimulate the body's energy flow and release the build-up of tension. It is not a massage or a manipulation, but a gentle process that encourages the body to heal itself.

Chiropractic

Chiropractic contends that an optimally-functioning nervous system enables the body to maintain its homeostasis and therefore its adaptability. It is the science of locating offending spinal structures and reducing their impact to the nervous system through restoring proper spinal biomechanics. Subluxation is the term used to describe the condition of bones that are out of alignment. It is this condition that gives rise to restricted mobility or excessive mobility and which affects the functioning of the nervous system. Practitioners use a specific force in a precise direction, applied to a joint that is fixated, locked, or not moving properly, and adjust it to its correct position and mobility.

Herbalism (Herbology)

Herbalism is a therapeutic system based on the use of herbs in the treatment of a wide range of ailments. Natural remedies are made from any number of substances taken from nature: leaves, roots, flowers or mineral deposits. In natural medicine, the proposition that the structure and appearance of the plant can be a clue to its therapeutic action is referred to as the Doctrine of Signatures. If a sick person's symptoms reflect this pattern or appearance, then a plant exhibiting the same pattern is used as a remedy for the disorder. Natural substances are chosen not to cure the client of his/her symptoms, but to correct an underlying problem.

Homeopathy

Homeopathy is a holistic therapy based on the principle that 'like cures like'. This is the belief that the agents that cause the symptoms of a sickness in a healthy person can cure the cause of those same symptoms in an unhealthy person, when used in extreme dilution. Homeopathy was first used by a German doctor, Dr Hahnemann, in the late 1700s and it has since developed into a respected and popular complementary therapy. Homeopathic remedies treat the cause of a disease rather than simply the symptoms, and are natural substances derived from plants, animal materials and natural chemicals.

Hypnotherapy

Hypnotherapy is a form of psychotherapy that can be used to improve both physical and mental health. It is believed that our minds consist of both conscious and subconscious parts. During a session, a therapist puts their client into a trance-like state and then makes suggestions to their subconscious minds, which rule their conscious minds. Through these suggestions our subconscious minds are able to reprogram our beliefs and patterns of behaviour and hypnotherapy is known to help with stress management, pain relief, phobias and addictions.

Indian Head Massage

With its roots in Ayurveda, Indian Head Massage is an ancient therapy which has been practiced for over 3000 years. Based on Ayurvedic 'shampooing' techniques, Indian Head Massage works on the scalp, face, neck, shoulders and upper arms of a person. It is a simple and versatile massage that can be given almost anywhere and is suitable for a diverse range of people from children to the very elderly.

Iridology

Iridology is based on the theory that an individual's health is reflected in the condition of their iris. It was developed by a Hungarian doctor, Ignatz von Peczeley, who as a child found an owl with a broken leg and noticed a black mark in its iris. Many years later he became a homeopath and when caring for a patient with a broken leg he noticed the same mark in the patient's iris. Today Iridologists examine people's irises to diagnose their health and their tendency towards disease.

Kinesiology

Kinesiology is a holistic therapy based on asking the body what it needs to return to optimum health. Its primary tool is muscle testing, which involves applying gentle pressure on a muscle and assessing the response. If the muscle locks, then the response is 'yes'; if the muscle is spongy, then the response is 'no'.

Kinesiology can be used to diagnose a disorder in an individual or to find the most appropriate therapy for that disorder. Kinesiology can be used in conjunction with a number of other therapies ranging from chiropractic to flower remedies.

Manual Lymphatic Drainage

Lymphatic fluid is moved through its vessels by muscular contraction or massage only and Lymphatic Drainage is a form of massage that focuses on manually moving the fluid. It was developed by Dr Vodder in the 1930s and it helps clear congestion, waste and fluid from the body. It is particularly beneficial to people suffering from disorders such as water retention or poor immunity.

Neurolinguistic Programming (NLP)

Developed in the 1970s by John Grinder and Richard Bandler, neurolinguistic programming is based on the idea that we can learn patterns of thinking that will positively influence our physical and mental behaviour. These patterns are modelled on how successful people communicate in terms of both verbal and body language. Grinder and Bandler noticed that successful people generally have successful attitudes which are, in a sense, self-fulfilling prophecies. Through an awareness of oneself and one's tools of communication, people can develop these positive attitudes and therefore succeed in life.

Oriental Facial Diagnosis (Chinese Face Reading)

Oriental facial diagnosis is an integral part of traditional Chinese medicine (TCM) but it can sometimes be used as a therapy in its own right to develop a picture of a person's health. Just as the hands, feet and ears of a person reflect their health and emotions, so too does the face. Figure 8.2 shows the face as a map of the body and in general the face is divided into three parts: the upper region reflects the nervous and mental functions of a person; the middle region reflects the circulatory activities; and the lower region reveals the digestive and reproductive health.

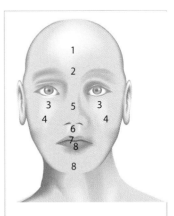

Key

1. Mind/Thinking/ Intellect
2. Liver
3. Kidneys
4. Lungs
5. Spine
6. Ovaries/ Testes
7. Stomach
8. Colon

Fig 8.2 Chinese face reading

Osteopathy

Osteopathy is a system of diagnosis and treatment which recognises that most of the pain and disability we suffer stems from abnormalities in the function of the body structure as well as damage caused to it by disease. It was founded by an American doctor, Dr Andrew Taylor Still (1828–1917).

Osteopaths use a highly developed sense of touch, called palpation, to identify points of weakness or excessive strain in the body. They then work with their hands, using a variety of techniques, to restore the body to its full structural and functional capacity and encourage it to heal itself.

Physiotherapy

Physiotherapy, or physical therapy, is the treatment of diseases and disorders through physical means such as massage, manipulations, exercises and the application of heat, cold, light or electricity. Its aim is to restore normal body functions and prevent disabilities that may result from injury, trauma or disease and it can help a person regain their posture, balance and mobility.

Reiki

The word Reiki is Japanese for 'universal life energy' and it was developed in Japan in the early 1900's by Mikao Usui. Reiki is based on the principle that the healer channels the universal life energy into the client's body. This energy creates a deep sense of relaxation, removes energy blockages and promotes general wellbeing.

Shiatsu

Shiatsu is a Japanese therapy that has its origins in Traditional Chinese Medicine. It is similar to acupuncture, but is performed without needles, and the Japanese name 'shiatsu' literally means 'finger pressure' (shi = finger, atsu = pressure). Shiatsu is a form of preventative, holistic healthcare in which the practitioner uses his/her fingers, elbows, palms, knees and feet to normalise the flow of Ki (energy) in the body. Shiatsu practitioners believe that congestion in the flow of Ki through the body will cause an imbalance or disorder in the body and so they apply pressure to specific areas that are congested with energy, or that are lacking energy. Through applying this pressure they encourage the flow of Ki which subsequently balances the systems, restoring health and vitality.

Spiritual Healing

Spiritual healing is 'hands-on' healing in which a healer channels energy, usually through their hands, into a person. This energy is of a divine, spiritual nature and can sometimes be felt by the recipient as heat, a draught, a tingling sensation or pins and needles. According to *The Hamlyn Encyclopedia of Complementary Health*, 'Spiritual healing provides the energy needed to crank our own healing mechanism back into action. When a healer lays his hands on you, he acts as a conductor or channel for the healing energy which he believes has the 'intelligence' to go where it is needed.'[7]

Stone Therapy Massage

Stone therapy is a highly relaxing, stress-relieving treatment that works on a deeper level than most other massages as one stroke with a stone is equal to six strokes with a hand. It is essentially the application of thermotherapy: the use of opposing extremes of temperature to stimulate the circulation and thus encourage healing.

Swedish Massage

Swedish Massage is the manipulation of soft tissue for therapeutic purposes. It is a very gentle, yet powerful method for treating, and preventing, pain and stress-related disorders. The massage technique consists of two main movements: pressure techniques that speed up the body's physiology, increases blood and lymph flow, pushes lactic acid out of stiff muscles and improves joint mobility; and slow, sweeping movements that have a soothing, relaxing effect that calm the nervous system and eliminate stress.

Yoga

Yoga is thought to have originated in India over 4000 years ago when yogis lived hermetic lives of meditation. Today it is a non-religious and non-cultural exercise system that benefits the body, mind and soul. There are three essential aspects to yoga: *pranayama* (breathing techniques), *asanas* (postures) and *dhyana* (meditation). Together they form the practice of yoga, which in Sanskrit means 'union'. Yoga benefits an individual on many levels. It relaxes the muscles, increases suppleness and fitness, relieves stress, improves concentration, helps one change negative thought patterns and instils a sense of serenity.

References

Chapter 1

1. Ted J. Kaptchuk, *Chinese Medicine, The Web that has no Weaver*, p23.
2. Nikki Bradford (Ed.), *The Hamlyn Encyclopedia of Complementary Health*, p30.
3. Sharon Stathis, *Ayurvedic Reflexology for the Feet*, p11.
4. Inge Dougans, *Complete Illustrated Guide To Reflexology*, p52.
5. Beryl Crane, *Reflexology – The Definitive Practitioner's Manual*, p25.
6. Eunice D. Ingham, *Stories The Feet Have Told*, p3.
7. Dwight C. Byers, *Better Health with Foot Reflexology*, p4.
8. T. McFerran (Consultant Editor), *Oxford Dictionary for Nurses* (4th Ed.)
9. Beryl Crane, Reflexology – *The Definitive Practitioner's Manual*, p14.
10. Eunice D. Ingham, *Stories the Feet Can Tell Through Reflexology*, p8.
11. Eunice D. Ingham, *Stories the Feet Can Tell Through Reflexology*, p1.
12. © 2005-2008 University of Alberta and Worth Publishers, www.psych.ualberta.ca
13. © 2009 www.PainClinic.org
14. © 2005–2008 University of Alberta and Worth Publishers, www.psych.ualberta.ca
15. S. Vedantam, *Against Depression a Sugar Pill is Hard to Beat*, © 2002, The Washington Post Company.
16. Dr Hilary MacQueen, *Is Reflexology Valid?*, © 2009 The Open University.
17. Eunice Ingham, *Stories the Feet Have Told Through Reflexology*, p6.
18. Beryl Crane, *Reflexology – The Definitive Practitioner's Manual*, p14.
19. Eunice Ingham, *Stories the Feet Have Told Through Reflexology*, p12.
20. Gerard Tortora & Sandra Grabowski, *Principles of Anatomy and Physiology (8th Ed.)*, p28.
21. Inge Dougans, *Complete Illustrated Guide to Reflexology*, p26.
22. Inge Dougans, *Complete Illustrated Guide to Reflexology*, p30.
23. Inge Dougans, *Complete Illustrated Guide to Reflexology*, p38.
24. Gerard Tortora & Sandra Grabowski, *Principles of Anatomy and Physiology (8th Ed.)*, p417.
25. Gerard Tortora & Sandra Grabowski, *Principles of Anatomy and Physiology (8th Ed.)*, p417.
26. Barbara and Kevin Kunz, *Reflexology Theory*, ©2003 Kunz and Kunz
27. Eunice Ingham, *Stories the Feet Can Tell*, p1.
28. Dr. Shweta Choudhary, *Reflexology Reduces the Requirement and Quantity of Pain Killers After General Surgery*, Reflexology Association of America, www.reflexology-usa.org/assets/dr_shweta_research_study.pdf
29. Dwight Byers, *Better Health with Foot Reflexology*, p9.
30. Peter Lund Frandsen, *Reflexology – An Energy Medicine*, www.washingtonreflexology.org
31. Beryl Crane, *Reflexology – The Definitive Practitioner's Manual*, Preface p xiv.
32. Dr Christiaan Barnard, *The Body Machine*, p162.
33. Clive O'Hara (Ed.), *Core Curriculum for Reflexology*, p52.

34. R.E. Allen (Ed.), *The Concise Oxford Dictionary (8th Ed)*, p1206.
35. Dr Rudolph Ballentine, *Radical Healing*, p5.
36. Clive O'Hara (Ed.), *Core Curriculum for Reflexology*, p129.

Chapter 2

1. Chris Stormer, *Teach Yourself Reflexology*, p6.
2. Peter Lund Frandsen, *Reflexology – An Energy Medicine*, www.washingtonreflexology.org
3. Ted J. Kaptchuk, *The Web that has no Weaver*, p56.
4. Dr Rudolph Ballentine, *Radical Healing*, p329.
5. Dr Rudolph Ballentine, *Radical Healing*, p391.

Chapter 3

1. Dr Rudolph Ballentine, *Radical Healing*, p161.

Chapter 4

1. Laura Norman, *The Reflexology Handbook*, p270.
2. Dr Christiaan Barnard, *The Body Machine*, p48.
3. Dr Rudolph Ballentine, *Radical Healing*, p189.
4. Inge Dougans, *Complete Illustrated Guide To Reflexology*, p78.
5. Dorthe Krogsgaard and Peter Lund Frandsen, Denmark, www.touchpoint.dk
6. Dwight Byers, *Better Health With Foot Reflexology*, p139.
7. Susanne Enzer, *Maternity Reflexology Manual – Part 1*, p48.
8. Dwight Byers, *Better Health with Foot Reflexology*, p140.
9. Inge Dougans, *Complete Illustrated Guide To Reflexology*, p52.
10. Inge Dougans, *Complete Illustrated Guide to Reflexology*, p68.

Chapter 5

1. Inge Dougans, *Reflexology – A Practical Introduction*, p189.
2. Ted J. Kaptchuk, *The Web that has no Weaver*, p10.
3. Ted, J. Kaptchuk, *The Web That Has No Weaver*, pp34–47.
4. Inge Dougans, *Reflexology – A Practical Introduction*, p205.
5. Jon Sandifer, *Acupressure*, p26.
6. Ted J. Kaptchuk, *The Web That Has No Weaver*, p54.
7. Ted J. Kaptchuk, *The Web That Has No Weaver*, p54.
8. Ohashi, *Reading the Body – Ohashi's Book of Oriental Diagnosis*, p104.
9. Ted J. Kaptchuk, *The Web That Has No Weaver*, p54.
10. Ohashi, *Reading the Body – Ohashi's Book of Oriental Diagnosis*, p104.
11. Ohashi, *Reading the Body – Ohashi's Book of Oriental Diagnosis*, p104.
12. Ted J. Kaptchuk, *The Web That Has No Weaver*, p55.
13. Inge Dougans, *Reflexology – A Practical Introduction*, p247.
14. Ohashi, *Reading the Body – Ohashi's Book of Oriental Diagnosis*, p171.
15. Ted J. Kaptchuk, *The Web That Has No Weaver*, p57.
16. Ted J. Kaptchuk, *The Web That Has No Weaver*, p58.
17. Inge Dougans, *Reflexology – A Practical Introduction*, p224.
18. Ted J. Kaptchuk, *The Web That Has No Weaver*, p67.
19. Ohashi, *Reading the Body – Ohashi's Book of Oriental Diagnosis*, p103.
20. Beryl Crane, *Reflexology – The Definitive Practitioner's Manual*, p183.
21. Ohashi, *Reading the Body – Ohashi's Book of Oriental Diagnosis*, p98.
22. Ted J. Kaptchuk, *The Web That Has No Weaver*, p55.

23. Ted J. Kaptchuk, *The Web That Has No Weaver*, p56.
24. Ted J. Kaptchuk, *The Web That Has No Weaver*, p65.
25. Ohashi, *Reading the Body – Ohashi's Book of Oriental Diagnosis*, p102.
26. Ted J. Kaptchuk, *The Web That Has No Weaver*, p59.
27. Ted J. Kaptchuk, *The Web That Has No Weaver*, p61.
28. Inge Dougans, *Reflexology – A Practical Introduction*, p249.

Chapter 6

1. Clive O'Hara (Ed.), *Core Curriculum for Reflexology in the United Kingdom*, p112.

Chapter 7

1. Vicki Pitman, *Reflexology – A Practical Approach*, p31.
2. Ohashi, *Reading the Body*, p116.
3. Menna Buckland Kleine, *Sterilization & Hygiene – A Practical Guide*, p4.
4. Ohashi, *Reading the Body*, p16.
5. Clive S. O'Hara (Ed.), *Core Curriculum for Reflexology in the United Kingdom*, p33.
6. Ohashi, *Reading the Body*, p18.
7. Vicki Pitman, *Reflexology – A Practical Approach*, p30.
8. Clara Davies and Tony Lowe, University of Leeds: http://www.webducate.net/cpdspot/kolb/
9. Gibbs G (1988) *Learning by Doing: A guide to teaching and learning methods*. Further Education Unit. Oxford Polytechnic: Oxford.

Chapter 8

1. G. Saint-Pierre & D. Shapiro, The Metamorphic Technique, p4
2. N. Bradford (Ed.), The Hamlyn Encyclopedia of Complementary Health, p20
3. G. Saint-Pierre & D. Shapiro, The Metamorphic Technique, p2
4. G. Saint-Pierre & D. Shapiro, The Metamorphic Technique, p3
5. J. Williamson, A Guide to Precision Reflexology, p11
6. L. Booth, Vertical Reflexology, p21
7. N. Bradford (Ed.), The Hamlyn Encyclopedia of Complementary Health, p134

Multiple choice answers

Chapter 1
1.a 2.c 3.b 4.c 5.b 6.b 7.c 8.a 9.d 10.b

Chapter 2
1.c 2.b 3.b 4.a 5.d 6.c 7.b 8.a 9.c 10.d

Chapter 3
1.b 2.a 3.d 4.c 5.a 6.d 7.c 8.a 9.b 10.d

Chapter 4
1.b 2.c 3.b 4.a 5.a 6.a 7.c 8.a 9.c 10.d

Chapter 5
1.c 2.d 3.a 4.d 5.a 6.c 7.b 8.c 9.b 10.a

Chapter 7
1.c 2.d 3.a 4.b 5.b 6.a 7.c 8.a 9.d 10. d

Bibliography

Allen, R. (1990). *The Concise Oxford Dictionary of Current English*. Oxford: Clarendon Press

Ballentine, R. (1999). *Radical Healing*. London: Rider Books

Barnard, C. (ed.) (1981). *The Body Machine*. Willemstad: Multimedia Publications Inc.

Beers, M. (ed.) (2003). *The Merck Manual of Medical Information (2nd Home Ed.)*. New Jersey: Merck & Co., Inc.

Booth, L. (2000). *Vertical Reflexology*. London: Judy Piatkus Ltd

Bradford, N. (Ed.) (1996). *The Hamlyn Encyclopedia of Complementary Health*. London: Hamlyn

Byers, D. (2001). *Better Health With Foot Reflexology*. St Petersburg: Ingham Publishing Inc.

Crane, B. (1997). *Reflexology – The Definitive Practitioner's Manual*. Shaftesbury: Element Books Ltd.

Dougans, I. (1992). *Reflexology – A Practical Introduction*. London: Element Books Ltd.

Dougans, I. (1996). *Complete Illustrated Guide To Reflexology*. Shaftesbury: Element Books Ltd.

Enzer, S. (2003). *Maternity Reflexology Manual*.

Faure-Alderson, M. (2007). *Total Reflexology*. Vermont: Healing Arts Press

Hall, C. *Reflexology Course Training Manual*.

Holdford, P. (1997). *The Optimum Nutrition Bible*. London: Piatkus Books

Hull, R. (2009). *Anatomy & Physiology for therapists and healthcare professionals*. Cambridge: The Write Idea Ltd

Ingham, E. (1938). *Stories the Feet Can Tell Thru Reflexology, Stories the Feet Have Told Thru Reflexology*, St. Petersburg: Ingham Publishing Inc.

Kaptchuk, T. (1983). *Chinese Medicine – The Web That Has No Weaver*. London: Rider Books

Kolster, B. & Waskowiak, A. (2003). *The Reflexology Atlas*. Rochester: Healing Arts Press

Kunz, B. & Kunz, B. (2006). *Hand Reflexology*. London: Dorling Kindersley Ltd.

McFerran, T. (ed.). (1998). *Oxford Dictionary for Nurses (4th Ed.)*. Oxford: Oxford University Press

Mortimore, D. (2001). *The Complete Illustrated Guide to Vitamins and Minerals*. London: Harper Collins Publishers Ltd.

Norman, L. (1988). *The Reflexology Handbook*. London: Judy Piatkus Publishers Ltd.

O'Hara, C. (Ed.) (2006). *Core Curriculum for Reflexology in the United Kingdom*. London: Douglas Barry Publications

Ohashi. (1991). *Reading the Body – Ohashi's Book of Oriental Diagnosis*. New York: Penguin Compass

Pitman, V. (2002). *Reflexology – A Practical Approach*. Cheltenham: Nelson Thornes Ltd.

Putz, R. and Pabst, R. (ed.) (2008) *Sobotta Atlas of Human Anatomy*. Munich: Elsevier GmbH.

Saint-Pierre, G. & Shapiro, D. (1982), *The Metamorphic Technique*. London: Vega

Sandifer, J. (1997). *Acupressure For Health, Vitality and First Aid*. Shaftesbury: Element Books Ltd

Stormer, C. (1996). *Teach Yourself Reflexology*. London: Hodder Headline

Thie, J. (1973). *Touch For Health*. Marina Del Rey: De Vorss & Company Publishers

Thomson, D. *Acupressure Massage Practitioner Training Manual*.

Tortora, G. and Grabowski, S. (1996). *Principles of Anatomy and Physiology (8th Ed.)*. Harper Collins

Williamson, J. (1999). *A Guide to Precision Reflexology*. Salisbury: Mark Allen Publishing Ltd.

Glossary

Please note that the terms below have been defined in relation to the subject of reflexology and the definitions given here may differ to those you find in a dictionary.

Adrenaline and noradrenaline	Hormones secreted by the adrenal medulla that function in the flight-or-fight response.
Anterior	At the front of the body.
Antiseptic	Substance that prevents or inhibits microorganisms on living tissue.
Aponeurosis	A flat, sheet-like tendon that attaches muscles to bone, to skin or to another muscle.
Autonomic nervous system (ANS)	Part of the nervous system that controls all processes that are automatic or involuntary.
Ayurveda	Ancient form of medicine developed in India. The word ayurveda is a Sanskrit word meaning the 'science of life' and it encompasses not only physical health, but also spiritual and emotional wellbeing.
Bacteria (sing. bacterium)	A group of unicellular micro-organisms that lack organelles and an organised nucleus.
Bactericide	Substance that kills bacteria only.
Body relation lines	See Transverse zones/lines.
Carpals	The bones of the wrist. They are the: trapezium, trapezoid, capitate, hamate, scaphoid, lunate, triquetrum and pisiform.
Continuing Professional Development (CPD)	Training that enables you to continually develop your skills.
Contraindication	A condition for which reflexology should be given with caution or not given at all.
Cortisol	Hormone secreted by the adrenal cortex that functions in the stress response.
Crystals/crystalline deposits	Granular (sandy) deposits that indicate congestion in a reflex.
Disinfectant	Substance that destroys or inhibits microorganisms.
Distal	Further away from a centre of attachment (e.g. the toes are distal to the ankle).
Dorsum/dorsal surface	The top of the foot.
Endorphins and enkephalins	Neurotransmitters that act as the body's natural painkillers.
Evert	Turning the sole of the foot outwards.
Fungi (sing. fungus)	Simple organisms that lack chlorophyll.

Grounding techniques	Techniques used to prevent yourself from picking up your client's negative energy or allowing your client to drain your own energy.
Hallux	The big toe.
Healing crisis	A latent disorder may be brought to the surface before the body can improve.
Holistic health	The idea that health is the result of harmony between the body, mind and spirit.
Homeostasis	Process by which the body maintains a stable internal environment.
Hygiene	The science and practice of preserving health.
Informed client consent procedure	Procedure of client signing to confirm that he/she understands the reflexology treatment and its effects and that he/she has given you all necessary medical information.
Integumentary system	System of the skin and its derivatives (hair, nails and cutaneous glands).
Invert	Turning the sole of the foot inwards.
Lateral	Away from the midline of the body (towards the small toe side of the foot).
Lateral longitudinal arch	Arch running longitudinally down the lateral length of the foot. It consists of the calcaneus, cuboid and the lateral two metatarsals.
Leverage	This is the pressure provided by the rest of your working hand, and sometimes your support hand, in opposition to your working thumb or finger.
Longitudinal line	A vertical line (runs from the top to the bottom of the body or vice versa).
Longitudinal zones	Ten energy zones/pathways running the length of the body from the toes to the top of the head and then down into the fingers (or vice versa) with five zones running either side of the median line.
Malleolus	Ankle bone.
Medial	Towards the midline of the body (towards the big toe side of the foot).
Medial longitudinal arch	Arch running longitudinally down the medial length of the foot. It consists of the calcaneus, navicular, all three cuneiforms and the medial first three metatarsals.
Meridian	Energy pathway used in traditional Chinese medicine.

Metacarpals	The five bones of the hand that connect the wrist (carpals) to the fingers (phalanges).
Metatarsals	The five bones of the foot that connect the ankle (tarsus) to the toes (phalanges).
Microorganism/ microbe	An organism too small to be visible to the naked eye (includes bacteria, viruses and fungi).
Nei-jing	Chinese medical text Huang-di Nei-jing, or the Inner Classic of the Yellow Emperor, that forms the basis of traditional Chinese medicine (TCM).
Organs of elimination	Organs/systems that eliminate waste from the body. These are the lungs, liver, kidneys, large intestine, lymphatic system and skin.
Parasympathetic nervous system	Nervous system that opposes the actions of the sympathetic nervous system by inhibiting activity, thus conserving energy.
Pathogenic	Disease-causing.
Phalanges	Toes/fingers.
Placebo	A completely ineffective substance, for example a sugar pill, that has no pharmacological action on the body.
Plantar	The bottom or sole of the foot.
Posterior	At the back of the body.
Prana	Sanskrit term for life force/life energy.
Proximal	Closer to a centre of attachment (e.g. the ankle is proximal to the toes).
Qi (Chi, Ch'i or Ki)	Eastern term for life force/life energy.
Referral areas	Areas of the upper body that correspond to areas of the lower body and vice versa. These include the hands/feet, wrists/ankles, elbows/knees, shoulders/hips.
Reflex	A reflection in miniature that, when stimulated, stimulates the organ or structure which it reflects
Sanitation	A process in which conditions are rendered and maintained clean and healthy.
Scope of practice	The limitations of the qualification.
Solar plexus	In reflexology this is an important reflex to work for calming and relaxing a person. Anatomically, the solar plexus (also called the coeliac ganglion or plexus) is a network of autonomic nerves that is located in the abdomen and that innervates the digestive organs.
Sterilisation	A process in which all living microorganisms are destroyed.
Stress	A physical or mental demand that can be caused by a wide variety of factors, often differing from person to person

Support hand	This hand is always close to the working hand and supports or holds the foot.
Sympathetic nervous system	Nervous system that responds to changes in the environment by stimulating activity and using energy. It prepares the body for 'fight or flight'
Tarsals	The bones of the ankle and foot. They are the talus, calcaneus, cuboid, navicular, medial cuneiform, intermediate cuneiform and lateral cuneiform.
Traditional Chinese Medicine (TCM)	A vast system of Chinese medicine covering acupuncture, massage, diet, herbalism and exercise.
Transverse arch	Arch running transversely across the foot. It is formed by the cuboid, all three cuneiforms and the bases of the five metatarsals.
Transverse line	A horizontal line (runs from side to side).
Transverse zones/ lines	Zones/areas running horizontally across the body that help you to locate the different organs and structures of the body. The transverse lines are the shoulder line, the diaphragm line, the waist line and the pelvic line. Also called body relation lines.
Viruses	Pathogenic microorganisms that consists mainly of nucleic acid in a protein coat and that can only multiply when inside another living cell.
Working hand	This is the hand that is applying pressure and working a reflex.
Zone therapy	Theory that the body can be divided into zones and that imbalances in one part of the zone can be addressed through working another part of the zone.

Index

NB: *f* = figures, *b* = boxed information, *t* = table.

Picture Credits

We would like to thank the following for granting permission to reproduce copyright material in this book:

Page 9 Photo of William Hope FitzGerald, MD courtesy of Diana Demms Reddington

Page 10 Photos of Eunice Ingham and Dwight Byers courtesy of the International Institute of Reflexology (727) 343-4811, www.reflexology-usa.net.

All photos of diseases and disorders courtesy of the Wellcome Trust Photo Library

All the anatomical illustrations are reproduced from Sobotta: Atlas der Anatomie des Menschen, 22nd edition © Elsevier GmbH, Urban & Fischer Verlag München

All other photographs are copyright © The Write Idea Ltd 2011.